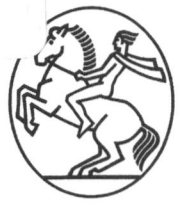

# Stereotactic Techniques in Clinical Neurosurgery

### D. Andries Bosch

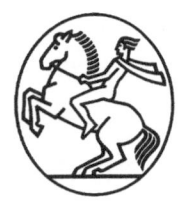

Springer-Verlag Wien New York

D. ANDRIES BOSCH, M.D.

Department of Neurosurgery,
St. Elisabeth Hospital,
Tilburg, The Netherlands

© 1986 by Springer-Verlag/Wien
Softcover reprint of the hardcover 1st edition 1986

With 216 partly colored Figures
Drawings by DOUWE BUITER

Library of Congress Cataloging-in-Publication Data. Bosch, D. A. Stereotactic techniques in clinical neurosurgery. Bibliography: p. Includes index. 1. Stereoencephalotomy. I. Title (DNLM: 1.Neurosurgery—methods. 2. Stereotaxic Technics. WL 368 B742s). RD 594. B67 1986. 617'. 48. 85-22260.

ISBN-13:978-3-7091-8809-5    e-ISBN-13:978-3-7091-8807-1
DOI: 10.1007/978-3-7091-8807-1

# Preface

Various textbooks on stereotactic neurosurgery have been published during the last few years (Riechert 1980, Schaltenbrand and Walker 1982, Spiegel 1982), all of them dealing with functional stereotactics as the major subject in the field. Diagnostic and therapeutic stereotactic interventions are only briefly described, whereas localization techniques are not yet mentioned.

Since 1980, however, an increasing number of reports has been published on CT guided and computer monitored stereotactic performances which enable the surgeon to combine diagnostic and therapeutic efforts in one session.

With recent progress in scanning techniques, including high resolution CT, NMR, and PET imaging of the brain, it has become possible to study and localize any brain area of interest. With the concomitant advances in computer technology, 3-dimensional reconstruction of deep seated lesions in stereotactic space is possible and the way is open for combined surgery with stereotactic precision and computer guided open resection. This type of open surgery in stereotactic space is already being developed in some centers with the aid of microsurgical, fiberoptic, and laser beam instrumentation.

With these advances stereotactic techniques will rapidly become integrated into clinical neurosurgery. Stereotactics has become a methodology which enables the surgeon to attack deep seated and subcortical small tumors. Neurosurgeons may abandon therapeutic nihilism, still frequently seen in glioma treatment, in the near future when stereotactic resection will be feasible and remaining tumor cells may be killed by adjuvant treatment modalities still in development.

This comprehensive guide to stereotactic principles, methodology, and possibilities is presented for use by general neurosurgeons who feel that stereotactics and computer aided surgery deserve clinical attention. Schematic drawings illustrate the principles of target positioning and calculation.

Stereotactic instruments in current use, including CT and NMR guided instrumentation, are discussed. Many photographs show the Leksell system, as this is the instrument in use in the author's department. Photographs of other instrumentation have kindly been presented to the author by various colleagues with permission for publishing. References have been collected and updated to June 1, 1985.

Tilburg, November 1985                                   D. Andries Bosch

# Acknowledgements

During the preparation of the manuscript many colleagues and friends offered invaluable help.

Mr. Douwe Buiter, Department of Neurosurgery, State University of Groningen, made the drawings.

Agfa-Gevaert, Antwerp, Belgium, generously provided support in the preparation of X-ray and CT pictures for publication.

Mr. H. Pattyn, Mr. R. van Hauthem, and Mr. M. van de Velde spent much time in selecting and skillfully reproducing the photographs. The neuroradiologist T. G. Tjan, M.D., provided many of the angiographic and CT scan studies.

The neuropathologist J. L. J. M. Teepen, M.D., examined specimens for histological diagnosis and prepared color photographs of illustrative cases.

Miss J. W. Adolfse, medical librarian, supplied the needed literature, corrected the list of references, and produced the final edition for printing.

Mrs. S. J. Baker and Miss J. S. de Smet were so kind to proof-read the manuscript.

# Contents

Chapter 1

# Introduction

Stereotactic neurosurgery was born in the mind of Robert Clarke, who in the early twentieth century (1906)—when he was convalescing from pneumonia in Egypt (Carpenter and Whittier 1952)—"used his genius to apply a simple principle out of its usual context", and gave the impetus to research into deep brain structures (Schurr and Merrington 1978). By that time clinical neurosurgery did not exist. Surgical neurology was performed by neurologists with some surgical training and consisted for a great deal of applied neurophysiology. It was, in fact, the ultimum refugium for neurologists to alleviate otherwise intractable disorders. Medical history describes three operations in which a burrhole was performed after localization of its site with the help of an "encephalometer". This instrument was constructed by Professor D. N. Zernov (Moscow 1892) and is the first apparatus based on mathematical principles that, after fixation on the skull, could be used for spatial orientation (Kandel and Schavinsky 1972). It was, however, employed mainly in surface topography for localization of the cranial sutures and cerebral sulci. Therefore it seems justified to state that the modern era of stereotaxy began in 1906 when Clarke and Horsley published work on a new method of brain research using a Cartesian tricoordinate system.

## I. Stereotaxy in Experimental Brain Research

### A. Clarke's Instrument

The original idea to apply geometry to the study of the brain came to Clarke when he collaborated with Victor Horsley in experimental work on the function of the cerebellum. Horsley tried to destroy deep tracts and nuclei to discover their function and felt an inability to be sure about the positioning of his electrodes with which he made electrolytic lesions. He recognized the problem and Clarke's idea brought the solution. Of course, the composition of the brain had occupied the minds of many people for centuries and its fine structure necessitated the development of very precise ways of investigation. But to make use of the cranium as a *platform* for localizing intracranial targets, to use it as a tool to a better understanding of

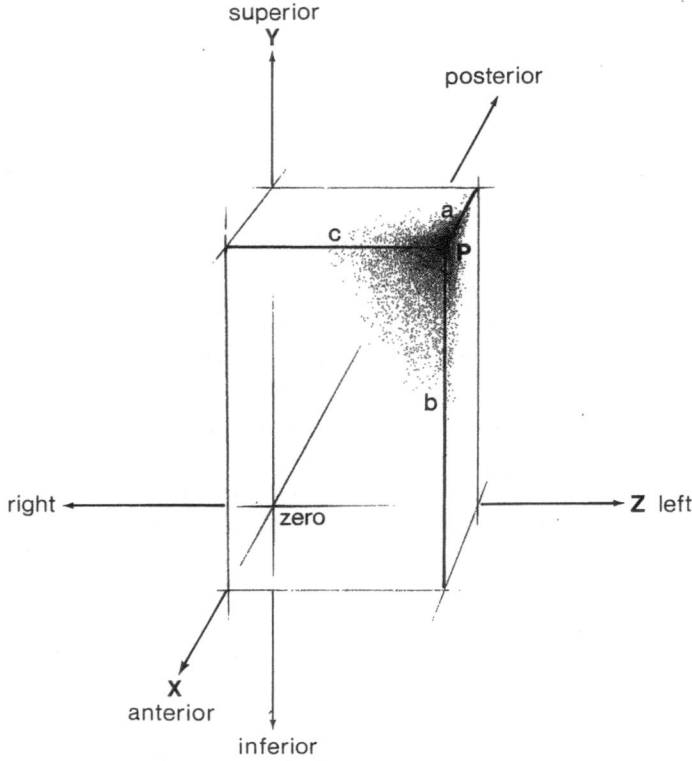

Fig. 1. Cartesian tricoordinate system for spatial orientation. P is given by:
x = a mm anterior to zero, y = b mm superior to zero, z = c mm lateral to
zero (to the left), XZ—plane is horizontal or axial plane, YZ—plane is frontal or
coronal plane, XY—plane is sagittal plane

brain function, is to the merit of Clarke. He realized also that there is no
constant relationship between the skull and the intracranial structures and
that the only way to find out where to place a needle tip in a given internal
part was to construct a map on which every target could be related to three
"zero planes", perpendicular to each other. Herewith Clarke introduced a
Cartesian coordinate system with which calculations could be made and any
point could be described by its coordinates x, y and z (Fig. 1). Clarke's
original apparatus was made in 1905 by Mr. J. Swift in London and
consisted of a frame of brass which was applied to the head of the animal by
means of rods attached to plugs inserted into the external auditory meati
and adjustable bars which rest on the nose and orbital margins. It was fixed
to the skull by pins which were screwed in laterally. The electrode was
supported by another bar that could be moved in three planes at right angles
to each other. With knowledge of the various types of stereotactic apparatus

available today, it is remarkable to see how its simplicity in construction has been preserved and only refined in these up to date instruments. Based on his instrument Clarke (and Henderson 1911, 1914 and 1920) published stereotactic maps of sections of the brain of the cat and monkey. Once again, one is struck by the timeless value of a good idea!

## B. Clarke's Idea

Although the stereotactic techniques were only applied in experimental brain research during the following years (1907–1947), as stereotaxy was intended for standardizing lesions in various structures to study the topographical and nosological composition of the brain, Clarke already anticipated in 1920 the therapeutic possibilities of his invention in human neurosurgery. He thought his instrument would enable brain tumors to be treated by electrical means or by the implantation of radium, and that it might be possible to relieve pain by coagulating tracts within the brain through a 5 mm hole in the skull (Jefferson 1957). Inspired by Clarke's animal device, A. T. Mussen, who collaborated with Horsley and Clarke, designed the first stereotactic apparatus for use on humans. This instrument was built by an instrument maker in London in 1918 (Picard *et al.* 1983), but never used "because at that time no one was interested in it" (quote from a letter by Mussen to his son in 1971).

## II. Stereotaxy in Man

The stereotactic method developed by Horsley and Clarke received little attention until E. A. Spiegel, who had had contact with Clarke shortly before his death in 1926, to ask permission to construct another apparatus by Mr. Swift for use in Vienna, emigrated to the United States and joined H. T. Wycis. In 1947 Spiegel (*et al.*) reported the first human stereotactic operation. So after forty years the big step from animals to man was taken, and within some years a "hausse" could be noticed in the development of stereotactic devices for application in man (Spiegel and Wycis, Leksell, Riechert, Talairach). In the early years of stereotaxy in man, however, a stereotactic map of human brain anatomy was not available. The first atlas of the human brain for stereotactic surgery was edited by Spiegel and Wycis in 1952, in which the posterior commissure was used as a single intracerebral reference point in combination with several external cranial references. In the beginning of the era of stereotactic neurosurgery the main interests lay in functional surgery. Since brain surgery for tumors and other space occupying lesions had a high mortality rate in these years and was—if at all—performed with one goal in mind, to treat by extirpation or bulk resection, it is evident that the profit of stereotactic techniques was not realized by the surgeons. The link between experimental and human stereotactic surgery was laid by the neurologists, who studied the effects of different ablations and destructions of parts of the brain to alleviate otherwise intractable syndromes. So first of all attention was paid to stereotactic possibilities in the treatment of convulsive disorders, intractable pain, hyperkinesias and parkinsonism. Even psychosurgical interventions were extensively studied and tried out. The first attempts to treat peatients with stereotactic operations were made in cases of intractable pain. Instead of the formerly used leucotomy (Moniz 1936) or even cortical extirpations to manage pain, stereotactic destruction of targets deep inside the brain were performed with the help of guided instruments. This meant a great progress in surgical possibilities and a significant reduction in mortality, due to the precise localization of the targets with the help of a ventriculography that gave the reference points needed (posterior commissure and sagittal plane).

## A. Functional Stereotactics

This development opened the way to treat by applying the same method other disorders, such as Parkinson's disease, the hyperkinesias and convulsive syndromes; these being illnesses in which open neurosurgical ablations were carried out formerly with considerable side-effects. During the two decennia after the introduction of stereotactic techniques in neurological surgery (1947–1967) clinical research flourished in this field and functional neurosurgery became closely related to stereotactic neurosurgery. After Hassler had published in 1955 (a–c) his results dealing with stimulation and coagulation in the human thalamus, this target became the lesion site of choice for the alleviation of various types of movement disorders. Spiegel and Wycis and also Cooper in America, Talairach and Guiot in France, Riechert and Mundinger in Germany and Leksell in Sweden brought their results with thalamic surgery over large groups of patients to the attention of everybody interested in neurological diseases and introduced improvements in stereotactic instrumentation and in the mapping of deep brain structures. Their results proved to be the most satisfactory in Parkinson's disease (tremor and rigidity) and in the various pain syndromes. New developments in neuropharmacology, which led to the introduction of dopamine drugs for the treatment of parkinsonism by Cotzias (et al. 1969) meant, however, a considerable drag on further progress of stereotactics in functional neurosurgery.

## B. Mass Lesions Stereotactics

The next leap forward—surprisingly enough originally thought of by Clarke in 1921—was made by the further progress in clinical neurosurgery. Mortality rate and complications after craniotomies decreased markedly by modern anesthesia, brain edema protection, and technical advances in instrumentation. Therefore neurosurgeons also became interested in deep seated brain lesions. Diagnostic possibilities increased surprisingly with the introduction of computerized tomography (Hounsfield *et al.* 1973) and even small lesions inside the brain could be detected. Neurosurgeons felt the need to discover and disclose the lesion's nature and had to decide again and again between exploration (including approaches with the microscope) and a biopsy through a burrhole. Stereotactic instruments could make a biopsy procedure a safe and reliable performance. Neuropathological investigation of the tissue specimen could give insight into the nature of the lesion and thus in the prognosis of the illness. In case of brain tumor the increasing number of treatment modalities made histological diagnosis imperative once and for all. Therefore, in otherwise inaccessible lesions of the brain stereotactically guided biopsy instruments came into use. Pioneers in stereotactic surgery (Leksell and Backlund in Stockholm; Riechert and Mundinger in Freiburg) utilized their talents to develop the necessary equipment and performed the first stereotactic biopsies. Herewith a technical solution was given to the problem of histological diagnosis in any case of neuroradiologically demonstrated brain lesion. In recent years histological diagnosis is becoming even more important, as radiation therapy and chemotherapy can offer substantial improvement in various types of brain malignancies. Today, stereotactic biopsy is more and more widely performed, and it is generally believed that, in the near future, this type of surgery can no longer be neglected in the treatment of tumor patients. Progress in neuro-oncology, which is a rapidly expanding field of interest and research, offers increasing possibilities for diagnostic and sometimes therapeutic stereotactic procedures. Possibilities, which are available to the neurosurgeon who has had a basic training in them. Moreover, in up to 10% of the cases suspected to have a tumor, stereotactic biopsy reveals the lesion to be no tumor at all, but a vascular or infectious disease, which should be treated in an appropriate way: especially the increasing group of immunocompromized patients shows a tendency to opportunistic infections (after cancer treatment or organ transplantation).

## C. Stereotactic Localization

The newest branch of stereotactic neurosurgery is formed by the localization stereotactics. The indication is given by small subcortical lesions, which could be treated perfectly by microsurgical means, but are not easily found. In the first place small arteriovenous malformations and hematomas, but also small tumors and abscesses, can be reached safely and without lesioning overlying brain tissue after stereotactic localization. Moreover, the shortest trajectory can be calculated and a minimal exposure of brain can be used. In this field of stereotactics the area of interest is

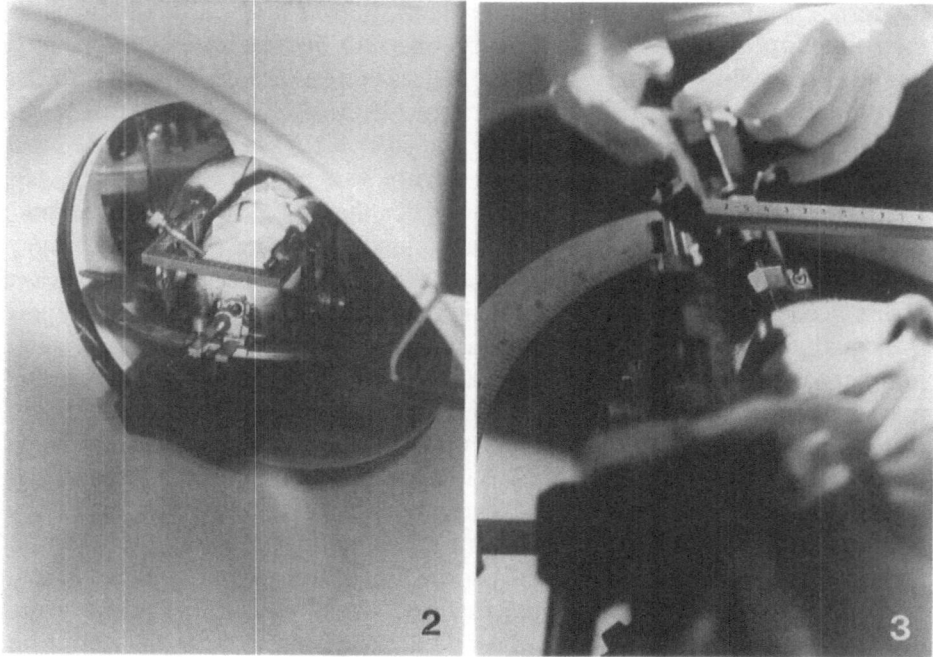

Fig. 2. Stereotactic surgery within the CT scanner (Leksell instrument)

Fig. 3. Stereotactic biopsy of a brainstem tumor with CT-guidance

marked (eventually with the help of intraoperative angiography) by the tip of a small silastic tube that is introduced along the preferential trajectory. With minimal damage to the brain and therefore even in as vital cortical areas as the parietal lobe, surgical intervention becomes acceptable. In case of deep seated small lesions stereotactic localization is the first step to adequate treatment, modalities for which are being developed nowadays with the use of isotope implantation, neurosurgical endoscopic designs with fiberoptically transmitted laser instrumentation and various types of external stereotactic irradiation (Apuzzo and Sabshin 1983, Edwards *et al.* 1983, Backlund 1979).

## III. Stereotactic Methodology

The advent of computed axial tomography has not only provided new insights into intracranial disease, but has also instigated a true revival of the neurosurgeon's interest in the utilization of stereotactics. CT guided stereotaxy with calculation of stereotactic coordinates from the computed tomographic scan (Gildenberg *et al.* 1982) has been available for some years and forms an integrated part of already existing stereotactic instruments (Leksell and Jernberg 1980, Mundinger *et al.* 1978 a, b), or has led to the construction of new stereotactic systems (Brown *et al.* 1981, Kelly *et al.* 1982 a, b). Devices for CT guidance may be divided into two groups: those with which the operation is performed within the scanner (Figs. 2 and 3) and

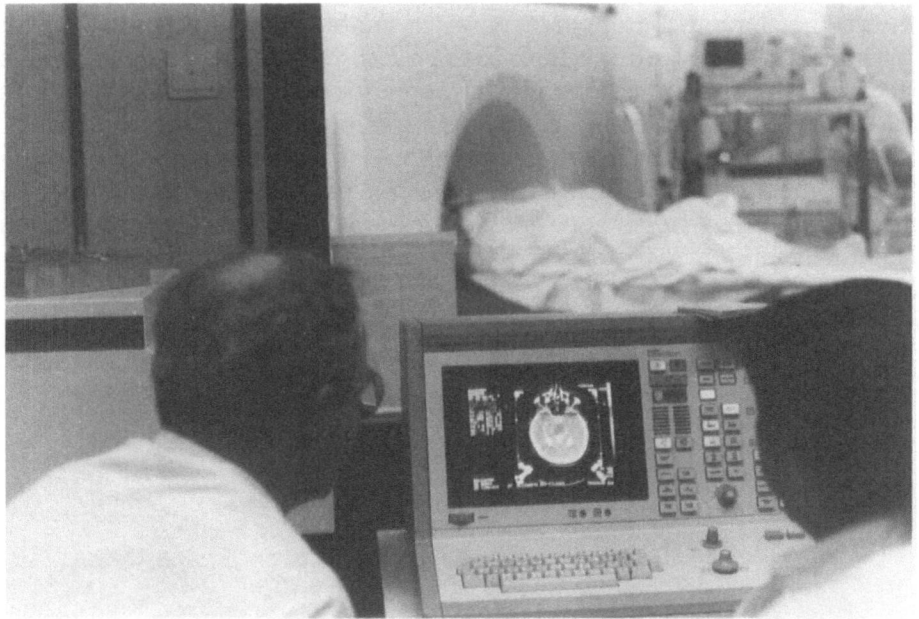

Fig. 4. CT scanning with stereotactic instrument fixed to the skull. Positive contrast is seen in the ventricles and around the brainstem for better visualization of the target

those that allow the translation of scanning data to the operating room (Fig. 4). With this instrumentation any intracranial point can now be reached with great accuracy (error is less than 1 mm). The stereotactic method therefore is a safe and rapid tool in the management and evaluation of mass lesions. By this method novel areas of interest can be explored, high risk craniotomies can be avoided and hospitalization periods can be reduced. Also by obtaining a tissue diagnosis the further strategy in the treatment of the individual patient can be planned better and subsequent craniotomy will be reserved for cases which benefit by open surgery. Stereotactic technique that originally has been presented as a method has matured to a methodology, a way of thinking and of treating the neurosurgical patient.

## IV. Integration of Stereotactics in Clinical Neurosurgery

Precision resection of intracerebral mass lesions (vascular malformations and tumors) can be achieved with computer monitored instruments
within a stereotactic system. With the help of computer graphics a three-
dimensional reconstruction of the lesion in relation to the instrument's
coordinate system can be made with continuous monitoring of instrument
positions as to the target area. Stereotactic craniotomy (Kelly *et al.* 1983)
stands for stereotactic localization of the target followed by craniotomy
within the stereotactic apparatus, which enables the surgeon to aim his
instruments (biopsy forceps, laser beam, microscope) stereotactically and to
resect or vaporize the lesion with intraoperative computer monitoring. In
the management of deep seated lesions a stereotactic retractor can be used,
which is attached to the instrument. Although the benefit is questionable in
the treatment of malignancies, the impressive technical facilities offered by
the computerized stereotactic method are obvious. With high resolution
scanning and the early detection of mass lesions there is no doubt, that in the
near future stereotactics will be integrated into clinical neurosurgery as an
important, if not sometimes essential, surgical adjuvant.

# Chapter 2

# Stereotactic Principles

## I. Development

Development of stereotactic principles in neurosurgery wouldn't have been possible if the brain wasn't soft in consistency and easy to penetrate—with the exclusion of vessels and meninges—without serious dysfunctions developing. Nevertheless many neurologists think puncture is hazardous and forget the ample evidence, derived from numerous stereotactic interventions, that puncture with guided (instead of free-hand) instruments of small diameter (preferably less than 4 mm) and with a blunt tip eliminates any real danger. The author has punctured once in case of emergency with a blunt, guided, 2 mm needle through the mesencephalon, pons and medulla to reach an intramedullary hematoma; after the evacuation functions restored and the patient recovered without any vital dysfunction. On the other hand, stereotactic techniques could only be developed due to the fact that the skull forms a firm envelope for its contents. The bone of the skull convexity provides the foundation for any stereotactic equipment and makes it possible to construct an apparatus that can be fixed to the skull with screws. This enables the neurosurgeon to introduce any stereotactic instrument that is supported by a bar, which is connected to the apparatus, just by sliding the guided instrument (needle, forceps, electrode) slowly through a burrhole into the brain. Penetration of surrounding brain structures by this guided technique is made even less dangerous by the high number of degrees of freedom that a modern apparatus possesses. So, after calculations have been made and the coordinates established, the instrument bar is adjusted in such a way that the tract towards the target is the preferable one (the shortest or the safest) according to the surgeon's opinion.

## II. Definition

*Stereotaxis* means a *spatial* (i.e. three-dimensional) *arrangement*, that is: fixing any point in space by application of mathematical principles. To apply these principles to the study of the brain, as is Clarke's invention, it is necessary to introduce a reference system that is generally accepted and extremely reliable. In the early days of stereotactic surgery Horsley and Clarke used a system of skull landmarks for the determination of the target. They were aware of the fact that there is no constant relationship between the skull landmarks and the intracerebral structures (except for the sella turcica and its contents). Nevertheless they used in their instrument as reference points the external auditory meati and the orbital margins. By now, these landmarks are only used as temporary fixation points during the adjustment of the instrument, before it is fixed with screws to the skull. A fundamental modification was brought into practice by Spiegel and Wycis (1947) with the use of intracerebral reference structures. It is their merit to have introduced the most reliable structure for the geometrical localization of the target, namely the third ventricle. They recommended that operations on selected areas of the thalamus would be preferable to the standard leucotomy operations (Egas Moniz 1936) in the treatment of psychic disorders. To reach their—selected—thalamic nucleus there was a strong need for precise localization, and their reference to the contours of the third ventricle has proven to be very reliable. Unwanted side-effects, which brought Moniz' psychosurgery into disrepute, were not seen with their stereotactic technique, in spite of the fact that Spiegel and Wycis didn't yet have a map of normal (standardized) brain anatomy during the first years of surgery on man.

## III. Stereotactic Atlasses

In 1952 the first atlas of the human brain for stereotactic surgery was edited (Spiegel and Wycis 1952), in which the posterior commissure was used as a single intracerebral reference point with several external cranial landmarks (the interaural plane which runs through both external auditory meati and is perpendicular to the so-called line of Frankfort). Talairach (*et al.* 1957) pointed out the necessity for at least two intracerebral reference points: the anterior and the posterior commissure (AC and PC). He demonstrated that the line connecting AC and PC has a very variable position relative to the formerly accepted and commonly used skull landmarks. For example, the angle between the AC—PC-line and the line of Frankfort (which runs through the lower orbital edge and the midportion of the upper margin of the external meatus) varies from 11.5 to 18.5 degrees (Van Manen 1967), as shown in Fig. 5. In this figure both the system of axes according to Spiegel and Wycis and its variability regarding the AC—PC-line are demonstrated. In his atlas, Talairach (*et al.* 1957) related deep brain structures to the AC—PC-line and two perpendiculars erected on it through these points (Fig. 6). Herewith, he introduced a system of axes that lies completely intracerebral, which implies the least variation in the topographical anatomy of the basal ganglia, thalamic nuclei and mesencephalic tracts

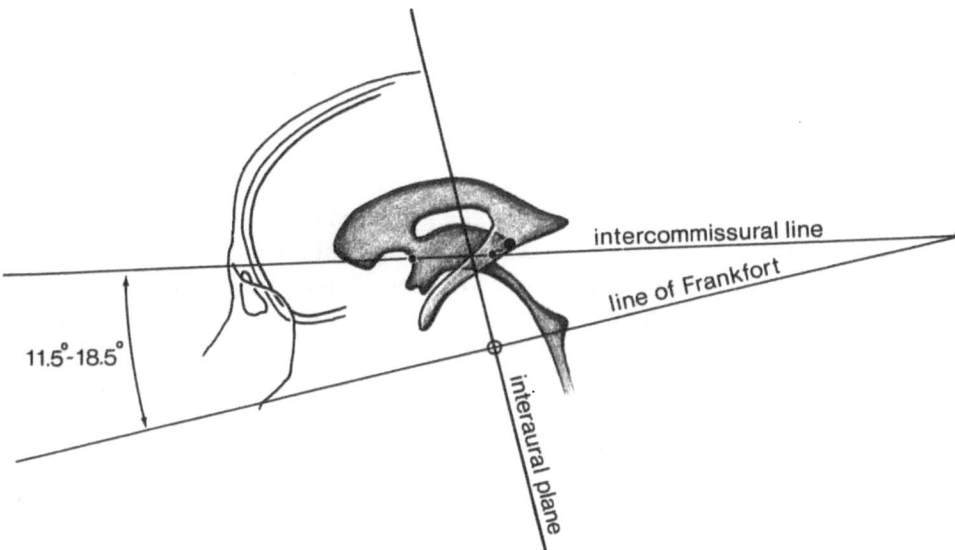

Fig. 5. System of axes according to Spiegel and Wycis (posterior commissure and interaural plane), with variability between intercommissural line and line of Frankfort. The distance between pineal gland and interaural plane also varies considerably (4–20 mm). Lateral view

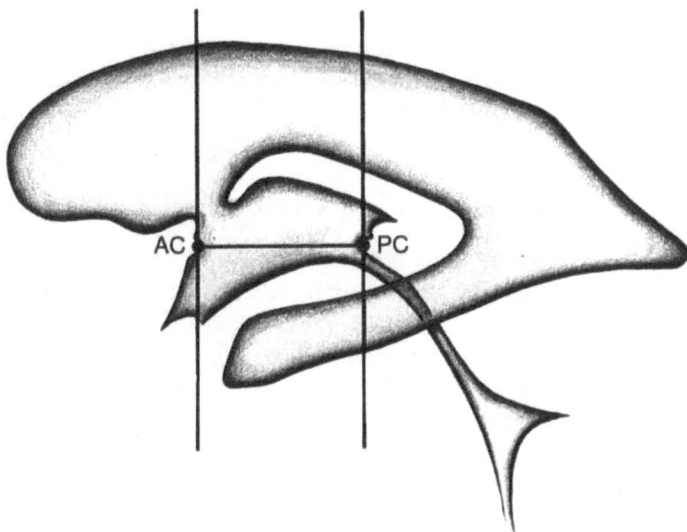

Fig. 6. Intracerebral reference points according to Talairach: anterior and posterior commissure (AC and PC) with perpendiculars erected on the line AC—PC (intercommissural line). Lateral view

as to the system of reference. Two years later, the atlas of the human brain by Schaltenbrand and Bailey (1959) simplified this system by taking as axes the AC—PC-line, lying in the median (sagittal) plane, and a perpendicular erected on it in the middle point between the two commissures. This middle point is the zero point of their system of axes (Fig. 7). The system of Schaltenbrand and Bailey became the most employed among neurosurgeons all over the world and is generally accepted as very reliable. It should be pointed out here that so far only intracerebral structures are described which serve supratentorial targets: the basal ganglia, thalamus, hypothalamus and mesencephalon. More recently, stereotaxy has started to involve also the rhombencephalon (i.e. the brainstem and the cerebellum), and therefore in the second edition of Schaltenbrand and Bailey's Atlas (Schaltenbrand and Wahren 1977) sections of the brainstem and cerebellum are also included. In 1978 Afshar, Watkins and Yap published an Atlas of the Human Brainstem and Cerebellar Nuclei, in which as infratentorial references were used the fourth ventricle floor plane and a perpendicular erected on it that runs through the fastigium, in combination with the sagittal (median) plane. Another important atlas was published by Emmers and Tasker in 1975 on the human thalamus, which gives extensive information on patients responses to electrical stimuli. All these Stereotactic Atlasses give microscopical sections of "normal" brains, cut in three different (X, Y and Z) planes. They give a better understanding of the topographical anatomy of deep brain structures and place them into a Cartesian system of axes, which enables the neurophysiologist and the neurosurgeon to find them with the aid of stereotactic principles. In this way, it is made possible to determine any target of interest (for example: the ventrolateral nucleus of the thalamus in cases of parkinsonian tremor) by the calculation of its coordinates x, y and z.

## IV. Invisible and Visible Targets

Later on, these target points, which represent nuclei or fiber tracts, were called the *invisible* targets to distinguish them from the targets formed by pathological lesions. In case of such lesions, which are visualized by CT scanning and angiography, the target is *visible*. This means that nearly always a visible target is present in patients who undergo a biopsy: a situation, in which no intracerebral reference system of axes is needed to calculate its position. To underline this important difference in the stereotactic management of invisible and visible targets, it is necessary to discuss briefly the main points of distinction. In the stereotactic determination of an invisible target the surgeon makes use of two completely *unrelated* Cartesian systems: first the system of axes, which is erected in the cerebrum to determine the position of the target in relation with these axes.

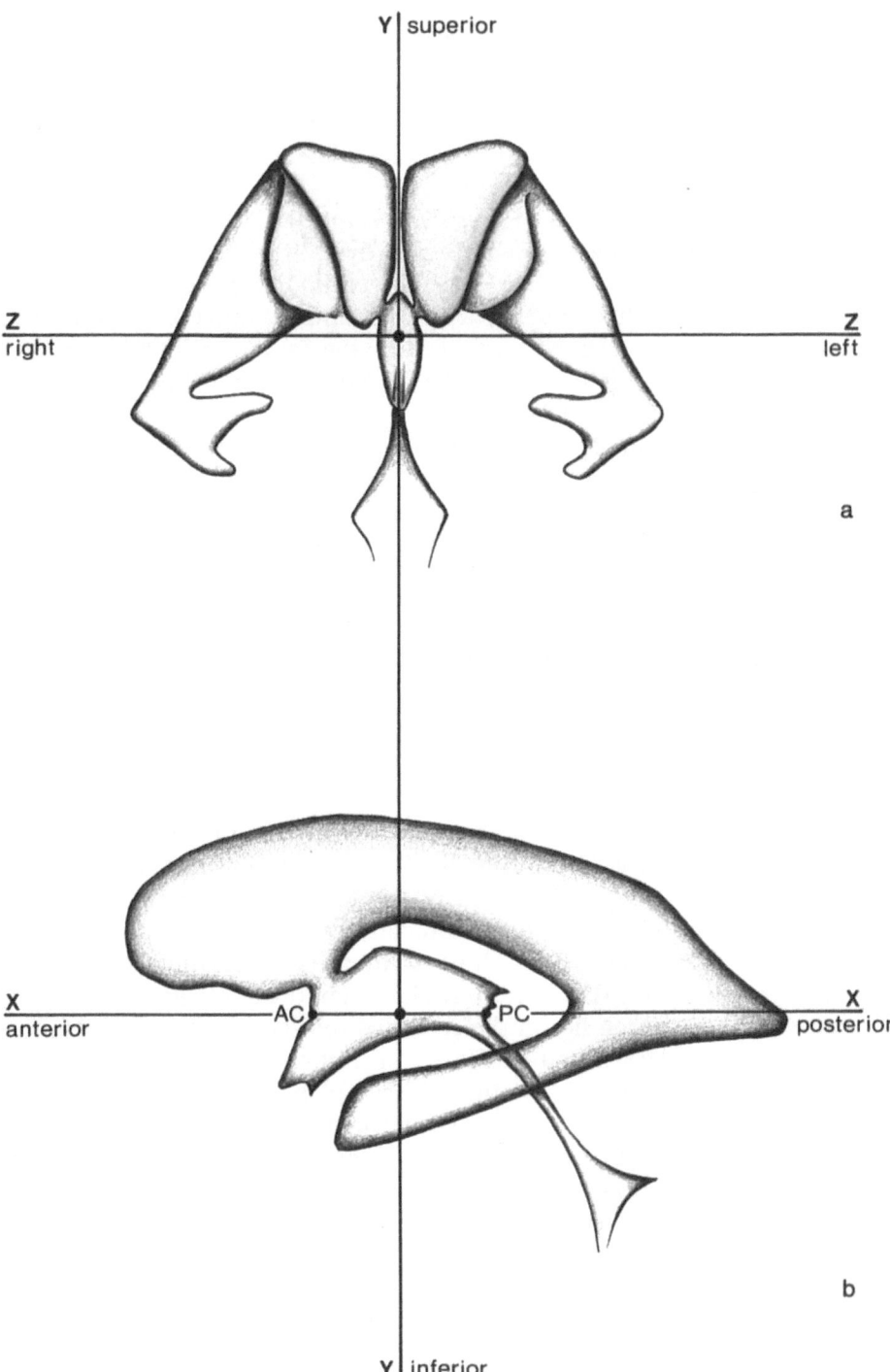

Fig. 7. Intracerebral reference points according to Schaltenbrand and Bailey: AC and PC with a perpendicular erected on the middle point of the intercommissural line. Middle point is zero point of system of axes. a) Anteroposterior view. b) Lateral view

This system of axes should be the same as the system used in the stereotactic atlas that informs the surgeon about the position of the target of interest (Figs. 6 and 7 in combination with respectively the Atlas of Talairach or of Schaltenbrand and Wahren).

*This manoeuvre makes the target visible,* because by then the target can be indicated on the X-ray pictures which already show the erected system of axes. Secondly, the system of axes that is embodied by the stereotactic instrument; this is illustrated in Fig. 8 a and b for the lateral and anteroposterior projection. The relation of the target of interest to this second system of axes is of course the actual coordinate setting for the planned stereotactic intervention.

In the determination of a visible target the surgeon makes use of only the latter system of axes, because the target of interest is present on the X-ray pictures or can be easily transferred to them from the already available radiological films. Fig. 9 a and b show the coordinate setting for a deep seated left temporal tumor.

## V. Preparation of the Stereotactic Intervention

### A. The Positioning of the Target with X-ray Pictures

#### 1. The Invisible Target

The positioning of the invisible target with help of X-ray pictures is done with a ventriculography, which fills the ventricles, and especially the third ventricle, with contrast. X-ray pictures are taken in a lateral and anteroposterior projection, strictly perpendicular to each other. In this way the lateral X-ray picture (Fig. 10) will show the line AC—PC, which lies in both the inter-commissural and the midsagittal plane of the brain, and the central perpendicular line, which lies in the so-called mid-commissural or frontal plane. The coordinates x and y of any target point can be read from a stereotactic atlas that uses the same reference planes, as does the Atlas of Schaltenbrand and Wahren (1977), and marked on this X-ray picture. On the anteroposterior picture the midsagittal plane can be drawn and the third coordinate z can be marked relative to this plane to the left or the right (Fig. 11). Marking on both X-ray pictures is done after proportional correction for X-ray magnification. In case the AC—PC distance in the patient is markedly greater than in the standardized brain atlasses (25 mm), an extra correction may be introduced given by the factor $\dfrac{AC—PC \ patient}{AC—PC \ atlas}$, for example $30/25 = 6/5$.

Now the situation is reached that mathematical calculations should be performed, which greatly depend on the type of stereotactic apparatus used.

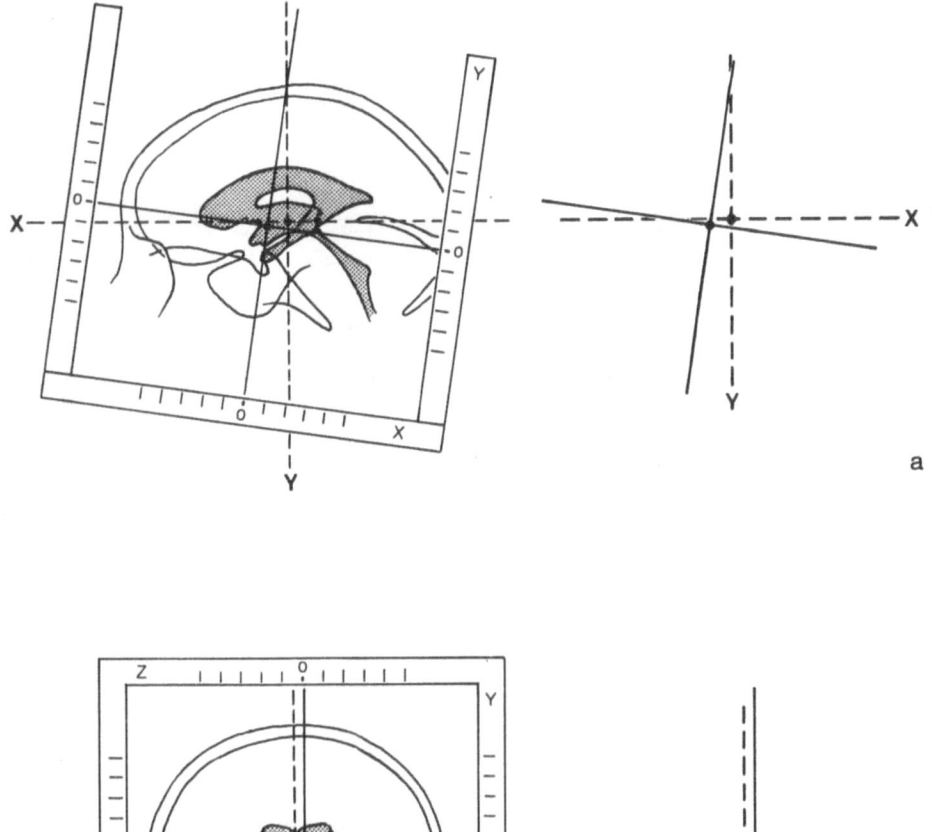

Fig. 8. Positioning of invisible target: two unrelated Cartesian systems of axes are needed. First the intracerebral system of axes according to Schaltenbrand and Bailey, and second the system of axes embodied in the stereotactic instrument. a) Shows the lateral view and b) the anteroposterior view for *different* instrument positions. Note that in the anteroposterior view of position a) the instrument system of axes would have been under the intracerebral system

## 2. The Visible Target

The positioning of the visible target with the help of X-ray pictures needs no ventriculography, as no intracerebral reference structures are necessary

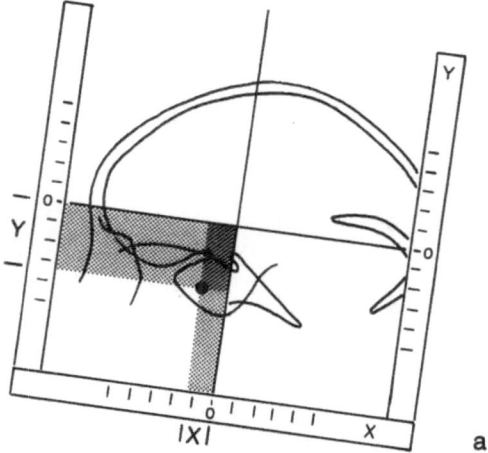

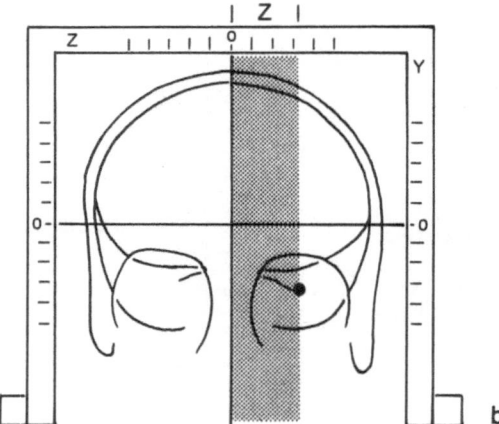

Fig. 9. Positioning of visible target: only the system of axes embodied in the stereotactic instrument is needed. Target is a left temporal tumor. a) Shows the lateral and b) the anteroposterior view with target determined by $x$ mm anterior, $y$ mm inferior, and $z$ mm left to various zero planes

for the determination. The target has already been visualized by conventional skull X-ray pictures (for example: a bullet in the brain), or by any other type of neuroradiological X-ray film (for example: a pinealoma in ventriculography, an intracerebral tumor in cerebral angiography). The only problem is, how to *transfer* this target from the pictures available onto the X-ray pictures taken with the stereotactic apparatus, which are again a

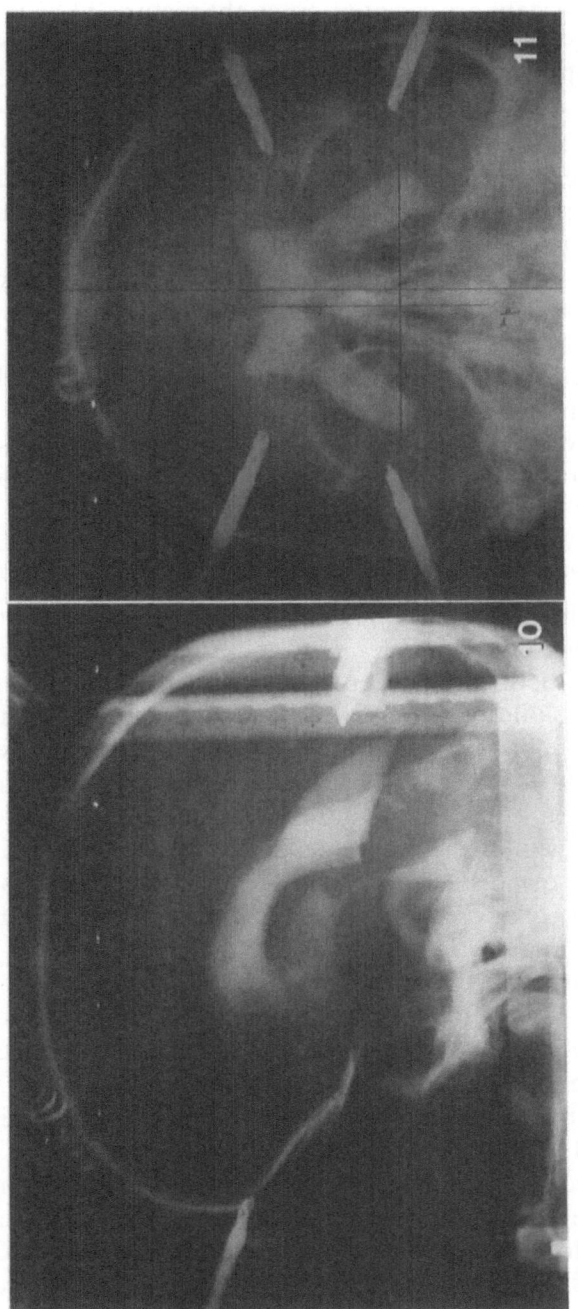

Fig. 10. Stereotactic ventriculography (Leksell instrument). Lateral view showing the 3rd ventricle and the commissures AC and PC

Fig. 11. Anteroposterior view, with midline shift of instrument to the left. mp—midsagittal plane of cerebrum

lateral and an anteroposterior projection, strictly perpendicular to each other. The following steps are essential. First, the pictures already available should show the lesion (= target) in the strictly lateral and anteroposterior projection. Secondly, the magnification should be the same as that used in the X-ray pictures with the stereotactic apparatus (i.e. the same focus-object-film distances). In the case of different magnification factors a proportional correction is to be calculated. This procedure is illustrated in Fig. 12 a and b for a deep seated left parietal lesion T. It is obvious, that in the calculation of proportional correction both skull- and intracerebral landmarks have exactly the same value. Frequently used landmarks are: the sutura coronaria, the sella turcica and a calcified pineal gland. The precision of transfer increases with less difference in magnification and moreover with landmarks closer to the target (so, in the posterior fossa the clivus and protuberantia occipitalis are prefered).

Now the situation is reached that mathematical calculations should be performed which greatly depend on the type of stereotactic apparatus used.

## B. The Positioning of the Target with Computerized Tomography

Positioning of the target (visible or invisible) with help of *computerized tomography* has become possible more recently. *Magnetic resonance imaging* of brain structures has been developed even more recently, and leads to similar possibilities of computer guided positioning of targets of interest. In both types of high resolution brain scanning use can be made of their computer facilities, which can be extended with software that enables the stereotactic surgeon to determine the target coordinates directly from the scan. Some mathematical systems have been described, which provide the surgeon with the real distances x, y and z of any target, visible or marked on CT pictures, in relation to the stereotactic instrument. Instrument adjustments are available for both CT and MR scanning of the skull contents with the stereotactic instrument fixed to the skull (Fig. 13). The visible target is directly related to the stereotactic apparatus and its system of axes by the scan computer. The invisible target is marked by the computer on the appropriate CT picture as soon as the computer is fed with the knowledge of any atlas that is based on CT slides of the human brain or even the commonly used stereotactic brain atlasses (Hardy *et al.* 1983). This type of computer assisted stereotactic surgery is in continuous development and will in the future enable any neurosurgeon to perform stereotactic interventions. With mid-sagittal CT scanning the line AC—PC can be visualized, which is the standard reference line in functional stereotactics. Reformatted horizontal, frontal and sagittal planes with CT of the patients brain should conform to anatomical sections of standard stereotactic atlasses. Future possibilities in stereotactic neurosurgery with the use of

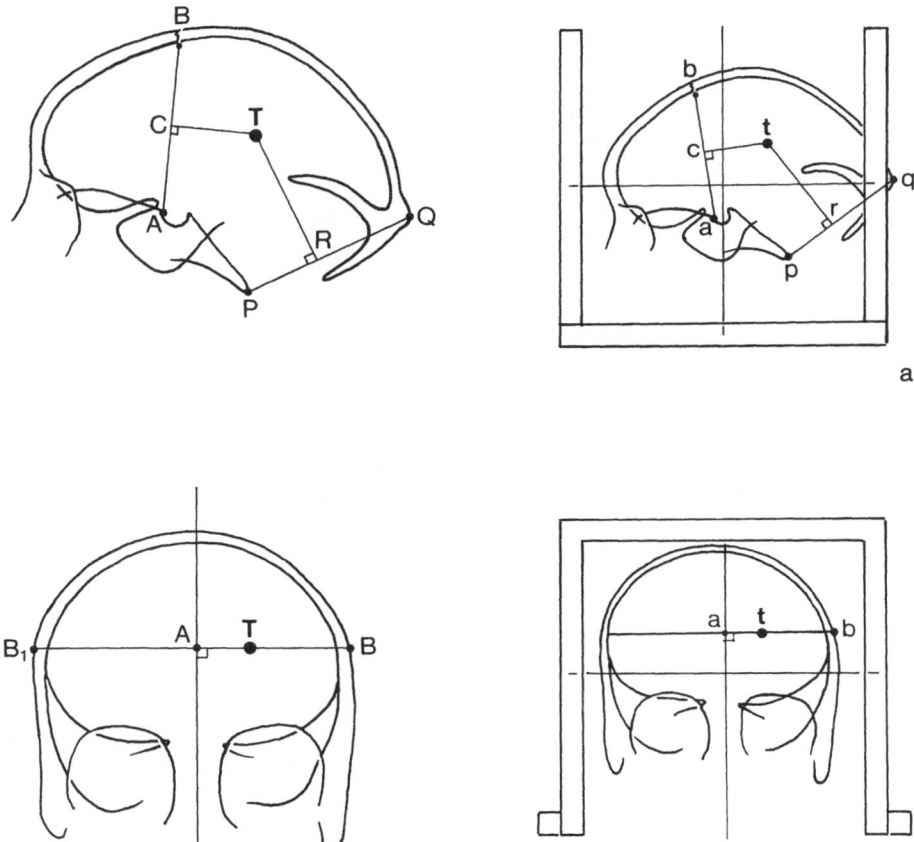

Fig. 12. Proportional correction in case of different magnification factors. a) Lateral view and b) anteroposterior view of position of deep seated left parietal lesion on angiographic (left) and stereotactic (right) X-ray pictures. Calculation:

$$AB:ab = AC:ac,\ ac = \frac{ab \times AC}{AB};\ AC:ac = CT:ct,\ ct = \frac{ac \times CT}{AC}.$$ The position

of target t may be checked with calculation based on the line PQ and the perpendicular through T on it (TR). To make the target visible on the ante-

roposterior view (b) the calculation is: $AB:ab = AT:at,\ at = \dfrac{ab \times AT}{AB}$. Note that

$AB = AB_1$ and that the midsagittal plane of the skull is not always identical with the midsagittal plane of the instrument. Moreover, the calculation of the z-coordinate could be more reliably done from the axial (CT-)view, due to differences in inclination

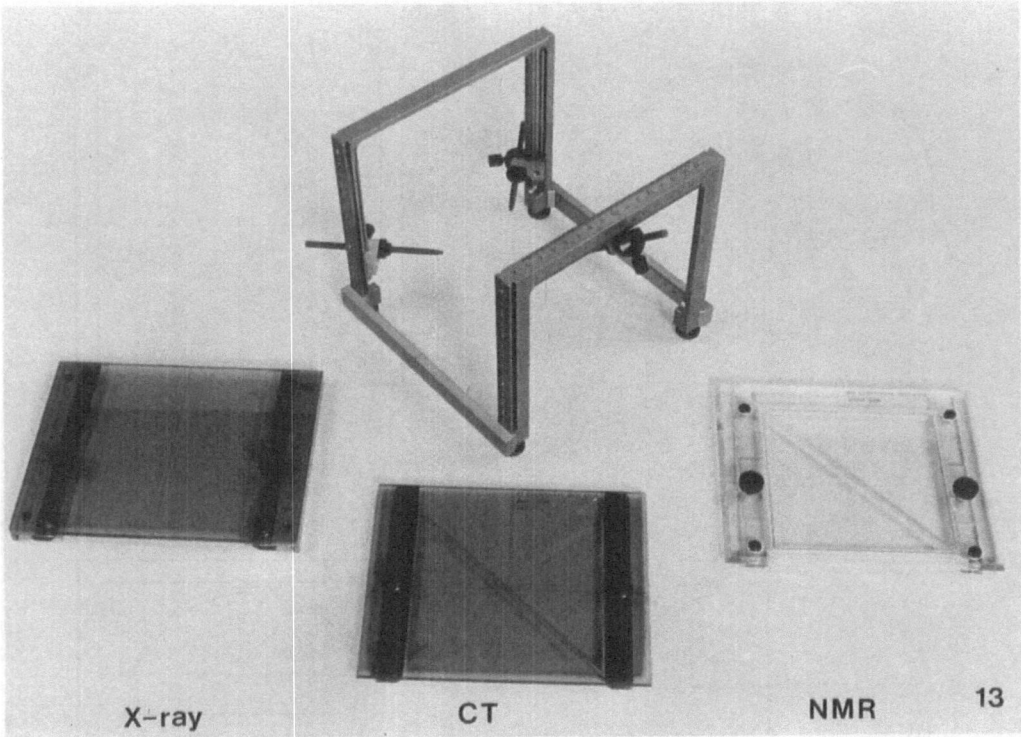

Fig. 13. Instrument adjustments in the Leksell system (by courtesy of Prof. Leksell). Conventional X-ray (left), CT (middle), and NMR (right) coordinate indicators

computerized tomographic scanning are illustrated by Kelly (1983) and Gildenberg (1983). Thus, in contrast with the positioning with help of X-ray pictures, mathematical calculations are not needed in CT-stereotactics, as the computer or any other simple ruling device (originally described by Leksell and Jernberg in 1980 for Leksell's apparatus), depending on the type of instrument used, produces the coordinates in relation to the system of axes of the stereotactic apparatus. In fact, some stereotactic head frames have been constructed, which are only applicable in CT-stereotactics and have a very special three-dimensional computer graphics approach to optimal target localization (Brown 1979, Brown *et al.* 1981, Kelly *et al.* 1982 a, b and 1983). In Applied Neurophysiology, issue 45 (1982), computer assisted stereotactic surgery is amply discussed.

## C. Calculation of Target Point

The position of the target point, relative to the stereotactic apparatus system of axes, is calculated with the aid of a mathematical method that is particular to the type of instrument used. Although therefore not accessible to a general discussion, some major points should be emphasized here because of the complexity of the matter. First of all the X-ray pictures are taken from a fixed distance to ensure constant X-ray enlargement of the object (i.e. skull + apparatus) on the film. To abandon X-ray enlargement, Talairach (1955) and Schaltenbrand (Riechert and Mundinger 1959) introduced *teleradiography,* which is based on an infinite focus-object distance (at least 6 metres).

This technique, however, is expensive and needs special building facilities. Most of the stereotactic centers therefore accept a constant enlargement that is standardized and make proportional correction by simple calculation (Spiegel and Wycis 1952) or by a special projection technique (Leksell 1957). Calculation of the enlargement is based on the formula:

$$\text{real distance} = \text{enlarged distance} \times \frac{\text{focus-object—distance}}{\text{focus-film—distance}}.$$

Fig. 14 illustrates in a) the lateral arrangement (taking a lateral X-ray picture) as seen from anterior and in b) the anteroposterior arrangement as seen from lateral; it is evident, that the nearer the object inside the stereotactic instrument is to the focus, the more enlarged it will be on the film. Objects that lie in the midsagittal plane of the instrument have the same enlargement in the lateral projection; for example the distance AC—PC on the lateral film should have the standard instrument enlargement (in Leksell's instrument the standard magnification for the sagittal plane is 40%). In Fig. 15 the projection of AC—PC on the film ($= AC'—PC'$) is indicated as well as the point of incidence of the central X-ray ($= O'$) where magnification is zero. As any distance is given by its end points, for a correct calculation each of these points should be corrected in relation to the zero point $0'$. In Fig. 16 the distance $T_1—T_2$, representing the size of the object T(umor) in lateral projection, will be more enlarged on the film than the same distance $H_1—H_2$, representing the size of the object H(ematoma) in lateral projection, because the tumor lies nearer to the focus.

When the object has only a virtual size (i.e. the target is represented by a point, as usually is the case in functional stereotactics), proportional correction is determined by the distance given by the target point and the zero point. Be it that the target does not lie in the sagittal plane, then these corrections will deviate from the standard instrument magnification and should be calculated precisely with the above mentioned formula or special instrument localizing equipment (as the spiral diagram for Leksell's instrument). Often a magnified ruler is available to read off the distances of interest in true millimetres for standard planes of magnification (the proximal and distal instrument planes and the midsagittal or midfrontal planes, as indicated in Fig. 14). Provided the X-ray tube is situated to the left

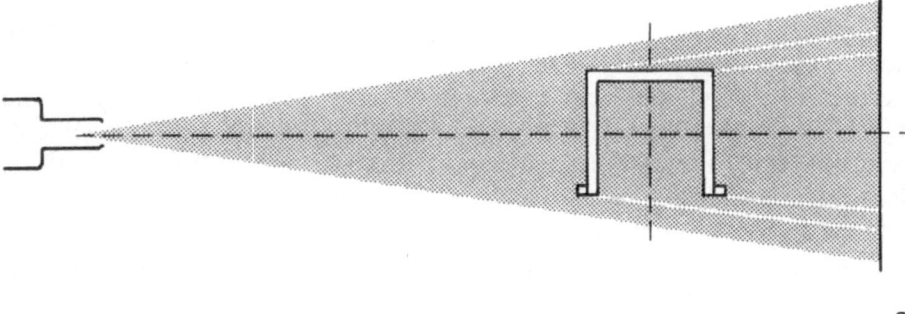

Fig. 14. Calculation of X-ray enlargement. Central X-ray running through the axial plane of stereotactic instrument. a) Is lateral arrangement as seen from ante-roposterior. b) Is anteroposterior arrangement as seen from lateral. The vertical midplane of the instrument [midsagittal in a) and midfrontal in b)] is the so-called plane of standard-enlargement. Note that the nearer the target inside the instrument is to the focus of the X-ray source, the more enlarged it will be on the film

of the patient in the lateral projection, and the film cassette to the right side, which is almost standard in stereotactic performances, a target with a true size is bigger when lying in the left hemisphere, and less big when lying in the right hemisphere in comparison with the standard enlargement of the midsagittal plane. Provided the X-ray tube is situated anterior to the patient in the anteroposterior projection, and the film cassette posterior, which is almost standard in stereotactic performances, a target with a true size is bigger when lying frontally, and less big when lying occipitally in

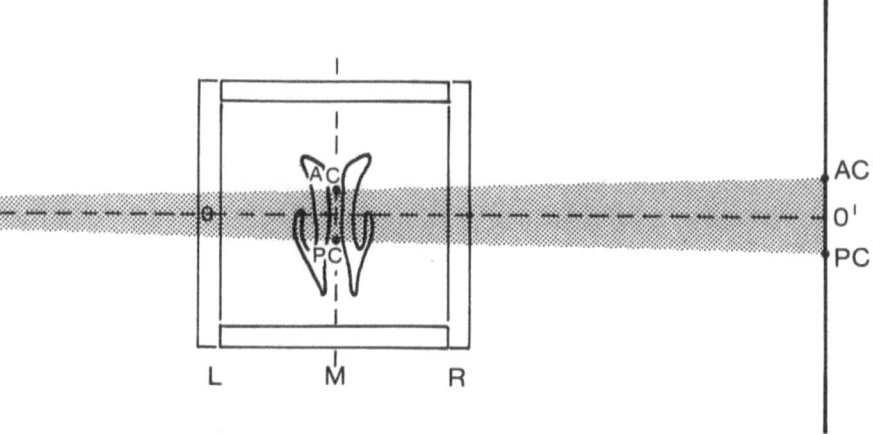

Fig. 15. X-ray enlargement illustrated with the lateral arrangement as seen from above. Targets in or near the midsagittal plane of the brain (the intercommissural plane with line AC—PC) will lie at a distance from $0^1$ on the film that is their real distance × the standard-enlargement (AC—PC × standard-enlargement = AC'—PC'). Note that the zero point of the system of axes erected intracerebrally only for the sake of clearness seems to lie at the zero point of the instrument system of axes

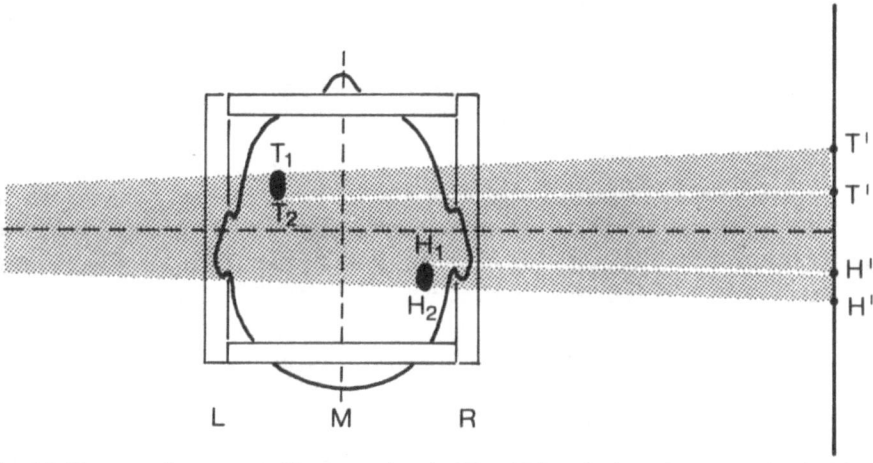

Fig. 16. X-ray enlargement illustrated as in Fig. 15 for various intracerebral objects. Left side tumor and right side hematoma with the same size. On the lateral stereotactic X-ray picture the diameter of $T_1T_2$ will be bigger than the diameter of $H_1H_2$, according to the formula: enlarged diameter = real diameter

$$\times \frac{\text{focus-film—distance}}{\text{focus-object—distance}}$$

comparison with the standard enlargement of the midfrontal plane, as is evident from Fig. 14b.

In the calculation of invisible targets that are related to the line AC—PC, it is logical that any deviation of the stereotactic apparatus to the left or the right produces a midline shift of the midsagittal plane of the instrument with respect to the midsagittal plane (with AC—PC) of the brain. This shift has also to be considered and included in the corrective calculations, as shown in Fig. 17.

Apart from these corrections, which are relevant to the lateral X-ray picture and are discussed above with the help of figures 15 and 16, similar corrections should be made for the anteroposterior X-ray picture. However, because the two coordinates x and y are already determined from the lateral picture, correction is much less critical. The z coordinate, standing for the distance between target and midsagittal plane, is seldom far from the midplane of the instrument in this projection (i.e. the midfrontal plane), and is therefore often assessed with the aid of the standard ruler of the instrument. Is the target lying far frontally or occipitally, however, this distance to the midfrontal plane of the instrument (= the already determined x coordinate) has to be taken into account and proportional corrections as described for the lateral picture should also be performed for this projection. The anteroposterior X-ray picture is essential to visualize any shift of the midsagittal plane of the instrument with regard to the brain's midsagittal plane (Fig. 17); not only in functional stereotactics, but also in the determination of visible targets any midline shift should be taken into consideration, because the transfer of a visible target from conventional to stereotactic X-ray pictures in the AP projection (Fig. 12b) is done in relation with the midsagittal plane of the brain, and not yet with the midsagittal plane of the instrument.

Because, especially in tumor biopsy, the target area does not necessarily lie in the midsagittal plane, the described method of calculation is rather time consuming. This in contrast to functional stereotactics, where thalamus and brainstem procedures are performed in the vicinity of the midsagittal plane. Much easier than the calculations based on the formula for X-ray enlargement is the use of Leksell's projection technique, which allows quick determination of the position of any intracerebral target with the aid of a diagram of concentric logarithmic spirals (Carlsson and Leksell 1971), that is based on a fixed ratio given by the position of the X-ray tube, the instrument and the film cassette. This projection technique is however only applicable to Leksell's stereotactic system.

Finally, it should be stressed that the above description of the calculation of the target point only holds for the positioning with help of X-ray pictures; in CT-guided stereotactics (discussed sub B) calculations are no longer

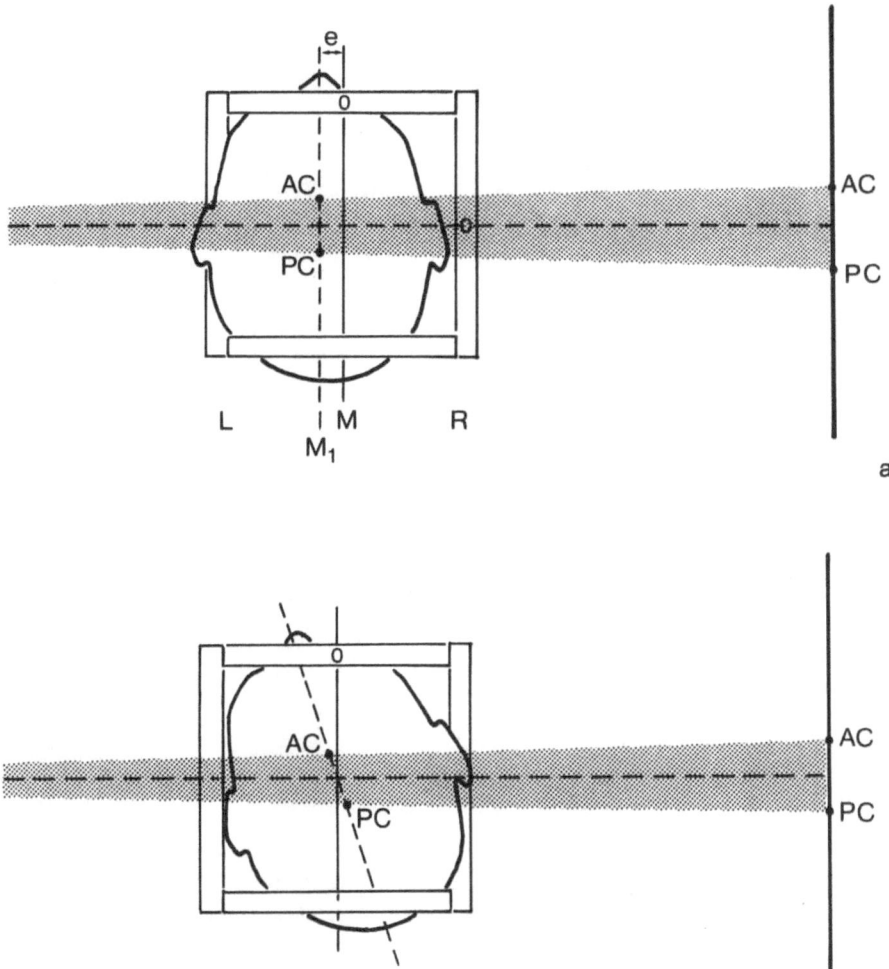

Fig. 17. Correction for midline shift of instrument. Illustrated with the lateral arrangement as seen from above. a) Shows midline shift of midsagittal plane of instrument (M) regarding midsagittal plane of brain ($M_1$). When the planes run (almost) parallel to each other this is acceptable, but needs correction. Shift to the right (as illustrated) leads to a $z$-coordinate, which is the true $z$ of the target + the error ($e$) with a target lying in the left hemisphere, and — the error with a target lying in the right hemisphere. b) Shows oblique positioning of skull in stereotactic instrument. This position is not acceptable and the instrument should be repositioned

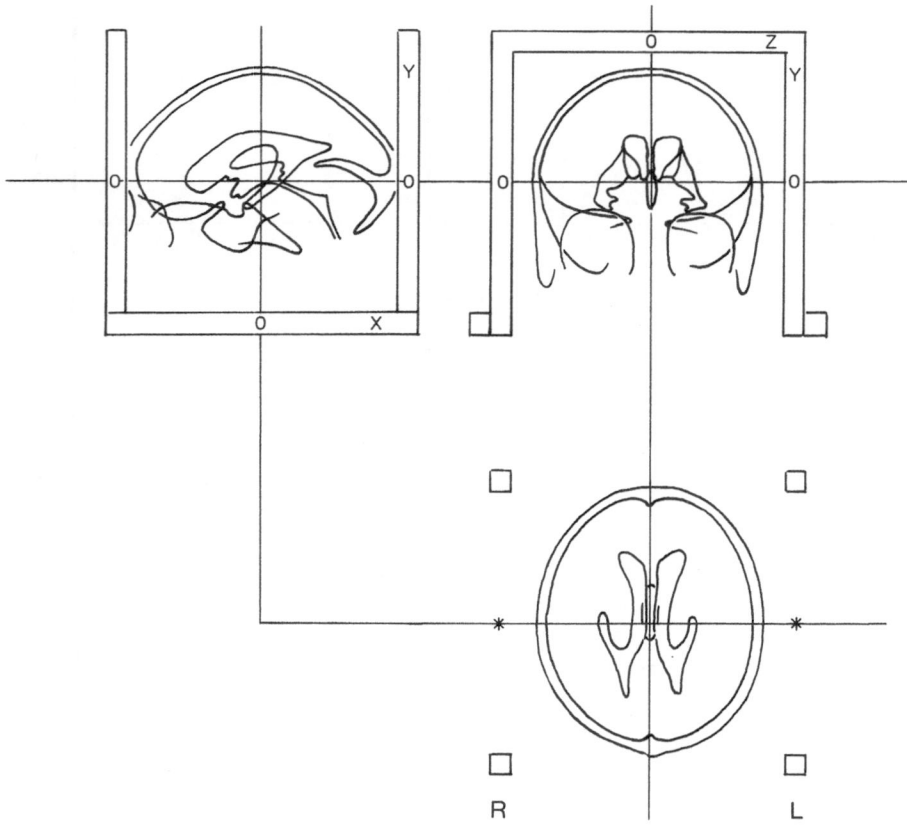

Fig. 18 a. Expression in coordinates of target position. Ventriculography for positioning of invisible target. For clearness no target indicated, but line AC—PC may be drawn. Spatial orientation with help of sagittal, frontal, and axial planes of stereotactic instrument. Coordinates *x* and *y* are derived from sagittal projection, coordinates *y* and *z* are derived from frontal projection, and coordinates *x* and *z* are derived from axial projection. Note that axial projection stands for CT-scan picture after positioning the instrument perpendicular to the scanner gantry

needed, as the computer is able to present the surgeon with real distances and therefore produces real coordinates.

## D. The Stereotactic Intervention

After having determined the position of the target point in relation to the stereotactic apparatus, one needs to express its position in coordinates. The x coordinate stands for the distance from zero to anterior or posterior, the y coordinate for the distance from zero to superior or inferior, and the z coordinate for the distance from zero to the left or the right (Fig. 18 a and b).

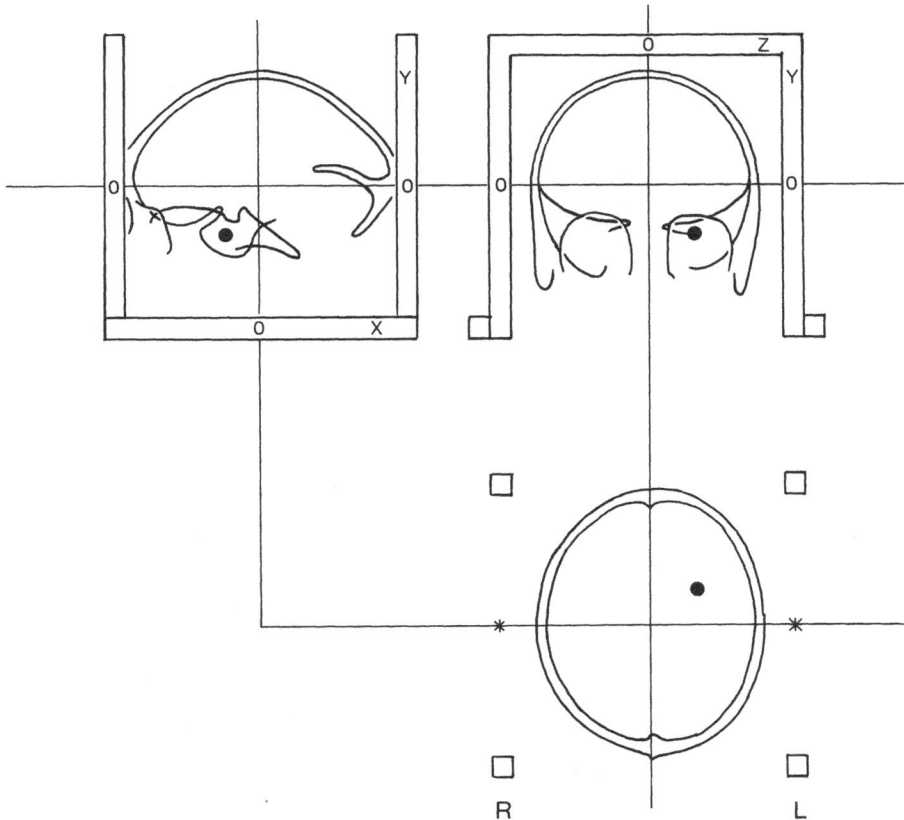

Fig. 18 b. Spatial orientation as in Fig. 18 a. Expression in coordinates of a visible target. Left temporal tumor is indicated. The axial projection (CT-scan picture) is well below the instrument's mid-axial plane that is shown sub a) (actually *y* millimetres), to visualize the lesion on the scan

However, with the new instrumentation designed for CT and MR imaging techniques (see chapter 4) the origin of the coordinate system may lie in the upper posterior corner of the right side of the frame due to international agreement on localizing standardization. Fig. 19 illustrates this important change in coordinates nomination. With this knowledge the stereotactic performance sensu strictiori can start. Aiming devices are mounted onto the head frame and a burrhole is made to introduce the stereotactic gadget needed (electrode, biopsy forceps, puncture needle et cetera). As the aiming devices are components of the different stereotactic apparatus available, it is unfeasable and uneffective to describe in detail all the types which have been constructed. In the period from 1947 to 1967 18 different devices were developed (Fox 1969)!

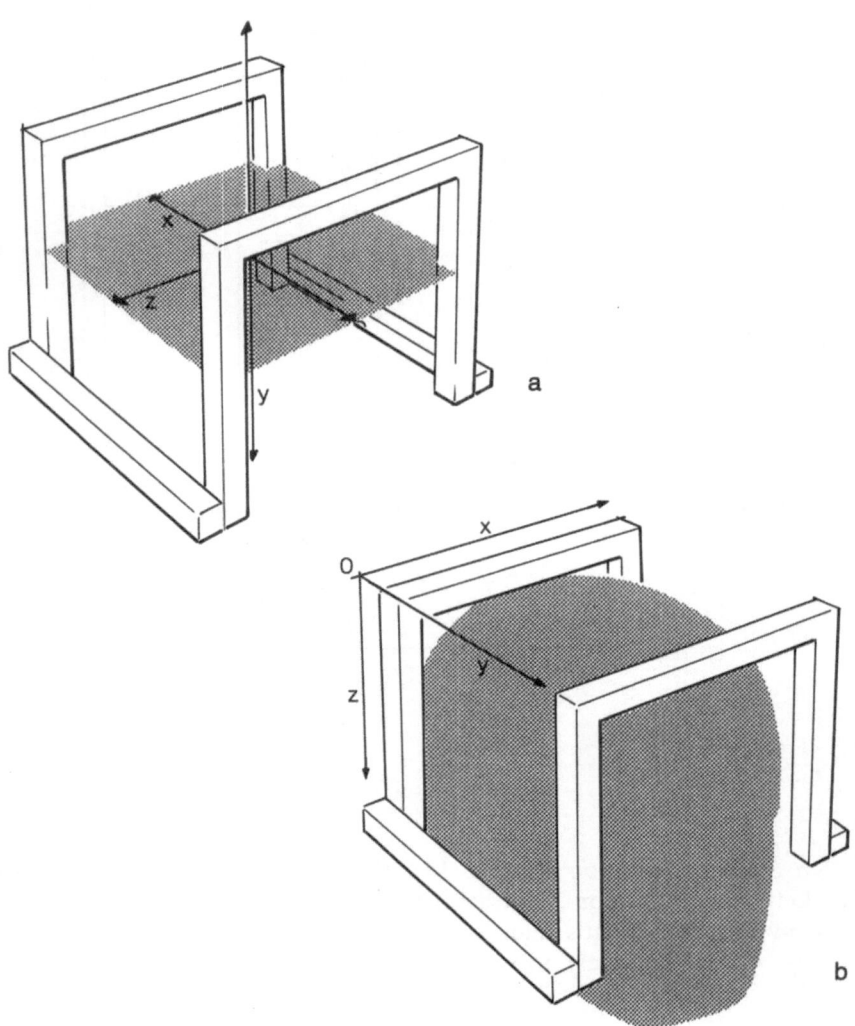

Fig. 19. Coordinate system of stereotactic instrument. a) Shows the system in use for stereotactic localizing with help of lateral and anteroposterior X-ray pictures. b) Shows the modern system for stereotactic localizing with help of computerized tomography (CT-guided localization)

We have no intention of passing judgement upon the many stereotactic instruments available. However, for the sake of clearness we will describe briefly four well-known devices, which are in current use throughout the world: the Talairach (*et al.* 1949), the Riechert-Mundinger (1955), the Leksell (1949, 1971), and the Todd-Wells (Todd 1967) apparatus. Computer-guided instruments will be discussed in the next chapter (4).

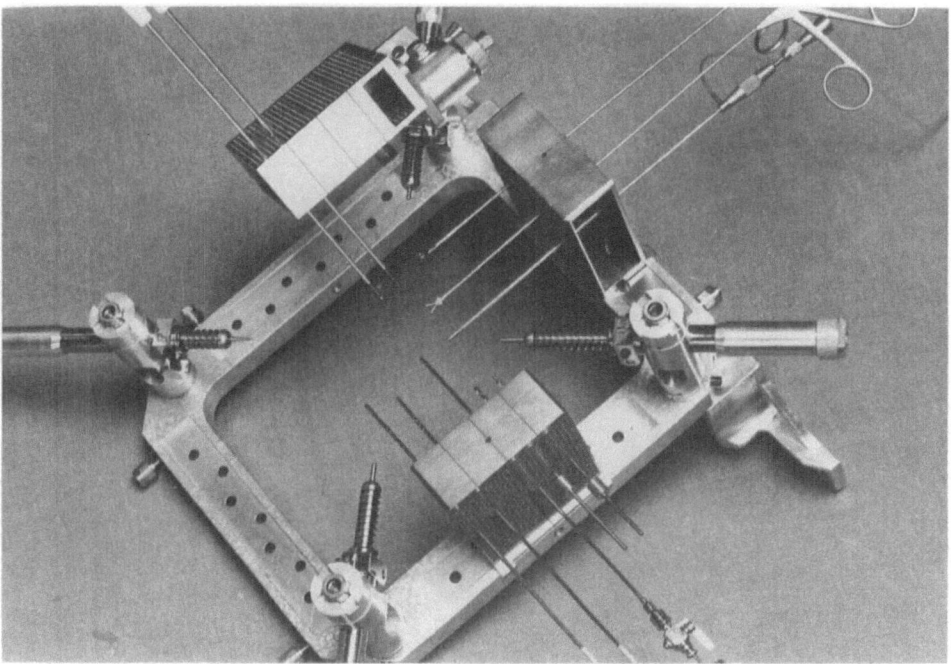

Fig. 20. Talairach system with various electrodes, cannulas, and biopsy forceps (by courtesy of Prof. Pecker)

## 1. Talairach System

The Talairach system consists of a rectangular headframe fixed to the skull with four pins. The frame is also fixed to the operating table. It is used with teleradiographic X-ray equipment with a tube-film distance of 5 metres. This means an enlargement of only 2.5% for the target studied. To reduce the enlargement factor still further, double grids of reference points are mounted on the headframe. Aiming of the X-ray beam is done with a parallel light beam, which ensures an orthogonal position of the X-ray beam as to the frame. The double grids are movable with help of a rectangular brace, which can rotate on a sagittal axis and guide the electrodes or biopsy forceps which are inserted through small trephine openings into the skull. This technique has the possibility of placing multiple electrodes in one target area (especially the temporal lobe in cases of epilepsy), but all the instruments introduced run a parallel course and have therefore their own trephine openings. Therefore the apparatus of Talairach (Fig. 20) is very suitable for clinical research of deep brain structures (f.e. stereotactic EEG recording) and for stereotactic cerebral angiography (Szikla 1979 b). A recent survey of possibilities in deep seated tumor management with this

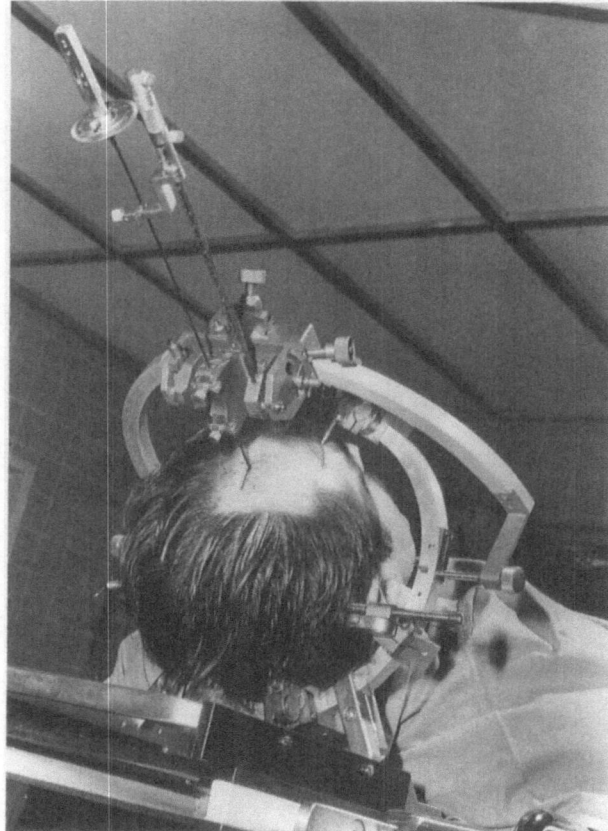

Fig. 21. Riechert-Mundinger system (by courtesy of Prof. Mundinger)

device is given in J. Pecker (*et al.* 1979 a): Démarche stéréotaxique en neurochirurgie tumorale. Scerrati (*et al.* 1984) described a modification of the Talairach orthogonal approach, which is also suitable for polar approaches. Their stereotactic device is basically a Talairach apparatus with the double grid system, to which two hemicircular supports for polar approach are added.

## 2. The Riechert-Mundinger System

This system is also based on the cartesian principle and consists of a circular basal ring, which is fixed to the skull with 4 to 6 holding pins. The frame is also fixed to the operating table and filmcassetteholder, but can easily be released when necessary during surgery. Similar to the system of Talairach, its main component is a basal head frame, thus leaving the skull convexity totally free for the case of combined stereotactic and open surgery

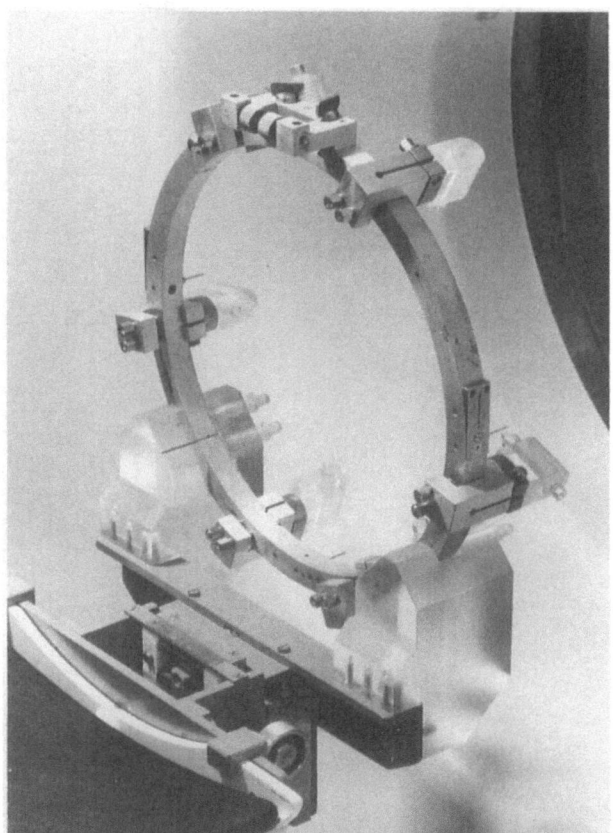

Fig. 22. Riechert-Mundinger system for CT-guided surgery (by courtesy of Prof.
Mundinger)

(craniotomy), as sometimes is advisable (e.g. in deep seated arteriovenous
malformations). It is used with teleradiography with a tube-film distance of
3–4 metres. The slight enlargement with this technique (3.5%) is further
reduced by the introduction of a metal ruler, which is marked in centimetres
and fixed to the skull convexity at about the target plane. Aiming of the X-
ray beam is also done with a parallel light beam. The aiming device for the
introduction of an electrode or biopsy forceps consists of an arc, that is fixed
in the mediotransverse (interaural) axis of the basal ring. It can be placed in
position at any desired angle within the range of 0°–180° as to the plane of
the basal ring (Fig. 21). In outline, Kirschner's apparatus (1933) for
puncture of the Gasserian ganglion through the foramen ovale has a similar
aiming device. After the determination of the position of the target point on
the stereotactic X-ray pictures the aiming device is first mounted on a
phantom device to determine the angle of incidence and the position of the

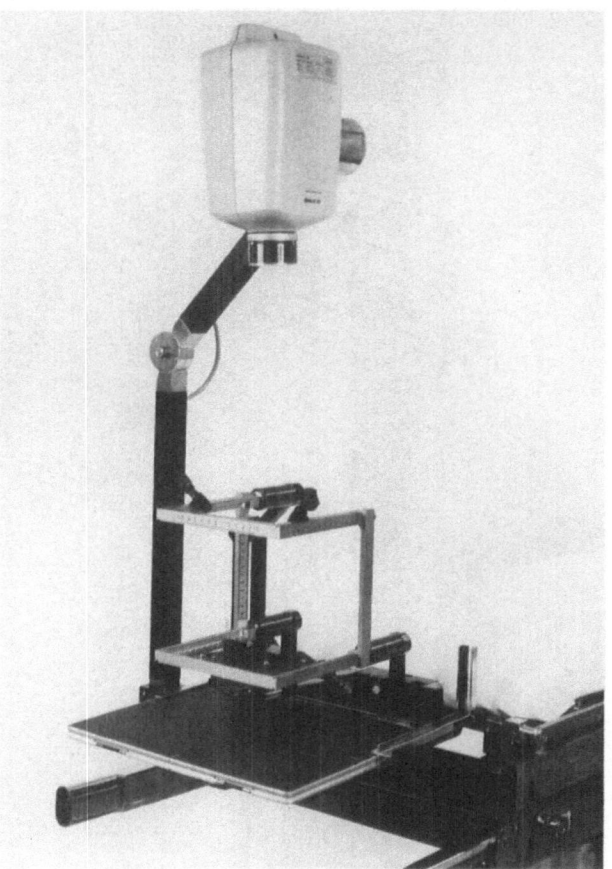

Fig. 23. Mechanical X-ray coupling arm for standardized X-ray enlargement in the
Leksell system (by courtesy of Prof. Leksell)

trephine opening in the skull. With this technique it is possible to reach any
point within the brain, also when the approach is made from the skull base
(e.g. transsphenoidal). For biopsy procedures a special forceps has been
developed by Riechert (*et al.* 1967). This apparatus and its applications are
extensively described by Riechert in 1980. The system is modified and
adapted for CT guided interventions by Mundinger (*et al.* 1978a, b);
Fig. 22.

### 3. Leksell System

The stereotactic system of Leksell consists of a cubical headframe, which
is fixed to the skull with 4 (formerly 3) pins that are drilled into the tabula
externa. The major difference with the other devices is, that this frame
constitutes a three-dimensional orthogonal coordinate system, which shows

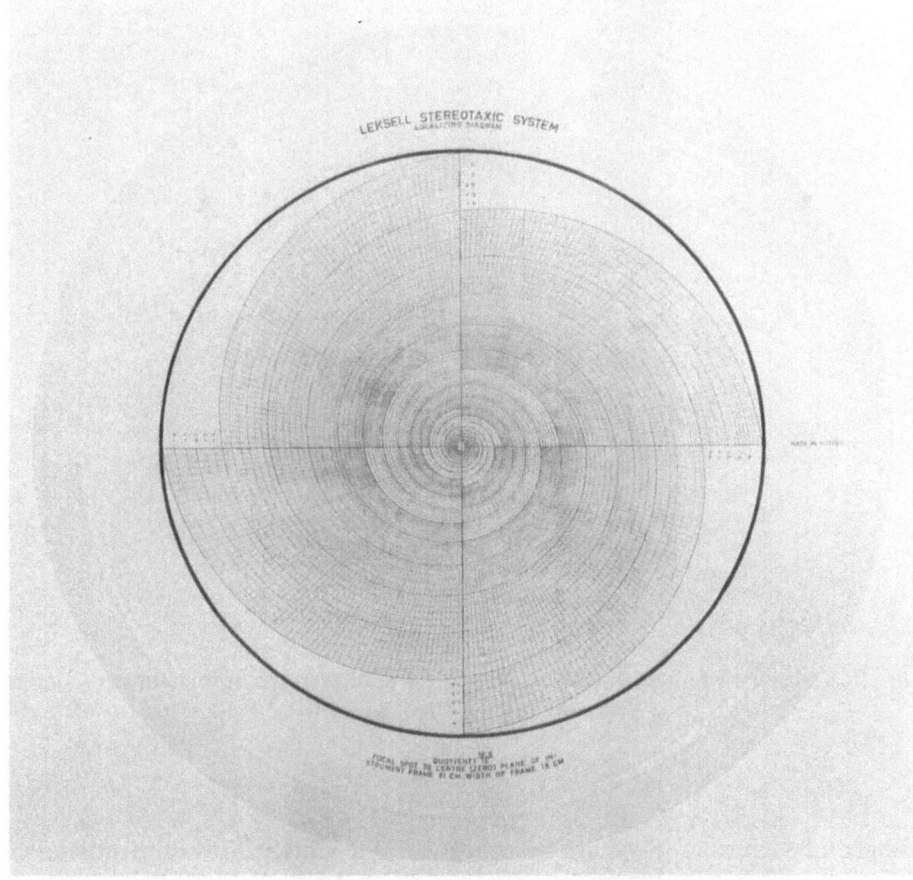

Fig. 24. Localizing diagram for calculation of coordinates from stereotactic X-ray pictures with standard enlargement (by courtesy of Prof. Leksell)

millimetre scales on all its edges. Although this instrument as to its applications will be described in more detail in another chapter (because it is the author's instrument, with which the stereotactic technique will be elucidated), in this overview some important points of difference with regard to the other systems are discussed. The headframe is not fixed to the operating table, but only onto the skull of the patient, who is either sitting conveniently in a chair (when operated upon without general anesthesia), or is lying on the table with his head supported by a neck rest. Although X-ray enlargement in the early years of development (1949) was reduced by long distance radiography, later on (1957) a mechanical X-ray coupling arm was constructed (Fig. 23) with the introduction of a geometric localizing diagram (Fig. 24). By this means X-ray enlargement was accepted (40%) and corrected by the projection technique, as already discussed. Thus an

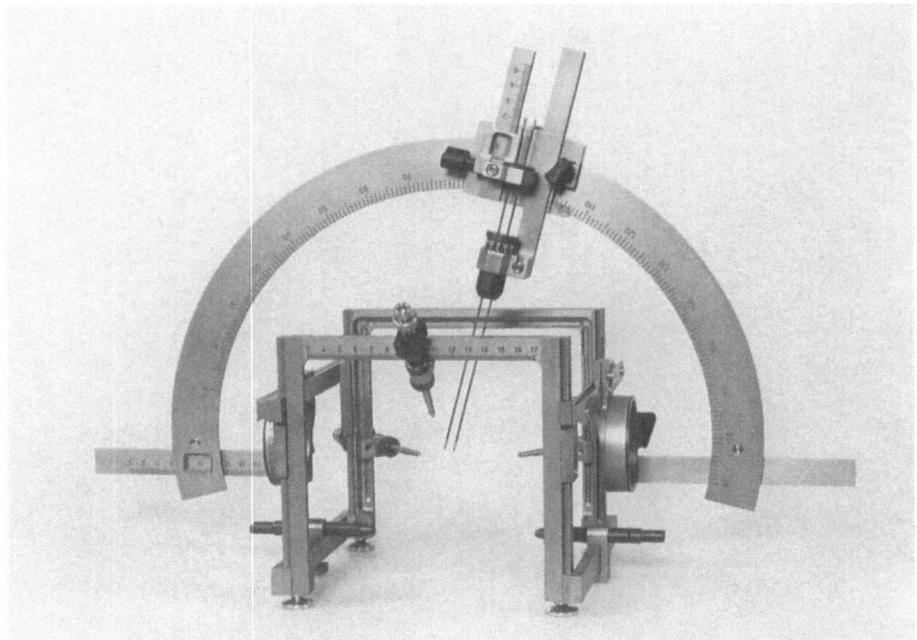

Fig. 25. Leksell system with semicircular arc and electrodes in instrument carrier
(by courtesy of Prof. Leksell)

integrated stereotactic system became available which allows short distance
exposure with X-rays (less expensive; no need for special building facilities)
and an elimination of time consuming calculations for correction of
enlargement (Leksell 1971). The aiming device with an instrument carrier
consists of a semicircular arc (Fig. 25), which is fixed to the headframe
according to the coordinates of the target in such a way that its center
corresponds to the target point. The arc can be rotated and the instrument
carrier moved along the arc, which enables the surgeon to introduce the
instrument into the brain through any trephine opening he wants. During
the operation X-ray pictures can be made of the target area for control of
positioning of the instrument tip (e.g. ventriculography to verify the needle
approaching a pinealoma; Fig. 26). As the device is very manoeuvrable it is
easy to perform more than one puncture (e.g. in both hemispheres) in one
session. Calculation of the coordinates of the different targets is then done
prior to the intervention which saves considerable time. Combined
stereotactic and open surgery is more difficult with the cubic frame, as it
only permits small craniotomies to be carried out with the headframe in
position (Fig. 27). However, for combined surgery a new frame has been

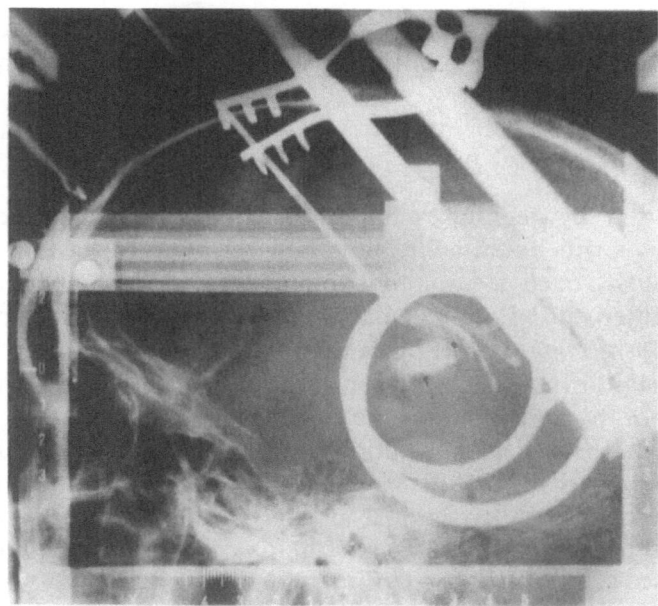

Fig. 26. Stereotactic biopsy of a tumor in pineal gland region. In the lateral view ventriculography shows the tumor at which is aimed

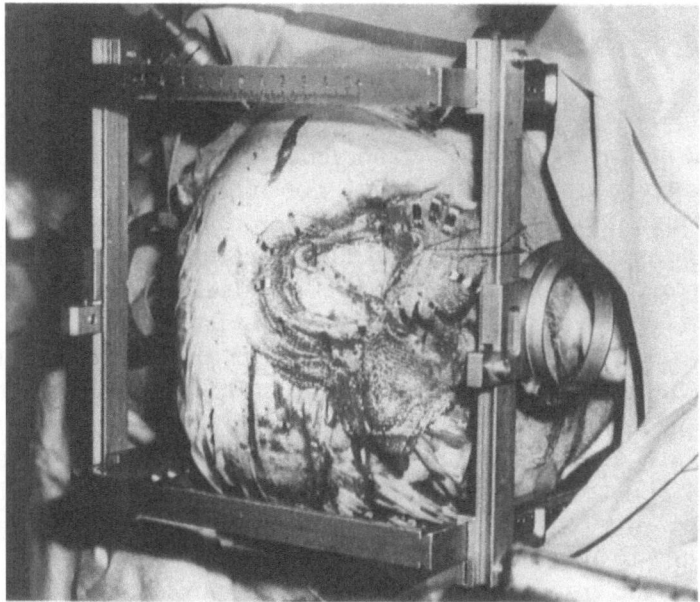

Fig. 27. Open surgery in stereotactic space. With the cubic Leksell headframe only small craniotomies can be carried out

constructed that can be attached to a Mayfield clamp and offers any positioning wanted for craniotomy (Leksell, personal communication 1985).

### 4. Todd-Wells System

The Todd-Wells stereotactic apparatus consists of a head holder with fixation screws, which is attached to a semi-permanent base that stands on the floor in such a fixed position that permanent X-ray alignment is secured. During the intervention only the patient's head with head holder is moved for target positioning. This apparatus involves a very simple principle, namely translation in x, y, or z motion of the patient's head until the target is at the center of the stereotactic frame, which is confirmed by X-ray. There is no need for mathematical calculations and no special X-ray equipment is necessary. The patient may also be placed in the prone position (e.g. in posterior percutaneous trigeminal or in pontine tractotomy). Aiming devices for different approaches include a transverse quadrant and a vertical quadrant, the use of each being dependent on the type of surgery wanted. X-ray pictures during the operation can be made of the target area as easy as with Leksell's system. For pure lateral approach (e.g. multiple epilepsy electrode implantation) a lateral micropositioner is available, which after removal of the transverse or vertical quadrant can be placed at the same coordinates. The Todd-Wells system, including many accessories, is documented by Radionics in various brochures (Fig. 28). Its equivalent for CT guided stereotactics will be discussed in chapter 4.

### 5. The Ideal Stereotactic System

For the neurosurgeon in general practice the ideal system should have all the particular instrument advantages. The aiming device of choice should possess a high number of degrees of freedom: i.e. it should be possible to readjust the aiming device quickly in all three cartesian planes. Besides these basic degrees of freedom (on which stereotactic surgery depends) it is a great advantage to have a free choice in the determination of the entrance site. Therefore, after adjustment of the aiming device according to the coordinates of the target, extra degrees of freedom are of utmost importance: i.e. the possibility of rotating the device and of moving the instrument carrier along the arc, and finally the sliding of the instrument stop in a parallel direction. The complete apparatus should be easy to handle, safely constructed (for repeated sterilization), exist of as few single parts as possible, and be reliable in its functioning with an aiming error less than 2 mm. As to the visualization of the apparatus plus skull on X-rays or CT scan, the construction should permit high quality pictures without artifacts. For conveniently performing open craniotomies with stereotactic control,

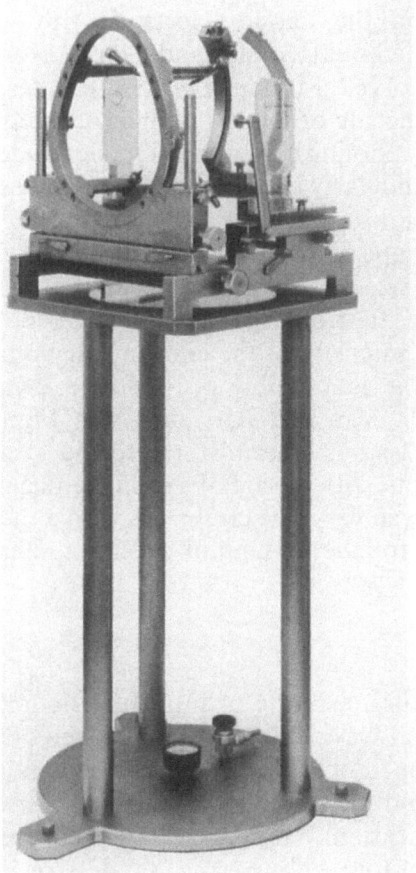

Fig. 28. Todd-Wells system (by courtesy of Dr. Cosman)

the frame should have most or all of its mechanical support structure outside the surgical field (Kelly 1983). Precise surgical control within threedimensional space needs computer assistance, that should be incorporated in the stereotactic system of the future. Technically speaking, an integrated and computer guided stereotactic system is within reach. Before long it will also become available to the general neurosurgeon.

## E. Stereotactically Guided Instruments

### 1. Electrode

The electrode was the first of instruments developed for stereotactic surgery. As neurophysiologists invented the stereotactic aiming technique for the selective destruction of intracerebral targets, the electrolytic lesion (with direct current on the anode—electrode tip) was the first well documented lesion carried out (Horsley and Clarke 1908, Sweet and Mark 1953, Spiegel and Wycis 1962, Mullan *et al.* 1965). Later on, to prevent gas formation to occur at the site of the lesion, neurosurgeons started making use of thermal lesions by cooling or heating. The electrode which produces a lesion by heating is particularly accepted as safe because of its predictable results. Only the temperature should not rise to 100 °C because of the formation of gas. The shape of the lesion depends on the electrode tip. Slight variations in the lesion size and shape are brought about by differences in vascularization (cooling effect of large vessels and cerebospinal fluid). With constant control of the intensity of the current, the voltage, the resistance and the temperature, it is possible to produce constant lesion sizes (Mundinger *et al.* 1960, Van den Berg and Van Manen 1962). Today, electrodes for thermal lesions (thermistor electrodes) can be purchased. Lesions are brought about with the aid of a radiofrequency lesion generator (Cosman *et al.* 1983). Even very fine electrodes with a thermocouple sensor in the tip are available for the making of precise and small lesions in the spinal cord.

## 2. Needle

The needle to puncture, aspirate or introduce liquids is an old tool in clinical neurosurgery and was easily adapted for stereotactic introduction. Puncture and aspiration alone is only of value in nonneoplastic cystic lesions, as an arachnoid cyst or a colloid cyst (Bosch *et al.* 1978). In cystic tumors, however, aspiration has to be repeated frequently or fluid accumulation should be stopped by means that destroy its production. For repeated aspiration of deep seated cysts a catheter is placed stereotactically and connected to a subcutaneous reservoir, which can be punctured easily (e.g. in recurrent craniopharyngioma; Gutin *et al.* 1980). To destroy the production of fluid in tumor cysts interstitial irradiation with $\beta$-emitters with short distance radiation is possible (e.g. Yttrium[90] with a halflife of only 64 hours). Backlund (1973, 1979) published his results with cystic craniopharyngiomas and shows the benefits of intracystic treatment with radionuclides. Endocystic $\beta$-irradiation of glioma cysts has also been reported, which proved to be successful in stopping secretion (Schaub *et al.* 1979). Concerning this subject of interstitial irradiation by stereotactic methods a Symposium has been held in Paris in 1979; the proceedings are edited by G. Szikla (1979 a).

## 3. Biopsy Instrument

The biopsy instrument to take tissue samples from deep seated lesions has become one of the most popular stereotactic tools. The first biopsies were carried out with fine needle aspiration and tissue smears for cytological investigation. Even in solid tumors it is almost always possible to collect some material by aspiration with a 10–20 cc syringe that is withdrawn to produce a vacuum inside the needle. Riechert (*et al.* 1967) developed a biopsy forceps of only 2 mm in diameter, which can be introduced through the electrode sheath. This instrument can excise small tissue specimens for histological examination. In 1971, Backlund described a new biopsy instrument, a spiral needle, which takes biopsies with a 12 mm length and a 1.2 mm diameter. This instrument is screwed into the target tissue, after which the outer needle with a sharp edge cuts it free by reverse rotation. Numerous slight modifications have become in use later on (Gildenberg *et al.* 1982). The Nashold biopsy needle is a side-window cutting type instrument and the Gildenberg instrument is a biopsy forceps and spring which both fit into a universal outer cannula.

### 4. Catheter

The catheter to drain stereotactically or to introduce fluids into the target area (antibiotics in abscesses; cytostatic agents in tumors) can be positioned correctly with the aid of a stereotactic introducer. It may be secured to the skull at the site of the trephine opening with the help of a fitting anchor.

### 5. Electrodes for Permanent Implantation

Electrodes for permanent implantation have been constructed during the last ten years for deep brain stimulation. In functional stereotactic neurosurgery permanent stimulation of various deep brain structures has become common practice as well as the single brain lesion in the effective treatment of various pain syndromes. Neurostimulation has also proven to be of some help in the management of spasticity. For details the reader is referred to "Advances in Stereotactic and Functional Neurosurgery" 4, section III (Gillingham *et al.* 1980), 6, section III (Gybels *et al.* 1984) and to "Functional Neurosurgery" (Rasmussen and Marino 1979). Various anchors for securing the electrodes to the skull are available today.

### 6. Archimedes Screw for Hematoma Evacuation

The Archimedes screw to evacuate intracerebral hematomas stereotactically is a special instrument designed by Backlund and Von Holst (1978). Although there was much debate among neurosurgeons as to the indications for stereotactic evacuation, it cannot be denied any longer that impressive results may be obtained with this technique. The instrument consists of an archimedes type of screw inside an outer cannula with distal side-window, which is rotated mechanically (about 100 cycles per minute) while irrigation and aspiration along its shaft help clear the clotted material. In this way it is easy to collect about 70% of the total volume of a gelatinous hematoma. Amano (*et al.* from Tokyo) and Kandel (*et al.* from Moscow) reported at the stereotactic meeting in Bratislava in 1983 on their results, which were satisfactory. The instrument outer diameter is 4 to 4.7 mm, depending on the type that is purchased. A slightly modified and innovated type of Archimedes screw is described by Higgins (*et al.* 1982) and is nowadays available as the Higgins Nashold hematoma evacuator. This technique should be applied to spontaneously developing hematomas that threaten to be fatal because of their size or position.

## 7. Endoscope

The endoscope is not yet fully employed in stereotactic surgery, although there are at the moment encouraging reports on the use of a fiberoptic device at the target site. For example, intraventricular inspection, exploration of cyst walls (eventually with biopsy from suspected areas) and inspection of the hematoma cavity after evacuation of the clot. A rigid type endoscope in which the transmission of images is achieved by a relay of lenses, is easy to introduce stereotactically, if the diameter is small. A flexible type endoscope requires a bundle of precisely aligned optical fibers and has the advantage that, after introduction through a stereotactic cannula, endoscopic inspection can be performed more freely.

## 8. Laser

Lasers are used as surgical tools through endoscopes for cutting and coagulation (Epstein 1980). If acute bleeding is present, it could be controlled by an argon or other type of laser beam under eye control (Edwards *et al.* 1983). In surgical use of the laser, radiant energy is targeted on endogenous chromophors, such as hemoglobin, or on tissue water to cause a thermal reaction. Photoradiation therapy (Dougherty *et al.* 1978) for tumors, which selectively retain photosensitizing agents (f.e. hematopor-phyrin derivative that is currently on trial), can be performed by laser light delivered safely via a fiberoptic probe. Laws (*et al.* 1981) published a phase I study in malignant brain tumors with use of a stereotactically placed fiberoptic instrument. Computer assisted stereotactic laser surgery is further discussed by Kelly (1983); a carbon dioxide laser beam is used to vaporize sequential slices of tumor and an argon or neodymium-YAG laser beam can be directed to vascular lesions or bleeding sites.

## F. Spinal Stereotactic Surgery

In their review on the Horsley-Clarke stereotactic instrument, Schurr and Merrington (1978) mention that in 1921 Clarke invented a similar instrument for use on the spinal cord, "though this has been of less significance in the development of physiology". Hitchcock (1969, 1970 a, b) developed a similar apparatus for spinal stereotactic interventions and published on stereotactic cervical myelotomy and trigeminal tractotomy. With the aid of a modified Hitchcock instrument Schvarcz (1976, 1978) performed a series of stereotactic cervical operations and discussed his results, which make spinal stereotactics a promising procedure in the treatment of intractable pain. Nádvorník (et al. 1983) has some experience with spinal cord stereotactics for the treatment of spasticity of the lower limbs, in which open surgery (laminectomy) is combined with stereotactic instrument positioning. A similar instrument for spinal stereotactic surgery has been developed by Nashold, who studied the effect of dorsal root entry zone lesioning for the relief of phantom pain (Nashold and Ostdahl 1979, Saris et al. 1985).

It should be mentioned here, that also the already discussed instruments of Riechert-Mundinger, Leksell and Todd-Wells can serve as a platform for spinal stereotactics, if performed at the $C_0$—$C_1$ level. The patients should then be placed in the prone position. Compared with the well established technique of percutaneous cervical cordotomy, that is carried out by free hand lateral puncture at the $C_1$—$C_2$ level, the open or percutaneous stereotactic cervical tractotomies are operations, in which the electrode is guided and held by an electrode carrier that is mechanically fixed to the stereotactic apparatus. Stereotactic tractotomies are performed in the posterior part of the cervical medulla and have therefore as reference the midsagittal plane that runs through the dens. The indications are completely different from those in percutaneous cordotomy, in which the spinothalamic tract is targeted on one side, giving relief from pains located on the other side of the body. Stereotactic tractotomy, or myelotomy, has the posterior commissure of the cervical medulla as target, giving relief of midline and sometimes even bilateral pains. Much of the effect is still poorly understood, as clearly described by Cook (et al. 1984), who spoke of "a challenge to traditional anatomical concepts". Stereotactic cervical trigeminal tractotomy can be considered as the stereotactic counterpart of the well known Sjöquist operation (1938) for trigeminal neuralgia. It is to be expected that in the near future more elaborated and significant reports become available on the value and indications for stereotactic spinal surgery (Gildenberg 1982 a). In anticipation of future indications Zlatos and Cierny (1975) have produced a stereotactic atlas and variability table of the identifiable spinal cord structures.

Chapter 3

# Expanding Field of Stereotactic Surgery

For ease of survey the continuously expanding field of stereotactic neurosurgery will be divided in three major subdivisions, namely:
— functional stereotactics
— mass lesions stereotactics
— localizing stereotactics + open surgery.

## I. Functional Stereotactics

The progressive expansion in our understanding of human neurophysiological mechanisms, coupled with the continual development of more refined and sophisticated equipment for recording the electrical activity of the nervous system and for stimulating nervous tissue electrically, has resulted in increasingly effective neurosurgical treatment of such conditions as movement disorders, pain syndromes, intractable epilepsy and spasticity. Was neurosurgery in the early years concentrated on the treatment of lesions, with this growing knowledge of neurophysiological processes surgery became involved in the treatment of *symptoms* of underlying lesions, that do not require treatment or are untreatable. This field of neurosurgery is generally called: functional neurosurgery. Although functional neurosurgery is not exclusively stereotactic, this link is becoming more and more evident at the present time. Both types of surgery are closely interrelated, which is evident from the denomination "Society for stereotactic and functional neurosurgery". This field has been extended in recent years to include even the lower brainstem, the cerebellum and the spinal cord. For reliable information and daily use stereotactic atlasses have been published, which include these structures (Schaltenbrand and Wahren 1979, Afshar *et al.* 1978, Emmers and Tasker 1975, Zlatos and Cierny 1975).

### A. Movement Disorders

In the late 1940s the application of the Horsley-Clarke stereotactic techniques on humans led to the effective treatment of a variety of motor disorders, such as parkinsonism, choreoathetosis, torticollis spastica, and hemiballismus, for which medical therapy had previously been relatively ineffective. In 1941 Russell Meyers published a lesioning of the caudate nucleus in a parkinsonian woman with a tremor whereas in 1949 he preferred a pallidotomy; both interventions still performed with the open technique (craniotomy) (Meyers *et al.* 1950). In 1955 (a, b) Hassler described his results on stimulation and coagulation in the human thalamus, the ventrolateral nucleus being the principal relay center of

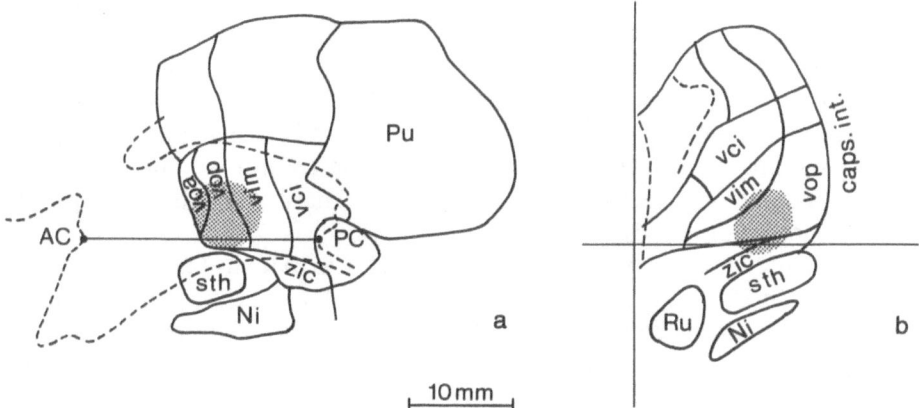

Fig. 29. Position of ventrolateral thalamic nucleus. a) In relation to line AC—PC in the lateral view, b) in relation to midsagittal plane in frontal view. Note that distance AC—PC is about 25 mm. Abbreviations used (according to Schaltenbrand and Wahren 1977): *Pu* pulvinar thalami; *voa* and *vop* nucl. ventrooralis ant. and post.; *vim* nucl. ventrointermedius; *vci* nucl. ventrocaudalis internus; *zic* zona incerta caudalis; *sth* corpus subthalamicum; *Ni* substantia nigra; *Ru* nucleus ruber; *caps. int.* capsula interna

pallido- and cerebellorubrofugal fibers towards the cerebral cortex. This nucleus of the thalamus became thereafter the target of choice for the treatment of a variety of movement disorders. Tremors (not only in parkinsonism, but also the essential tremor and the tremor of intention), torsion dystonias and some cases of cerebellar dyskinesia proved to be the most responsive (Schaltenbrand and Walker 1982, Riechert 1980; respectively the pages 503–563 and 272–276). In Fig. 29 the position of the ventrolateral nucleus (Vop and Vim) is shown in relation to the intercommissural line AC—PC in the lateral view (Fig. 29 a) and in relation to the midsagittal plane in the frontal view (Fig. 29 b). When dealing with chorea, athetosis, symptomatic dystonia and hemiballism, the results of stereotactic treatment are still poor (Molina-Negro 1979, Andrew *et al.* 1983). Posttraumatic movement disorders, however, may benefit from stereotactic thalamotomy, as reported by Bullard and Nashold (1984).

## 1. Parkinsonian Tremor

In parkinsonian patients tremor and rigidity can be treated successfully by stereotactic coagulation of the contralateral thalamic ventrolateral complex, as is clearly shown in extensive reports published by Cooper and Bravo (1958), Gillingham (*et al.* 1960), Krayenbühl (*et al.* 1961) and Van Manen (1967). In these early publications coagulations were often performed bilaterally with an interval of some months between the two procedures, but later on stereotactic neurosurgeons changed this practice because of the high risk of speech disturbances herewith evoked. In particular, coagulation on the dominant side carries with it the danger of a special type of dysarthria with lack of fluency, slurring and monotonous parlance (Petrovici 1980). Recurrence of tremor after a successful coagulation is seldom seen, but an aggravation of the tremor on the other (not treated) side occurs in about 44% of the cases (our own series in chapter 9; Van Manen *et al.* 1984).

Histochemical research of the basal ganglia led Hornykiewicz (1966) to the publication of his findings of dopamine deficiency in parkinsonian patients. This evidence led Cotzias (*et al.* 1969) to medical treatment with chronic administration of L-dopa. Clinical observation, however, revealed that the tremor responded only weakly to the institution of L-dopa therapy, which resulted in a renewed interest in stereotactic intervention. From an empirical point of view it is obvious, that both medical and stereotactic treatment have their own applicability and indication in the optimal management of parkinsonian patients. Because a life-long treatment with L-dopa has serious side-effects and a decreasing influence on the symptoms, there are advocates of early neurosurgical treatment (Siegfried 1980, Van Manen *et al.* 1984) before akinesia develops. Dopa therapy could be postponed until akinesia requires its institution. On the other hand, even patients treated for a long period with medical therapy can benefit from stereotactic surgery in the case of an otherwise untreatable and disabling tremor (Kelly and Gillingham 1980). As stated by Guiot (*et al.* 1976): "En bref, l'avènement de la L-Dopa et le progrès apporté par l'association d'inhibiteurs à la L-Dopa ont supprimé l'indication primitive de la chirurgie stéréotaxique. Mais la chirurgie et la pharmacologie peuvent être complémentaires dans certaines circonstances, celles en particulier d'un tremblement accentué et rebelle; une méthode ne réduisant nullement les effets bénéfiques de l'autre".

## 2. Essential Tremor

The essential tremor (or heredofamiliar tremor) that is autosomal dominant is related to striatal disease. This type of tremor is also treated by coagulation of the ventrolateral thalamic nucleus, but only if so distressing that the patient seeks relief through surgical therapy (Walker 1982 b).

This characteristic postural tremor of the upper limbs that has no other neurological abnormalities should first be treated medically. Medicines of choice are: propanolol (Jefferson et al. 1979 a, b), and primidone (O'Brien et al. 1981) which is almost as effective as alcohol.

## 3. Cerebellar Dyskinesia

Intention tremor of cerebellar dyskinesia can sometimes be relieved by stereotactic thalamic coagulation. Cooper (1965 b) describes a series of 110 cases operated upon, with a 90% success rate. Brice and McLellan (1980) communicate on the suppression of intention tremor on patients with multiple sclerosis by deep brain stimulation. Recently, Speelman and Van Manen (1984) published gratifying results with thalamotomy for intention tremor in 11 cases with multiple sclerosis. Our own experience with 2 patients, who had severe and completely disabling tremor of intention in MS, confirms that a substantial alleviation of the dyskinesia can be accomplished at the treated side. This also resulted in restoration of potentialities which enabled patients to take care of themselves again. The target for coagulation is the ventrolateral nucleus of the thalamus that is described (Narabayashi 1983) to be a relay centre for cerebellofugal fibers which run to the cerebral cortex (Eccles et al. 1967).

## 4. Torticollis Spastica

Torticollis spastica represents an exaggeration of the head's function of rotation resulting from a lesion of a structure, which normally inhibits this movement (Molina-Negro 1979). The vestibular system is the principle structure involved and the ascending vestibular pathways have a thalamic relay in the Vim nucleus (Hassler 1955 c). Therefore a stereotactic intervention (Hassler and Dieckmann 1970) may lead to marked alleviation of the torticollis. The lesion is to be made in the nucleus Voi and Voa, which is the integration centre of vestibular and cerebellar impulses and not in the nucleus Vim itself, because lesioning this target may lead to an undesirable motor neglect of the contralateral extremities (Hassler and Dieckmann 1982). Sometimes an additional lesion in the internal pallidum is required. The lesion should be carried out contralateral to the direction of head turning (Bertrand et al. 1978). Hassler and Dieckmann (1970) published a series on 92 patients with spasmodic torticollis with a follow-up of 1–14 years after stereotactic coagulation of 87 cases, in which 30 excellent and 28 good results were noted. Postoperative physiotherapy to achieve full benefit from the operation is mandatory, however.

## B. Pain Syndromes

### 1. Stereotactic Lesions to Alleviate Pain

Apart from percutaneous cordotomy, which is not essentially a stereotactic procedure, many types of stereotactic intervention have been developed and partly abandoned during the last 40 years. In fact, the first human stereotactic operation was done in a patient with trigeminal neuralgia by Spiegel and Wycis (1962) in 1948, who made a lesion at the level of the superior colliculus and relieved pain for the remaining 14 years of life. Later on, mesencephalotomy (even bilateral) became a promising and effective procedure in cases with pain caused by cancer of the head and neck (Leksell 1966, Nashold 1975, Whisler and Voris 1978). The lesion should be placed lateral to the aqueduct and between it and the medial lemniscus. In Fig. 30 the position of the lesion is illustrated in relation to the third ventricle with the line AC—PC in the lateral view (Fig. 30 a), and in relation to the aqueduct and the midsagittal plane in the frontal view (Fig. 30 b). Pain relief can be obtained in 90–95% of the patients without untoward sequelae. Vertical gaze paralysis and/or pupillary abnormalities may be a transient phenomenon (Nashold 1982). Hitchcock (1973) published on a pontine tractotomy for pain relief in malignant disease with similar results, as did Barberá (*et al.*) in 1979. It is clear, that such lesions compared with those obtained with cervical cordotomy have the advantage of relieving pain from head and neck and can be performed bilaterally, if necessary. Besides that, untoward side-effects from the motor system as is quite possible in cordotomy (Mooij *et al.* 1984) will not occur. Therefore, this type of brainstem stereotactic surgery has held its reputation especially in patients suffering from cancer pains. CT scan control both pre- and postoperatively may refine this surgery even more (Dettori *et al.* 1982).

The relief of chronic pain states is a completely different matter. As with cordotomy, mesencephalotomy may give pain relief for only one year, with some exceptions that are not representative. Before acquiring this knowledge, various lesions in the somesthetic thalamus (thalamotomies) were also carried out in chronic pain syndromes (Cooper 1965 a, Riechert 1960, 1966, Voris and Whisler 1975). Their results were disappointing in the long run, pain recurring after some months which is usual after all types of surgical intervention in chronic pain. This concept leads to the conclusion, that only cancer pain should be treated by stereotactic lesions, taking into account the fact that life expectancy is short. Even if the original pain does not recur, painful dysesthesias may occur, which are sometimes even more agonizing (Drake and McKenzie 1953, Nashold 1982).

So far a description is given of stereotactic pain surgery in the course of the spinothalamic tract and quintothalamic tract including part of the medial lemniscus (Fig. 30 b). This system terminates mainly in the

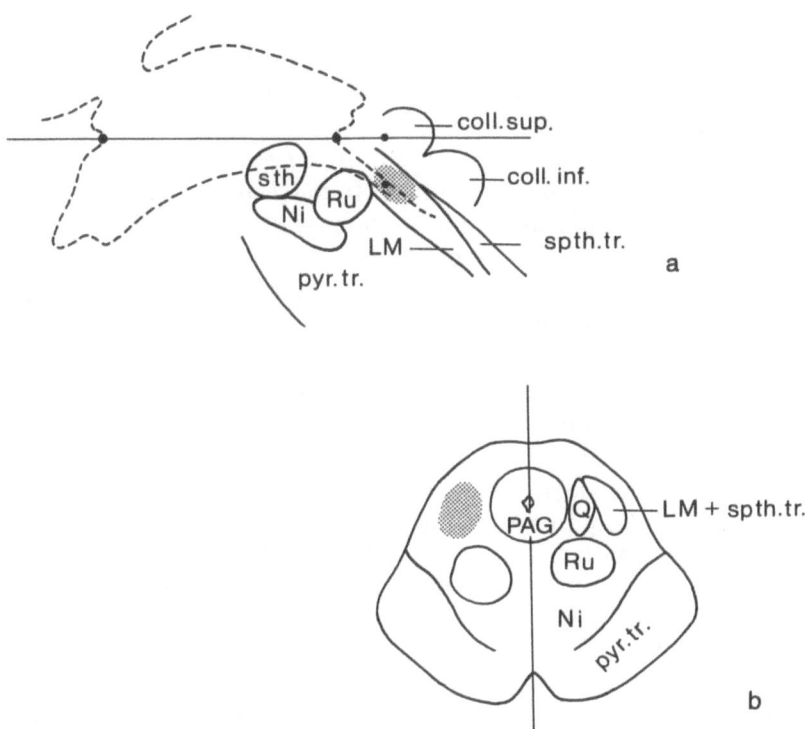

Fig. 30. Position of lesion in stereotactic mesencephalotomy. a) Lateral view with relation to third ventricle and AC—PC-line. Target for lesioning 5 mm behind and below PC. b) Frontal view with relation to midsagittal plane and aqueduct. Target for lesioning about 8 mm lateral. Abbreviations used: *spth. tr.* tractus spinothalamicus; *pyr. tr.* tractus pyramidalis; *LM* lemniscus medialis; *Q* tractus quintothalamicus; *PAG* periaqueductal grey matter; *sth* corpus subthalamicum; *Ru* nucleus ruber; *Ni* substantia nigra; *coll. sup.* and *inf.* colliculi superiores et inferiores

somesthetic part of the thalamus (nuclei VPl and VPm), according to Hassler (1960), and is generally called a specific, neospinothalamic pathway. The other system of afferent pathways for noxious stimuli is the paleospinothalamic, nonspecific group of tracts, which is referred to by Bowsher and Albe-Fessard (1963) as extralemniscal. These fibers run more medially and are situated in the periaqueductal grey at the outer edge. Extralemniscal stereotactic lesions for pain relief are also reported in the literature. Noordenbos (1959) considers this system to be a short fibre, slowly conducting pathway, organized as a multisynaptic net, which is phylogenetically an older system and projects to other thalamic nuclei (the pulvinar and the centromedianum-parafascicularis complex). A type of extralemniscal mesencephalotomy is described by Amano (*et al.* 1980), with the lesion placed more medially than in the normal mesencephalotomy. His patients belonged to the chronic pain group (most of them suffering from a thalamic syndrome) and relief was noted for periods ranging from 3 months to 5 years. In stereotactic myelotomies at the cervical level (Hitchcock 1970 b, Schvarcz 1978, Eiras *et al.* 1980) the target is also the extralemniscal system, leading to less loss of functions (almost no sensory loss) than with surgery of the neospinothalamic system (e.g. cervical cordotomy). In general, one might say that midline and trunk pain, as well as the pain suffering syndrome, benefit the most from extralemniscal surgery, while pain in extremities is relieved more by lesions in the neospinothalamic system.

Stereotactic chemical *hypophysectomy,* using the transsphenoidal route, has proven to be a reliable method for the treatment of pain due to diffuse metastatic malignancies (Katz and Levin 1977, Tindall *et al.* 1979, Levin *et al.* 1980). The mechanism by which pain relief is achieved is unknown, although metastatic pains from hormone dependent tumors (breast and prostate cancer) are the most sensitive. In this context it is surprising and very interesting to read the contents of a recent publication by Levin (*et al.* 1983) on the use of stereotactic chemical hypophysectomy in the treatment of the thalamic pain syndrome. Stereotactic instillation of 5 cc of absolute ethanol, delivered over three different targets inside the pituitary gland, resulted in unexpected complete pain relief (follow-up 19–58 months). Hypopituitarism after treatment required maintenance hormone therapy. It is tentatively suggested by the authors, that pain relief is the result of stimulation of a hypothalamic pain suppressing mechanism. Further research is needed to evaluate this technique of treating various chronic pain states.

To achieve pain relief in phantom pain after spinal root avulsion, Nashold and Ostdahl (1979) studied the effect of dorsal root entry zone (DREZ) lesioning at the cervical level. After laminectomy to expose the cord, the authors made small lesions with fine thermocouple electrodes, which may be guided by a special stereotactic instrument that is placed and fixed to the spine (Saris *et al.* 1985). Good results were obtained in 6 of 9 patients with phantom pain alone and in 5 of 6 patients with phantom pain due to traumatic amputation associated with root avulsion.

## 2. Stereotactic Stimulation with Electrodes to Achieve Pain Relief

Inductive electrical stimulation of deep brain structures to control chronic intractable pain was introduced by Mazars (*et al.* 1973), Delgado (*et al.* 1973), and Hosobuchi (*et al.* 1973). In a way, it is based on the "gate control theory" of pain, published by Melzack and Wall in 1965, which postulated a pain-inhibitory descending system that could be activated by electrical stimulation. In 1969, Reynolds observed powerful analgesic effects in the rat by stimulating the periaqueductal grey matter (PAG), which became one of the target structures for stereotactic stimulation. The other target of interest is the nucleus ventralis posterolateralis (VPl) of the thalamus which is the target used also in thalamotomies to alleviate intractable pain. Adams (*et al.* 1974) also stimulated in the posterior limb of the internal capsule to suppress severe spontaneous pain associated with lesions of the central nervous system (so-called central pain states). Adams and Hosobuchi (1977) differentiate between two anatomical systems for the control of pain: the thalamic sensory nuclei + posterior limb of the internal capsule for central or deafferentation pain, and the periventricular + periaqueductal grey matter for the pains of peripheral origin. Hosobuchi (1980) summarizes his results in deafferentation pain due to the thalamic syndrome, anesthesia dolorosa, post-herpetic neuralgia, phantom limb pain and central dysesthesia with a 16/40 success rate, and his results with pains of peripheral origin with a 16/22 success rate. Other authors, however, as Dieckmann (*et al.* 1979), disagree with this rather artificial distinction in two different anatomical control systems. The PAG is very rich in serotonergic cell bodies and electrical stimulation of the PAG fails to induce analgesia when the activity of the serotonergic cells is blocked (by LSD). Administration of 5-hydroxytryptophan, a serotonin precursor, reversed tolerance to stimulation, indicating a strong analogy between stimulation induced analgesia and morphine analgesia (Besson and Oliveras 1980).

The neurophysiological basis for these observations is still unknown, as is the reliability of this way of pain treatment. Meyerson (1980) discusses the possible role of endogenous opioid mechanisms in the stimulation of the periaqueductal area; he collected data from more than 200 patients subjected to intracerebral stimulation, which show that the outcome is still unpredictable. Nothing, until now, indicates such a role of opiates in the stimulation of the posterior thalamus. At the same time deafferentation pain responds poorly to the administration of opiates. The technical details of introducing stimulation electrodes into deep brain structures can be found in "La neurostimulation électrique thérapeutique" (Sedan and Lazorthes 1978). The implantation is done in fully awake and cooperative patients. The effects of the stimulation should be evaluated before the implant is made permanent. The permanent system may consist of an internal (electrode + receiver) and external part (transmitter + antenna) or a completely implantable system with a magnetic key mechanism. The most common complication is infection (about 3%); very seldom movement of the electrode is seen even after long periods of correct tip position.

## C. Intractable Epilepsy

In "Advances in stereotactic and functional neurosurgery 4" (Gillingham *et al.* 1980), a detailed survey is given of this (probably the oldest) field in functional neurosurgery. Although surgical resection (especially in temporal lobe epilepsy) is a favourite procedure (Rasmussen 1980), stereotactic electrode localization of the focal area (Talairach and Szikla 1980), a so-called stereo-EEG, is of the utmost importance as a preoperative investigation. But, when the pattern of seizures suggests a focal origin, which cannot be defined unequivocally by all commonly used methods, a stereotactic lesion that interrupts the conduction pathways is indicated (Gillingham *et al.* 1976, Gillingham and Campbell 1980). Since the work of Nádvorník (*et al.* 1974) it seems there is indeed a single pathway of conduction in the epileptic discharge, which is almost similar to that for the dyskinesias (the pallidum being one of the targets, according to Caveness (*et al.* 1980). Gillingham (*et al.* 1980) published a 50–75% reduction in seizure frequency after stereotactic lesions placed in the pallidum of the ipsilateral hemisphere. Narabayashi (1972, 1980) studied posttraumatic and postencephalitic epileptics (children and adults), treated with stereotactic medial amygdalotomy. He described in about 60% of his cases marked improvement both regarding the epileptic as the behavioral abnormalities. Often a bilateral lesioning is necessary. A long-term follow-up study (Heimburger *et al.* 1978) stresses the persistent relief of symptoms. On the other hand, Porter (*et al.* 1977) showed that in 70% of patients considered to have intractable epilepsy fits could be managed significantly better with careful revision of all nonsurgical antiepileptic regimens.

## D. Psychiatric Disabling Disease

Since the first paper on this subject by Egas Moniz (1936), surgical interventions have been discussed with high praise at one time (Moniz received the Nobel prize in 1949 for his prefrontal leucotomy) and with bitter criticism at another. At the moment open psychiatric surgery has been abandoned and stereotactic interventions have come in its place, at least in those countries which allow psychiatrists and neurosurgeons to do so in cases of otherwise intractable illness. Selection of patients is still a matter of debate, but there is general agreement, that individuals disabled by disorders of affect, such as depression, anxiety, obsessive-compulsive neurosis, and phobias are most likely to benefit (Wycis 1972). A United States Congress Commission published a Report in 1977 concerning the use of psychosurgery in practice and research (discussed by Ballantine and Giriunas in 1979). Stereotactic psychosurgery comprises bilateral anterior cingulotomy (Ballantine *et al.* 1967), and bimedial leucotomy, and is a much more precise and safe procedure than open surgery, such as Scoville's orbital undercutting (Scoville and Bettis 1977). Bingley (*et al.* 1973) described stereotactic anterior capsulotomy as a successful procedure; this work comes from the Leksell group of investigators and has a thorough psychiatrist's selection and follow-up of patients. Overall improvement in so-called well selected patients has been shown to be achieved in 60–80% of cases. This type of surgery also has been performed, with similar results, in cases of desperate drug addiction (Kanaka and Balasubramaniam 1978). The interested reader is referred to Spiegel's monograph (1982, pages 35–46) for a survey of the many target structures explored in stereotactic psychosurgery. Unbiased study of unwanted side-effects by psychologists (Teuber *et al.* 1977) revealed no serious neurological or psychiatric complications. On the other hand, as compared with the early years (before 1950), the indication is very seldom evident because of the introduction of potent neuroleptic drugs by that time.

## E. Spasticity

Spasticity is caused by an exaggeration of the myotatic reflexes; there is an abnormal muscle spindle stimulus because of a lack of descending inhibition. Already in 1908, Foerster introduced posterior spinal rhizotomy for the relief of spasticity. Later on more selective rhizotomies were published by Gros (*et al.* 1967) and Laitinen (*et al.* 1983). Interest for these modalities of treatment increased with the growing efforts to give some substantial help to patients with multiple sclerosis. Spinal cord stimulation with percutaneously introduced electrodes (Siegfried 1979) sometimes gives marked reduction of spasticity in those cases. Cerebral palsy (Little's spastic diplegia and hemiplegias) eventually develops into a condition in which conservative treatment completely fails and stereotactic destructive lesioning of the cerebellar nucleus dentatus should be considered. Heimburger observed moderate improvement in 46 of the 64 patients (Siegfried 1982). The effect, however, decreases over the years. Complications due to the stereotactic intervention are seldom reported.

In advanced cerebral palsy Zervas (1977) observed only initial improvement of the motor performance and considered the future use of dentatotomy in this condition unwarranted. Therefore, the position of stereotactic dentatotomy in future functional neurosurgery is questionable. Dorsal column stimulation is considered more promising in the treatment of spasticity.

## F. Spinal Stereotactic Procedures

Although Clarke (1921) already had described and constructed a spinal cord stereotactic frame for use in animals, spinal stereotactics in man was first reported in 1969 by Hitchcock. The object was to interrupt the spinothalamic tract at the cervical level, a procedure known in classic open neurosurgery as the anterolateral cordotomy. In 1963 Mullan (*et al.*)

published the first percutaneous cordotomy effected by the introduction under X-ray guidance of a strontium needle at the $C_1$—$C_2$ level by the lateral approach. Rosomoff (*et al.* 1965) introduced the radiofrequency lesioning with an electrode by the same route and technique. The stereotactic introduction of the electrode, however, needs another route and a special instrument for guidance; Hitchcock developed a special apparatus to exploit the suboccipital puncture route in the fully flexed head position. To reach the anterolateral cord segment it is necessary to traverse the substance of the spinal cord almost completely. No complications of that penetration are reported, but the technique is rather cumbersome and no longer exploited for reaching the spinothalamic tract, because free hand lateral procedures have become much more elegant and subtle. To reach the extralemniscal system, however, there are at present two stereotactic cervical procedures, which have proven to be successful in the management of pain, and are in fact a logical progression of the techniques for percutaneous cordotomy. The *first* is the extralemniscal myelotomy, which was thought to be helpful for pain relief confined to the upper cervical dermatomes, but was shown to give pain relief over large areas of the body without any substantial analgesia to painful stimuli (Hitchcock 1970 b, Schvarcz 1976). This accidental finding of bilateral pain relief after a single lesion in the central cervical cord region ($C_0$—$C_1$ level) made Hitchcock postulate a midline extralemniscal pathway throughout the spinal cord. This "challenge to traditional concepts" is beautifully discussed by Cook (*et al.* 1984) in an extensive overview on sensory consequences of commissural myelotomy. In 1974, Hitchcock published satisfactory results in 68.4% of his 26 cases and Schvarcz confirmed the usefulness in 1976. Mostly it concerned cancer pain patients, but some chronic pain cases also responded to this type of surgery. The lesion is made in the region of the central canal after threshold stimulation, which gives a consistent pattern of ascending paresthesias beginning at the soles of both feet. Gildenberg and Hirschberg (quoted by Gildenberg 1982 a) tried to aim at the postulated pathway at the level of the thoracolumbar segments by free hand introduction of the electrode and found excellent pain relief in the lower part of the body.

The *second* stereotactic spinal procedure is the trigeminal tractotomy at the $C_0$—$C_1$ level, made possible by Hitchcock in 1970 (a) with use of his spinal apparatus. In a way, it is the stereotactic counterpart of the open tractotomy of Sjöquist (1938). The electrode is introduced 6.5 mm from the midline and the lesion gives relief from pain of malignancy and pain of benign origin. In the largest series (104 cases) Schvarcz (1978) reported relief in 83% of malignant disease and 87% of postherpetic neuralgia of the face, versus 72% in cases of trigeminal dysesthesia after peripheral procedures for "genuine" neuralgia. Surgery is done in the sitting position with fully flexed head to fix the cervical medulla. Apparatus for spinal surgery are recommended, but the systems of Todd-Wells, Leksell and Riechert-Mundinger are appropriate too. However, in Todd-Wells spinal procedures the patient is in the prone position, as is described by Crue (*et al.* 1970). It is evident, that the stereotactic approach has its advantages in accuracy, safety and simplicity as compared with the open Sjöquist tractotomy. Serious complications, such as pulmonary or bladder dysfunction, have not been reported.

In dorsal root entry zone lesioning (DREZ) laminectomy is combined with stereotactic guidance of the electrode with the aid of a special stereotactic instrument (Nashold and Ostdahl 1979, Saris *et al.* 1985). The indication for DREZ lies mainly in pains from root avulsion and traumatic phantom pains.

## II. Mass Lesions Stereotactics

Although Clarke in 1921 already suggested applying the principles of stereotactic surgery to the treatment of pain and brain tumors, history shows a great lack between the beginning of functional and oncological stereotactics (1947 versus 1960). Even Leksell in his chapter "Gezielte Hirnoperationen" in the "Handbuch der Neurochirurgie" (1957) only mentioned the possibility of "die Einstellung von Kanülen zur Punktion von Hirntumoren". This obvious delay in application of stereotactics in neuro-oncology can only be explained by the very bad prognosis of patients with brain tumors in those days. According to Olivecrona (1967) tumors of the basal ganglia and brainstem "are surgically of little interest, they are all inoperable". Because of the lack of any other oncological treatment except surgery, this statement was correct at that time and biopsy without any further possible treatment seemed not justified. But at about the same time a lot of experience was collected from the surgical treatment of more peripherally lying brain tumors, the first conclusion being that a glioma cannot be totally resected, which led to trials with radiotherapy afterwards. The next conclusion was, that the results of surgery plus radiotherapy greatly depended on the type of brain tumor and the pathological grading of its malignancy. Progress in radiobiology and radiotherapeutic instruments increased the 5 years survival rate considerably and sometimes—depending on the tumor histology—even made cure attainable.

A big leap forward could be made in the field of neuro-oncology with the introduction of CT scanning by Hounsfield (*et al.* 1973), which for the first time gave pictures of the brain itself and a tremendously better insight in the position and the extent of any intracerebral mass lesion! Before the era of CT scanning only angiographic and encephalographic studies could be performed, but after 1955 this could be done in combination with brain scintigraphy. Brain scintigraphy, however, is only of value in pathological conditions and does not show normal anatomy (Penning and Front 1975).

The new generation CT scanners is able to visualize normal and pathological intracranial anatomy with a 2 mm resolution capability, which makes
them suitable for localization of stereotactic targets (Burchiel *et al.* 1980)
and the study of stereotactic accuracy (Hitchcock *et al.* 1978, Tampieri and
Bergstrand 1983, Passerini *et al.* 1978). Stereotactic biopsy of tumors was
introduced by Mundinger in Freiburg (1958, 1963, 1966), and all the
requisites to employ stereotactic techniques in neuro-oncology were
available by the time the CT scan came into use.

In 1953 Riechert had already started with stereotactic pituitary surgery
(Riechert 1955 b). Treatment of pituitary adenomas by stereotactic means
(Conway *et al.* 1969, Dashe *et al.* 1966) was temporarily performed, until
microsurgical techniques could take over using controlled removal. Mass
lesions stereotactics sensu strictiori, as described below, offer many
possibilities both in diagnosis and in treatment, and have been developed
mainly during the last ten years.

## A. Diagnostic Mass Lesions Stereotactics

Depending on the consistency of the lesion to be biopted, various
techniques have been described; all of them can be found in Backlund's
paper (1971), which presents a stereotactic tool that is based on a spiral
needle and is suited to take biopsies independent of the tumor consistency.
This needle can be applied to all types of stereotactic instruments. Besides
this biopsy tool one needs an aspiration needle to evacuate any present fluid
(as in cystic brain tumors). The first aim in stereotactic tumor biopsy is to
get a representative sample of tissue and to decide, with the help of the
neuropathologist, if the lesion is a tumor or not. It must be emphasized, that
in about 10% of early detected small brain lesions no tumor is found (Bosch
1980); Apuzzo and Sabshin (1983) report a series of 71 mass lesions, of
which 40 could be verified to be tumors, 20 to be infections/abscesses and 7
to be vascular lesions. Even with the newest generation of CT scanner
available and with a complete angiographic study, it sometimes occurs, that
a small infarction (with early filling vein) or a small hematoma (in its later
presentation with a halo of enhancement around it) or even an abscess or a
MS plaque (Fig. 31) is encountered. Especially nowadays, with an almost
routinely performed CT scan of the brain even in minor complaints (f.e.:
headache, vertigo, neuralgia) one should be prepared for the detection of
small lesions, which could be tumors (Fig. 32).

When the diagnosis of a tumor is made with neuropathological studies of
the biopsy tissue, a complete oncological treatment, including various
possible modalities, will be started and might give the most benefit to the
patient at a time when the lesion is still small. To illustrate the utmost
importance of taking a biopsy (preferably stereotactically) to confirm the

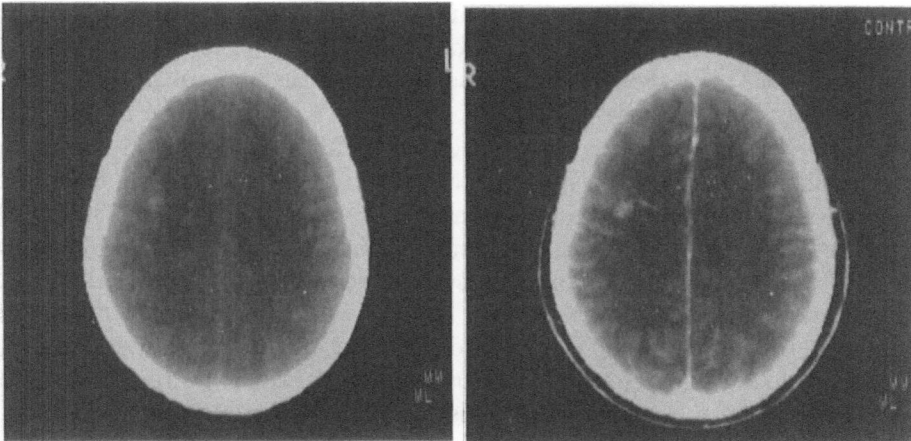

Fig. 31. CT scan pictures (right after contrast) show a plaque in multiple sclerosis (in the right hemisphere)

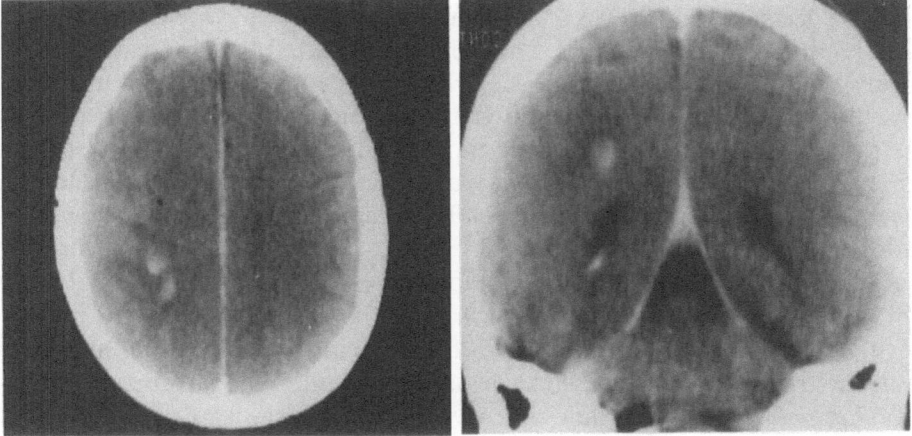

Fig. 32. CT scan pictures (with contrast) show a right parietal deep seated small lesion, that turned out to be a highly malignant oligodendroglioma (biopsy case)

lesion to be a tumor, we would like to refer to the paper of Wang (*et al.* 1983) on suspected lesions that turned out to be an acute demyelinating disease (MS) and to the publication by Lunsford and Nelson (1982), that describes an unsuspected brain abscess evacuation in a stereotactic performance which was planned to take a tissue biopsy. Discussing the value of stereotactic biopsies in deep seated mass lesions, Broggi and Franzini (1981) reported histological confirmation of a tumor in 25 out of 35 cases with a mortality rate of 0%. Ostertag (*et al.* 1980) published the largest series of biopsies in 302 patients, who underwent a stereotactic biopsy (including

Mundinger's cases) and reports 232 malignancies, 21 craniopharyngiomas, 3 pituitary adenomas, 4 plexus papillomas, 5 meningiomas, 1 neurinoma, 4 epidermoids, 3 colloid cysts, 3 abscesses and 26 miscellaneous cases (gliosis; cysts). Operative mortality was 2.3% and morbidity 3%. The other large series of biopsies has been reported from the Karolinska Hospital in Stockholm by Edner (1981), who presented 345 cases including 84 cystic lesions of which 19 cystic astrocytomas; this makes a total of 280 cases, which can be compared with the results of Ostertag. Edner's publication gives a 5% yield of non-neoplastic lesions, a mortality rate of less than 1% and a morbidity of 2.3%. Our own results, with more than 250 cases in which stereotactic biopsy was performed for a suspected mass lesion, resemble closely those reported by Ostertag and Edner: in about 10% no tumor was present, in about 3% no histological confirmation was achieved, in about 2% there was a fatal outcome and morbidity ranged up to another 3%. The percentages for the non-neoplastic group, however, tend to increase in recent years because of the continuous refinement in diagnostics that reveals suspected brain areas more frequently.

The decision to perform a stereotactic biopsy or an "open craniotomy" will be discussed in Chapters 5 and 6 in more detail, but indications have changed in more recent years remarkably because of progress in neuro-oncology. In the case of a supratentorial glioma, which is classified as an astrocytoma (the most common type of glioma), surgery alone ("bulk resection") will result in a 26% survival rate after 5 years for the histological grades I and II (Kernohan) and in a 49% 5 years survival, when followed by adequate radiotherapy (Bouchard 1966). For the grades III and IV (glioblastoma multiforme) surgery alone gives a 2% one year survival and a 40% survival after combination with radiotherapy. Although this impressive increase in survival due to radiotherapy can be achieved in malignant astrocytomas, the 5 years survival is almost nil. This suggests a higher sensitivity of the high grade astrocytoma but at the same time an only palliative effect on the disease, whereas the low graded group can sometimes be cured (Deeley 1974, Jones 1960). These data may serve as an example for our discussion on the changes in indications. Deep seated gliomas are inoperable in the sense of bulk resection, but a stereotactic biopsy may be performed without any harm to the patient. When the classification by the neuropathologist leads to the diagnosis of a low grade astrocytoma, radiotherapy will increase the survival for years and sometimes even cure the patient. In case the diagnosis reveals no glioma, but a metastasis or a germinoma (Fig. 33) or another tumor or may be no tumor at all, these possibilities lead to different kinds of treatment with great impact on the patient's prognosis. In certain types of tumor (malignant lymphoma, medulloblastoma, intracerebral manifestation of leukemia e. a.) the results of treatment (Fig. 34) can be improved by chemotherapy; an expanding

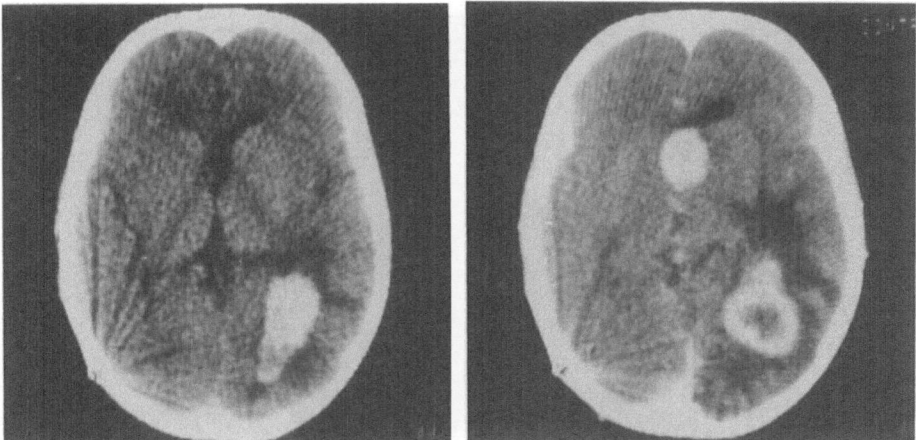

Fig. 33. CT scan pictures (contrast, with a 3 months delay). Tumor in a 11 years old boy, recurring after local irradiation for "pineal tumor". Biopsy revealed a germinoma, spreading intraventricularly after inadequate adjuvant therapy

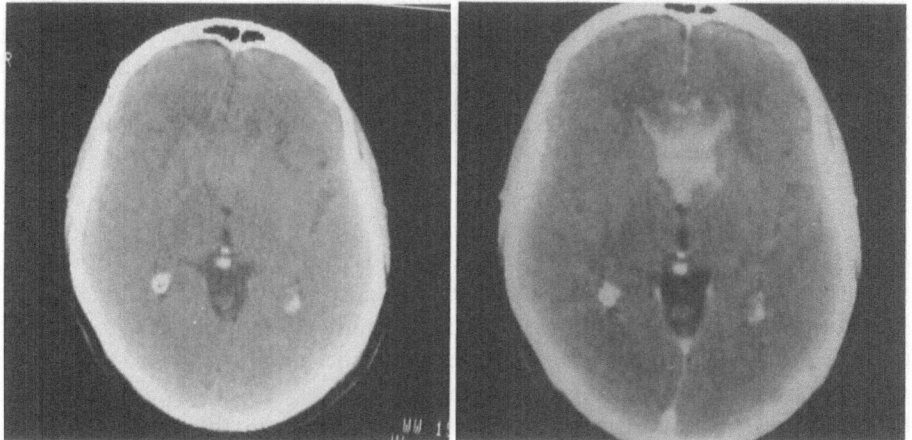

Fig. 34. CT scan pictures (right after contrast) show a strongly enhancing butterfly tumor in a 62 years old man. Biopsy revealed a malignant lymphoma and radiotherapy + chemotherapy cured the patient (follow-up 4 years)

field on its own. Some years ago a mass lesion was held to be inoperable when deep seated—i. e. independent on size. Nowadays very small lesions have become detectable and offer a challenge to the neurosurgeon to operate with the help of CT guided stereotactic aiming of his instruments. He may choose a biopsy forceps or microsurgical instruments, to perform a bulk resection (in malignancies) or a complete removal (in benign lesions).

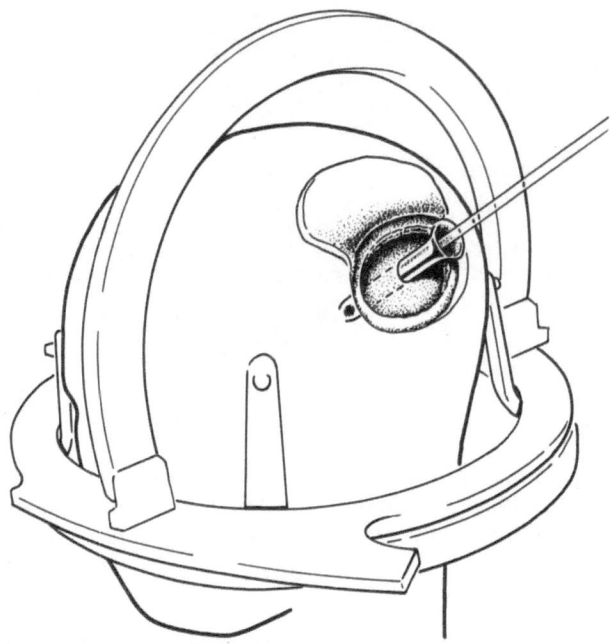

Fig. 35. Artist's impression of instrument positioning for performing a stereotactic craniotomy. After stereotactic localization of the target area exploration is carried out with guided microsurgical, fiberoptic or laser instrumentation. Guidance is given by CT based computer reconstruction in stereotactic space of the lesion

Using classical methods these small subcortical lesions are inoperable, because they are not found without causing extensive damage to the surrounding brain tissue. This applies especially to lesions in the parietal lobes. Stereotaxis offers technical equipment to reach these lesions by the route of choice, safely, and without any disturbance to the overlying brain. At the target the surgeon can first take a biopsy and have it examined. According to the histological diagnosis he thereafter can proceed with surgery or other treatment modalities (e.g. interstitial irradiation). Some clinics have already the technical equipment to perform stereotactic craniotomies (Jacques *et al.* 1980, Kelly *et al.* 1983), which makes it possible for the surgeon to continue after the biopsy with resection of the lesion with help of a stereotactic speculum to expose the target area. An impression of both computerized localization and open surgery to remove a lesion is given in Fig. 35. Modern instrumentation (Chapter 4) offers all potentials to resect any predetermined tissue volume.

There is no doubt, that these developments will open the way to a real integration of stereotactic aiming techniques into clinical neurosurgery. The interested reader is referred to the Chapters 4 and 13 for further information.

On the other hand, neuropathological entities also increase in number, leading to more subtle distinctions in histological and cytological diagnosis of mass lesions of the brain. Partly due to the longer survival of patients with systemic disease, including cancer, which leads to metastatic spread inside the central nervous system or to a high incidence of CNS infections (Chernik *et al.* 1973); partly because of the more frequently encountered immune deficiency syndromes (spontaneously as in AIDS or after immunosuppressive treatment as in organ transplant recipients or patients under chemotherapy for systemic cancer). A high incidence of intracerebral toxoplasmosis in these circumstances is reported by Handler (*et al.* 1983). Superimposed viral infection by herpes viruses (Whitley *et al.* 1981, Juel-Jensen 1980) may need proof by biopsy: Whitley reports, that brain biopsy for clinically suspected disease was only positive in 57%, which proves its value as only 5.4% false negative biopsies were found on a total of 182 patients. Also Lunsford (*et al.* 1984 b) stresses the usefulness of stereotactic biopsy in viral disease. Furthermore, second malignant neoplasms have been reported after chemical immunosuppression (Penn 1974 and 1976), which tend to arise in the brain (Schneck and Penn 1971). This means, that a patient cured from systemic cancer may develop a second tumor, not infrequently a malignant lymphoma, inside the brain; these cases can be expected in higher numbers in the future and may benefit from a stereotactic biopsy to evaluate the proper diagnosis and the radio- and chemosensitivity.

In the case of proper management of septichemia with antibiotics or of fungal disease with antimycotics some patients may develop intracerebral mass lesions, which might be of infectious origin. In the publication of Britt and Enzmann (1983) early stages of brain abscess (so called cerebritis) are described and neuropathological confirmation is shown after stereotactic aspiration of lesions which in the early stage of abscess formation resemble tumors. Their series of 14 patients includes 7 immunocompromized cases, which led to a large spectrum of causative organisms, including fungi and protozoa. As culture of the causative organism(s) has been shown to be mandatory for successful treatment of the cerebral lesions, a stereotactic biopsy is the only way to get a positive proof by a simple procedure. In the Aquired Immune Deficiency Syndrome (AIDS), only known since 1981 (Durack) and particularly observed among male homosexuals and intravenous drug abusers, many opportunistic infections have been described as well as an increased incidence of Kaposi's sarcoma. Among over 150 such patients seen in the New York University-Bellevue Medical Center 6 have come to neurosurgical attention because of intracranial mass lesions (4%) that proved to be toxoplasmosis (Handler *et al.* 1983). In 5/6 the lesions were multiple on CT scan and were not clearly different from abscesses or

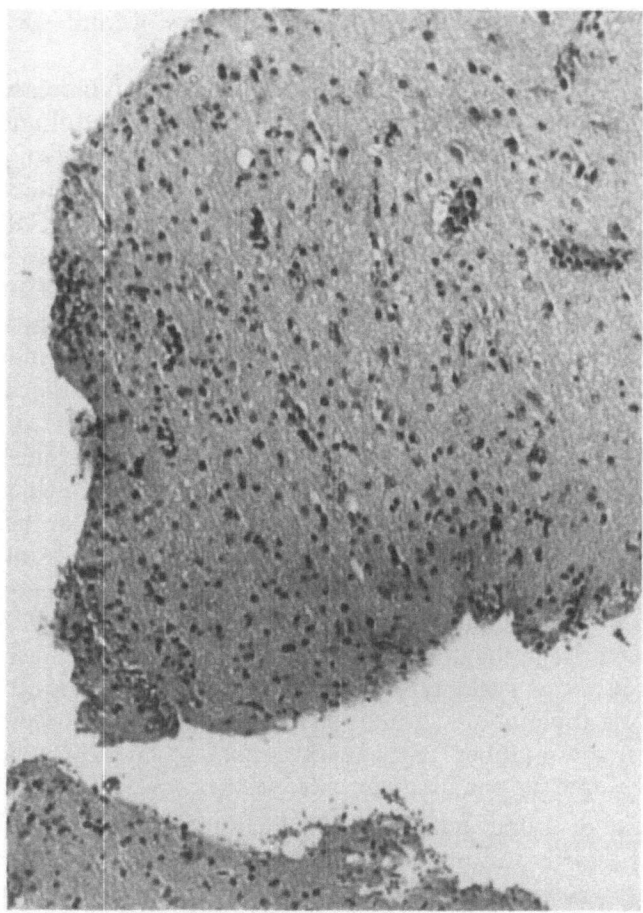

Fig. 36. Histological specimen (H & E) of temporal lobe biopsy in a girl of 15 years with encephalitis. Virological studies proved the causative agent to be a herpes simplex virus

metastatic disease, which makes the diagnostic value of brain biopsy evident. Levy (*et al.* 1984, 1985) discuss the value of brain biopsy in AIDS with mass lesions of the brain, and consider it to be critical for the evaluation and appropriate treatment. As toxoplasmosis is effectively treated with antibiotics, resection of the lesion(s) is not indicated. Therefore, not only for deep seated lesions which are clinically suggestive for tumors, but also for multiple lesions lying at random throughout the brain the biopsy technique is extremely useful. One should be prepared, however, for infections and try to aspirate some fluid, if tissue is not available at the target, to have it examined bacteriologically including cultures. When the illness is suggestive for herpes encephalitis, brain tissue (Fig. 36) should be prepared for virological and immunofluorescence studies, leading to proper diagnosis and the starting of treatment within some hours after surgery (Lunsford *et al.* 1984 b).

Finally, the stereotactic biopsy is so simple, that it forms an excellent alternative for an exploratory craniotomy in the elderly or seriously ill patients. This enables the surgeon to discuss the diagnosis with the patient

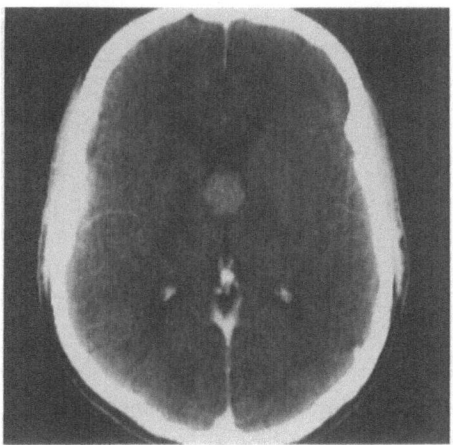

Fig. 37. CT scan after contrast shows a typical colloid cyst of the third ventricle that was evacuated stereotactically

and to reserve invasive surgery for cases that will benefit. As Apuzzo and Sabshin (1983) state, "preoperative strategic planning may be brought into sharper focus in certain cases".

## B. Therapeutic Mass Lesions Stereotactics

### 1. Aspiration and Evacuation of Fluids

In neuro-oncology many tumors have cystic components, which can be evacuated easily by stereotactic puncture and aspiration. In those lesions not amenable to open surgery, aspiration is performed and a biopsy of the adjacent tissue (the cyst "wall") is done. The fluid collected should always be sent for cytological and bacteriological examinations. Depending on the nature of the mass lesion, evacuation of the cyst's contents may be sufficient [as in colloid cysts of the third ventricle (Fig. 37); Bosch *et al.* 1978], or a drain should be left inside the cyst (as in cystic astrocytoma and craniopharyngioma), to make sure that future fluid collections can be

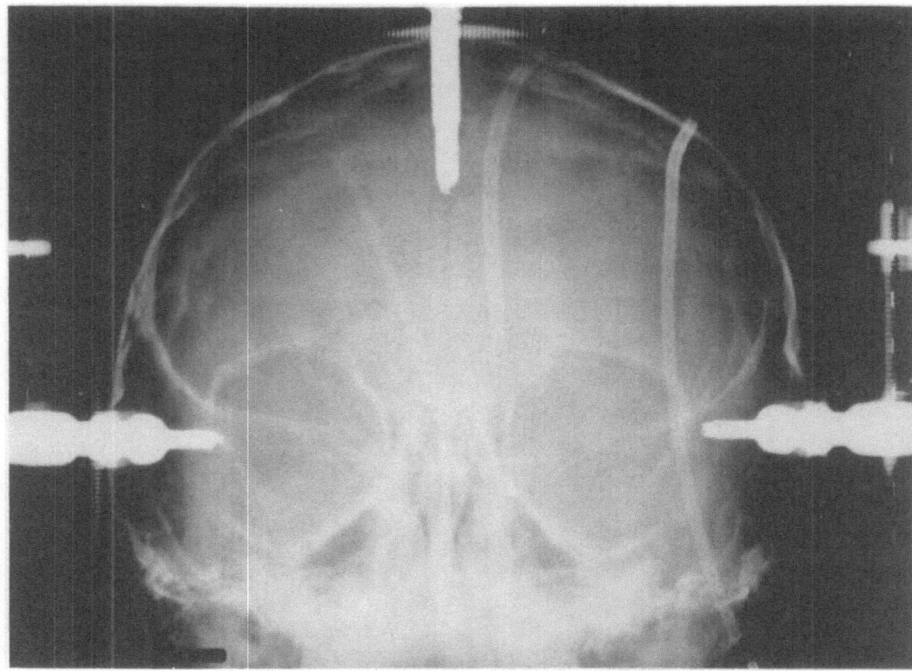

Fig. 38. Stereotactic placement of catheter inside cystic craniopharyngioma. Anteroposterior view with external CSF drainage through leftsided burrhole, and stereotactically introduced catheter through rightsided burrhole

evacuated simply (Figs. 38 and 39). An Ommaya reservoir may help for percutaneous aspiration (Gutin *et al.* 1980). Mann (*et al.* 1983) reports successful percutaneous sump drainage using a Rickham reservoir on eleven patients with cystic lesions (including 6 astrocytomas and 4 craniopharyngiomas) after open surgery. Postoperative radiotherapy was started and whenever symptoms of increased intracranial pressure recurred fluid collection was percutaneously aspirated by needle puncture of the reservoir (Fig. 40). Sometimes the drain will be blocked by high protein content of the cyst fluid and flushing with sterile saline may be required before re-evacuation. Leksell (1957) already described the stereotactic puncture of cystic craniopharyngiomas with aspiration of the fluid and subsequent administration of radioactive isotopes: the first case treated in this way was published by Leksell and Lidén in 1953, using $^{32}$P as isotope, which is a pure $\beta$-emitter. Later on, a special program for the stereotactic treatment of craniopharyngiomas was developed by Backlund, including intracystic $^{90}$Yttrium delivery and external stereotactic irradiation of the solid part with the stereotactic cobalt unit designed by Leksell (1971); the results of this combined stereotactic regimen were published by Backlund

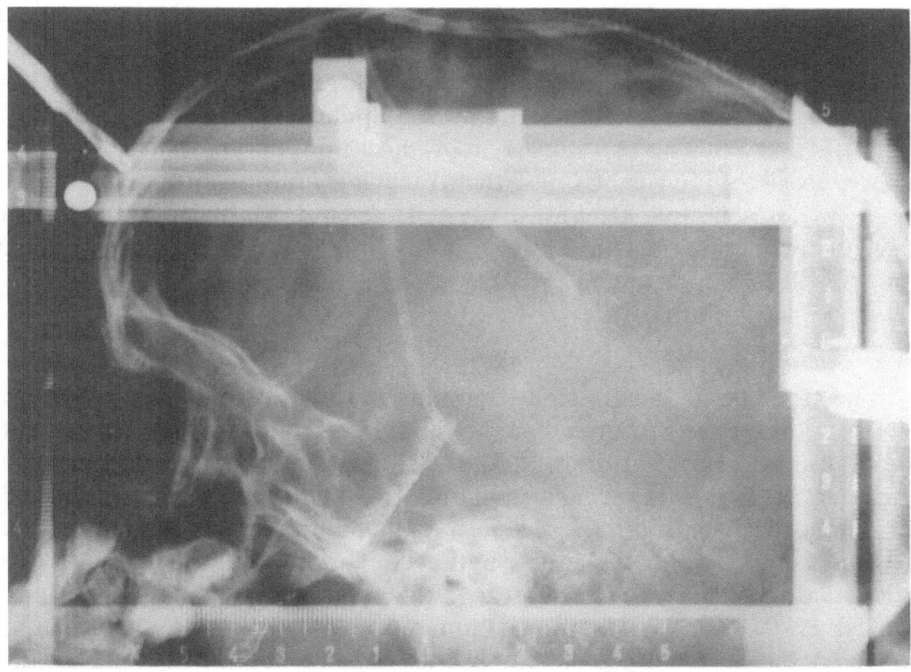

Fig. 39. Lateral view with catheter lying inside craniopharyngioma cyst. Boy aged 8 years

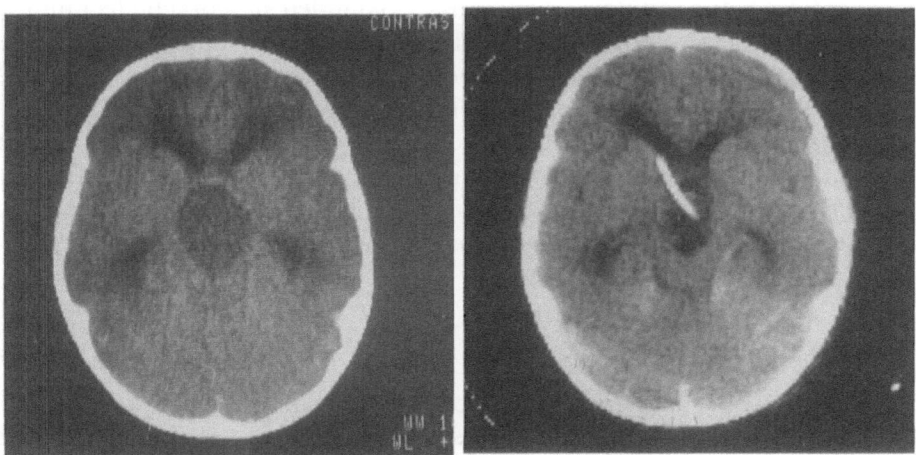

Fig. 40. CT scan pictures (same patient as in Figs. 38 and 39). (Left) cystic craniopharyngioma prior to, and (right) after the introduction of a draining catheter

(1972, *et al.* 1972, 1973, 1979). The treatment of choice in craniopharyn-gioma is still a matter of debate: there are advocates of total microsurgical resection and of subtotal removal followed by radiotherapy (Shillito 1980, Cavazzuti *et al.* 1983). Stereotactic treatment is restricted to the centers that possess stereotactic external radiation equipment (Boston, Los Angeles, Sheffield and Stockholm). Recurrent cystic craniopharyngiomas, however, offer a possibility to treat them with intracavitary radio-isotopes (Georgi *et al.* 1980, Bosch and Beekhuis 1979, Huk and Mahlstedt 1983). For stereotactic intraneoplastic irradiation in gliomas the reader is referred to the INSERM symposium 12 (Szikla ed. 1979a).

## 2. Interstitial Radioisotope Application

The stereotactic localization technique offers a method in which after biopsy radioactive isotopes can be implanted locally. For permanent implantation gold[198], iridium[192] and yttrium[90] are used. Mundinger in Freiburg started this approach to glioma treatment in 1958 and published his results in 1966. Solid tumors were treated with wires of iridium with a 0.3 mm diameter and a 4 mm length. The total radiation activity was calculated to be about 120 Gy at the outer tumor border (Mundinger and Metzel 1970). The philosophy behind this way of glioma treatment is twofold: the tumor dose is not limited by the tolerance limit of the surrounding brain, and early detection of recurrence by CT scan follow-up allows to implant the radioisotope again. Sometimes, a cure of a small tumor with this method has been achieved (Mundinger 1982a, b). The success of this so called curietherapy depends entirely on the exact localization of the radioactive implants. CT guided stereotactic techniques allow refined calculations of the lesion's position, configuration and volume. Dosimetry includes the choice of a suitable radioisotope in a suitable state (solid as a pellet or a wire; liquid), and the calculation of the total activity to be achieved with isodose distribution around the tumor center. Recently, this method which is actively being performed in Europe (Szikla 1979a, Mundinger 1982a, b) is evolving in North America too (Apuzzo and Sabshin 1983, Gutin *et al.* 1981, Kelly *et al.* 1978, 1984c, Mackay *et al.* 1982).

## 3. Stereotactic Radiosurgery

Although not suited to the treatment of malignancies, external stereotac-tic irradiation with gamma rays (Leksell 1951, 1971) or with heavy particles (Kjellberg *et al.* 1964, Lawrence *et al.* 1962), which are focused towards the target, has proved to give good results in small, nonmalignant, tumors as pituitary adenomas, craniopharyngiomas and acoustic neurinomas. Also arteriovenous malformations that are unsuitable for microsurgical treat-

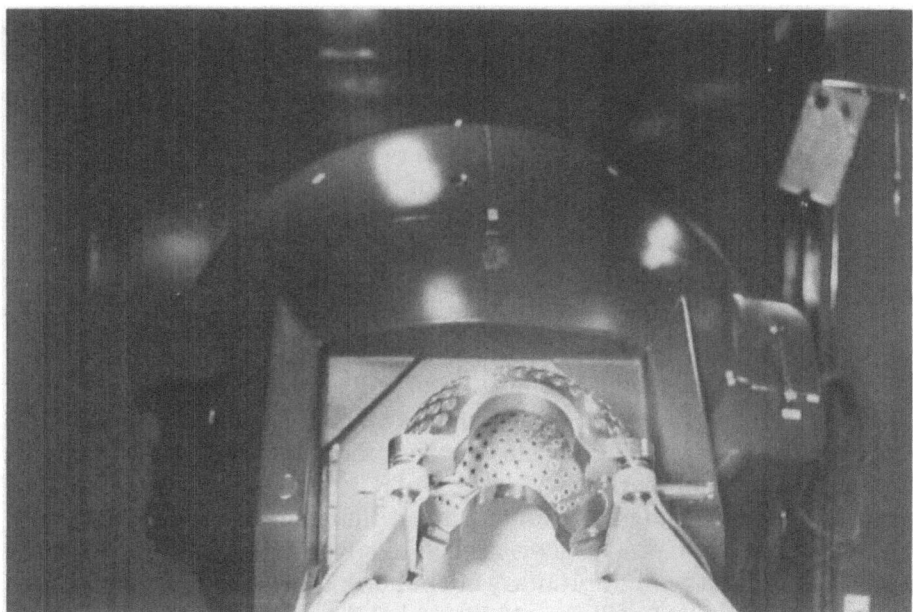

Fig. 41. Leksell's stereotactic Gamma Unit, with heavily shielded hemispherical central body containing the sources of radioactive cobalt

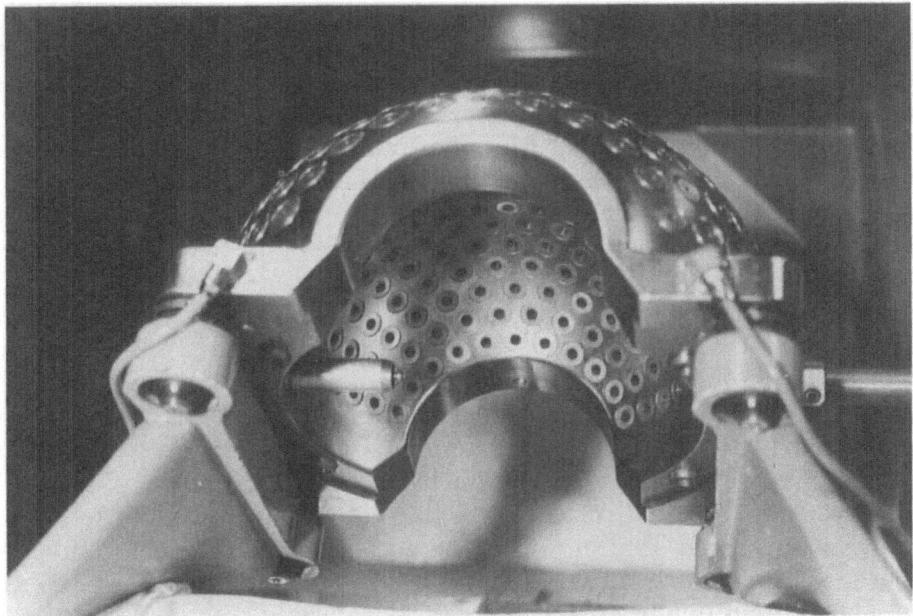

Fig. 42. The collimator helmet, that allows fixation of the patient's head in such a way that the target structure in the brain corresponds with the beam focus (by courtesy of Prof. Leksell)

ment have been treated successfully with these techniques (Backlund 1979, Kjellberg *et al.* 1983). These stereotactic irradiation units, however, are very expensive and only a few are operational: the stereotactic cobalt[60] Unit in Stockholm (Figs. 41 and 42), Los Angeles and Sheffield, and the Bragg-peak proton beam in Boston. Both types of instrument work according to the stereotactic principles, i.e. the head of the patient is secured by skeletal fixation and X-ray pictures are taken in anteroposterior and lateral projections to calculate the coordinates for the target of interest. The calculation of the coordinates may also be obtained by the CT scan computer. In the treatment of arteriovenous malformations only the small shunting vessel compartment is irradiated, which results in endothelial swelling and subendothelial deposition of collagen and hyaline substance, which narrows the lumens of the small vessels during the first 12 to 24 months after the procedure. This means, that definite results are only obtained after that period. All types of lesions, in which stereotactic radiosurgery is considered, should have a diameter of less than 25 mm; otherwise more than one target is needed to cover the whole lesion. On the radiosurgical treatment of pituitary adenomas reports have been published by Kjellberg (1979), Backlund (1979) and Rähn (1980).

## 4. Coagulation/Resection with Stereotactic Instruments

Radiofrequency thermal lesions—as commonly used in functional stereotactics to destroy a small target—have until now no application for the treatment of tumors. Only Conway (1973) described a few cases of pinealoma in which he tried to perform cryosurgery. Gleason (*et al.* 1978) reported details on a patient, who after radiotherapy for an astrocytoma had a recurrence that was treated with multiple RF thermal lesions. Although this field is entirely experimental, it seems justified to expect promising results from hyperthermia as a treatment mode for malignancies in general, and brain tumors in particular; preliminary preclinical studies have been successful, especially in combination with radiotherapy (Hahn 1982, in his monograph on "Hyperthermia and Cancer"). Recently Silberman (*et al.* 1984) reported on both animal and human experiences with brain malignancies. The patients suffered from recurrent chordoma and glioma after surgery with radiotherapy and were treated with a combination of BCNU and a brain hyperthermia protocol, which was approved by the UCLA Human Subject Protection Committee. The authors concluded that non-invasive localized radiofrequency hyper-thermia to the brain is feasible and can be performed safely in the presence of a solid brain tumor.

Stereotactic resection of mass lesions inside the brain has become possible with the development of neurosurgical lasers. Hara (*et al.* 1980) discusses the first group of patients treated with the carbon dioxide laser for mass lesions, including gliomas, meningiomas, metastatic tumors, a hemangioblastoma and an arteriovenous malformation. These authors, however, made use of a craniotomy without stereotactic techniques. Kelly (*et al.* 1982 a, b) and Alker (*et al.* 1983) have developed a system of three-dimensional, computer simulation guided, stereotactic $CO_2$ laser resection with help of computerized tomography. With this system they have treated deeply located cerebral lesions such as gliomas, metastatic tumors and arteriovenous malformations with promising preliminary results. This type of performance is called a stereotactic craniotomy, i.e. a craniotomy with the head of the patient still in the stereotactic frame after thorough CT scanning of the lesion in relation to the stereotactic instrument. The lesion is then approached using the laser and the operating microscope. With computer guidance precise positioning of the instruments relative to the lesion is ensured and a self-retaining retractor is placed at the lesion's surface, whereafter the lesion is vaporized slice by slice. The different laser types that are suited to neurosurgical use are reviewed by Edwards (*et al.* 1983). Transposition of volumetric information derived from computed tomography scanning into stereotactic space is described by Kelly (*et al.* 1984 b).

### 5. Intraneoplastic Drug Delivery with Stereotactic Instruments

The idea to treat malignant gliomas with intraneoplastic drug delivery came from Ommaya (*et al.* 1979), who designed a tumor cyst device to maintain a cavity at the tumor site after partial resection by open surgery. The reasoning was twofold: to circumvent drug delivery problems in the central nervous system due to the blood-brain barrier, and to provide the most direct method to prevent local regrowth. Tator (1977) studied intraneoplastic injection of CCNU in an animal brain tumor model and found increased survival and less systemic toxicity than after the i.p. route. Morantz (*et al.* 1979) studied bleomycin in a similar model and reported prolonged survival too. These studies are very interesting, because the ability to cross the blood-brain barrier seems to have no importance in intraneoplastic delivery: CCNU passes the barrier easily whereas bleomycin does not. In 10 patients with malignant astrocytomas, Garfield (*et al.* 1975) injected BCNU into the tumor bed after partial removal by craniotomy. He found no systemic toxicity, although the drug was delivered in total doses of up to 1,050 mg by daily repeated injections. There were only 2 long term survivors (3 and 4 years).

Kroin and Penn (1982) studied chronic microinfusion of cisplatin in rat brains and showed that a platinum concentration of 2 ng/mg tissue, wet weight, can be maintained over a 1 cm region of brain. They discussed the extension of these results to human brain neoplasms and the possibility of stereotactic placement of the cannula for infusion. Until now the only publication concerning stereotactic drug delivery is of bleomycin in glioma patients (Bosch *et al.* 1980): 1 patient survived for 3 years (on a total of 3 cases). To summarize, there are some promising results from both preclinical and clinical pilot studies, but no real progress has as yet been made in this field of—stereotactic—neuro-oncology.

## III. Localizing Stereotactics + Open Surgery

### A. Interventional Stereotactics

Although surgical intervention is always part of the stereotactic procedure, the term interventional stereotactics applies to those stereotactic actions, which are performed to eliminate something (f.e. an aneurysm or a bullet). The stereotactic removal of intracranial foreign bodies is reviewed by Hitchcock and Cowie in 1983. It is a common opinion, that low velocity missiles when left inside the brain may give rise to infection (Hagan 1971). Conventional approaches to the removal of missiles carry the risk of further injury, especially when the bullet is lying in vital brain. Therefore, with stereotactic aiming techniques the foreign body should be extracted with a type of biopsy forceps whenever there is a real danger of infection (Sugita *et al.* 1969). Riechert (1955 a) published the stereotactic extraction, in combination with a small craniotomy to clean the entrance wound. A complete description, including many photographs, is published by Riechert (1980: pages 84–89).

Stereotactic clipping of intracranial aneurysms has been developed and exploited almost exclusively by Kandel and Peresedov in Moscow (1977). They designed a special device for clipping of aneurysms and feeding vessels of AVM's to be able to handle these lesions through an ordinary burrhole. Although avoiding manipulation of blood vessels and brain retraction seems to be an advantage, impressive results made with microsurgical techniques during the last decade make direct and open surgical attack of aneurysms highly preferable. On the other hand, there may be some intracranial aneurysms, which might even be considered inoperable by open surgery nowadays; in these aneurysms stereotactic induced thrombosis has been performed with good results by Mullan (1974) and Smith and Alksne (1977). Mullan developed a method to induce thrombosis in giant aneurysms and carotid cavernous fistulas by the introduction of a very fine copper wire through a needle that punctures the aneurysm. His report discusses both stereotactic and open techniques and presents much information about the indications for open and stereotactic thrombosis of these vascular anomalies. Smith and Alksne (1977) used the injection of a polymerizing iron compound into otherwise inaccessible aneurysms with help of a stereotactic puncture needle. This needle penetrates the aneurys-

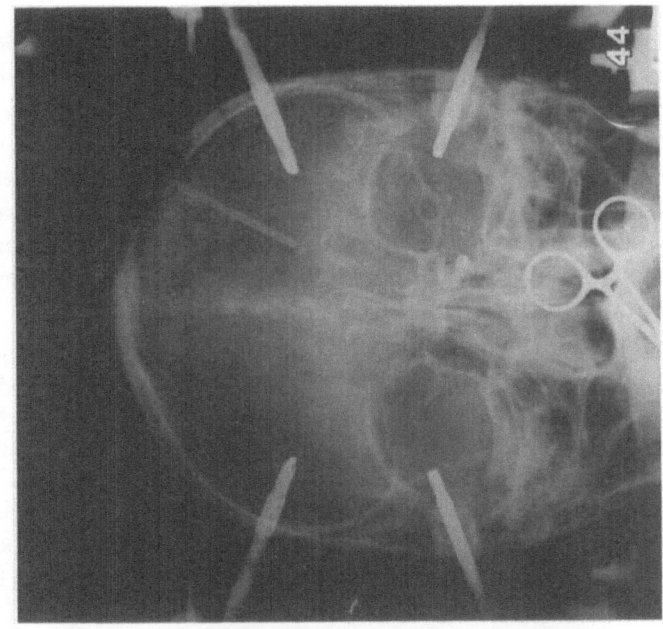

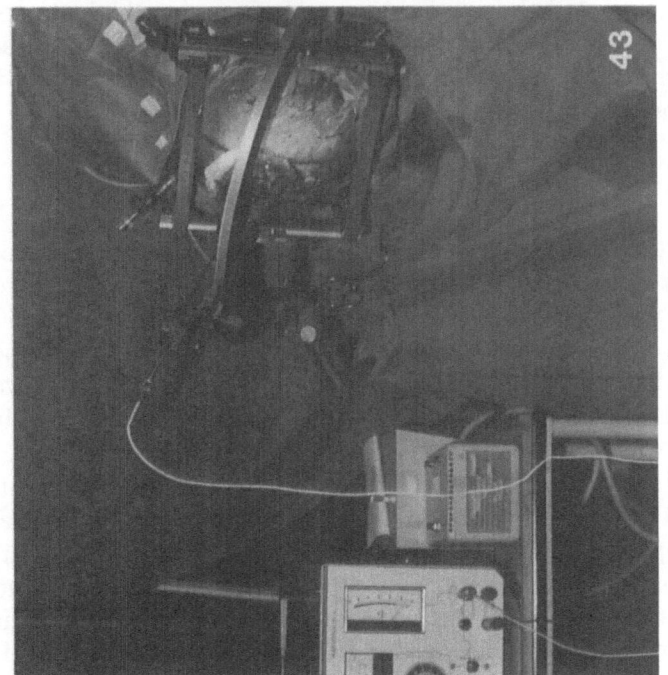

Fig. 43. Stereotactic performance for coagulating a tiny paraventricular arteriovenous malformation

Fig. 44. Angiogram during the stereotactic coagulation attempt, which was unsuccessful. Open resection with stereotactic guidance was necessary

mal fundus, whereafter magnetically controlled metallic thrombosis is achieved with a stereotactic magnetic probe. It is interesting to note, that those aneurysms which are inaccessible with microsurgical techniques—intrasellar, intracavernous and ventral to the brainstem lying basilar ones—can be occluded using this technique (without opening the dura) with the magnetic probe positioned through the transsphenoidal or transclival route. Sheptak (*et al.* 1977) treated aneurysms by injection with the tissue adhesive IBC (isobutyl-2-cyanoacrylate); 2 of their 20 cases were treated by stereotactic injection. There were, however, more than 50% incomplete occlusions, which makes this technique unreliable unless a method for monitoring aneurysm thrombosis during injection is developed.

In arteriovenous malformations the shunt is sometimes very small and could be occluded easiest by interventional stereotactic technique. Cahan and Rand (1973) describe a case of stereotactic coagulation of a little paraventricular malformation, but our own experience with a similar case led us to believe that it is not always successful. After four attempts (Figs. 43 and 44) to coagulate the shunt with a thermistor electrode, which was lying with its tip at the site of the shunt—controlled with intraoperative angiography in 2 directions—,we finally decided to resect it after having made a small craniotomy for microsurgical exposure.

This approach is called the combined technique, in which stereotactic localization is done prior to craniotomy for microsurgical resection. Advocates of this combined technique, as far back as the sixties, were Guiot (*et al.* 1960) and Riechert and Mundinger (1964).

## B. Localizing Stereotactics

To use the stereotactic procedure with its precision and target accuracy for the surgical treatment of deep seated angiomas and arteriovenous malformations was the idea of Riechert (1962) and Guiot (*et al.* 1960). By that time, after stereotactic localization, the operation was continued by craniotomy and classical surgical principles. It is evident, that nowadays many cases will be treated without this stereotactic aid, because occluding the feeders of the malformation is no longer the sole objective to be pursued. The nidus itself should be resected for which microsurgical instrumentation is mandatory. Those AVM's, that are easily localized do no longer require stereotactic approach. On the other hand, new indications for this combined technique have appeared. All lesions that are small and not localized without stereotactic aiming should be approached according to stereotactic principles to minimize damage to surrounding brain during microsurgical resection. This applies particularly to the paraventricular (Fig. 45) and subcortical malformations and also to those small mass lesions (tumor, hematoma and abscess), that are only detected with CT scanning.

Here is a challenge for the neurosurgeon to do surgery with modern equipment (operating microscope, endoscope or laser beam), but, nertheless, the aiming is the crucial point. Stereotactic localization is then needed for proper exploration and the calculation of the most harmless transcortical approach. Recently papers have been published which emphasize the benefits of this method (Garcia de Sola *et al.* 1980, Kelly *et al.* 1982 b) and our own experience with 4 cases (small subcortical AVM's) confirms the correctness of this combined surgical approach.

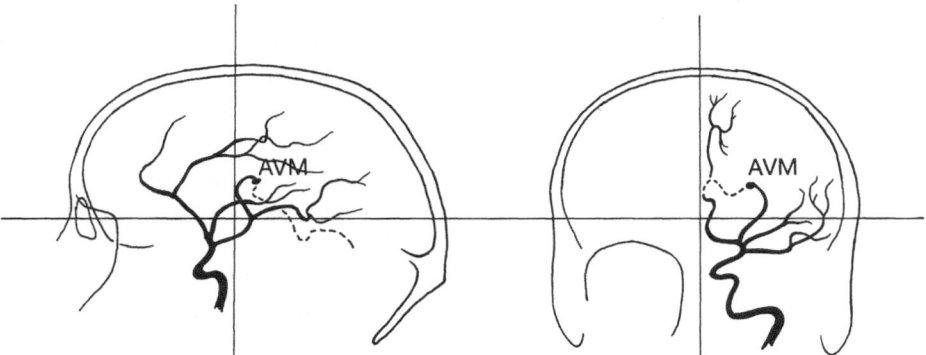

Fig. 45. Deep seated paraventricular arteriovenous malformation in stereotactic space. This schematic drawing shows, that very small and/or deep seated malformations cannot be resected without the aid of stereotactic localization

In small tumors similar experience is gained with the combined technique (Shelden *et al.* 1980, Sugita *et al.* 1975). Jacques (*et al.* 1980) made use of a newly designed tumorscope, which is introduced through a 4 mm cortical opening and is opened at the appropriate coordinate settings to expose the lesion. Lunsford (*et al.* 1982, 1984 a, and Martinez 1984) started stereotactic surgery with the patient placed in the CT scanner, which offers direct assessment of therapeutic results.

CT guided localization with stereotactic principles is also used to treat deep seated brain abscesses (Wise and Gleason 1979, Lunsford and Nelson 1982). Because CT repeatedly demonstrates clinically indiscernable lesions, including brain abscess, stereotactic localization (with or without CT guidance) offers a simple method to treat the deep seated abscesses by aspiration, culture, and subsequent treatment with a course of antibiotics. For extensive information on CT scan and clinical correlations of brain abscesses, including neuropathological staging, the reader is referred to the publication by Britt and Enzmann (1983).

Primary intracerebral hemorrhage resulting in intracerebral hematoma has been treated successfully by stereotactic evacuation, after Backlund and

Von Holst (1978) published their results using an Archemedian type of screw, which was constructed according to their design. By the same time, the general opinion regarding the effect of surgery versus conservative treatment changed: formerly, surgery in the acute stage was thought to be contraindicated and craniotomy was only performed after some delay, when the hematoma due to vascular spasm and cerebral edema acted as a space occupying lesion (McKissock et al. 1961). In 1977 however, Kaneko (et al.) published their results with microsurgery in the acute stage (within 7 hours after the attack) with impressing results: 34 out of the 38 patients became selfsupporting again after 6 months. Recently, the same group of investigators (Kaneko et al. 1983) described a long-term evaluation in 100 cases: 50 were selfsupporting and 33 needed partial care at home. A thorough review of publications, relating to the natural history of primary intracerebral hemorrhage and to the comparative efficacy of surgical and nonsurgical modalities of treatment, leads to the conclusion that large and medium sized (20–40 cc) lobar hematomas benefit from surgical treatment (Kase et al. 1982), whereas small lobar hematomas do well with conservative treatment. Deep seated small (and larger) hematomas, however, result in serious neurological deficit and often require surgery. According to Kaneko, primary hypertensive putaminal hematoma is an indication for microsurgical removal and may also benefit from stereotactic evacuation (Matsumoto and Hondo 1984, Broseta et al. 1982). Primary brainstem hematoma has been successfully evacuated stereotactically by Beatty and Zervas (1983) and Bosch and Beute (1985).

The indications for stereotactic evacuation are an established diagnosis of primary deep seated hematoma with impairment of mental status and depressed level of consciousness (Higgins et al. 1982). Relative indications form those hematomas that can be approached just as easily with microsurgical techniques. Amano and Kandel, at the Bratislawa conference in 1983, demonstrated satisfactory results with stereotactic evacuation of all sizes of primary intracerebral hematomas. Higgins (et al. 1982) modified Backlund's instrument for easy aspiration of both liquid and solid hematomas; the original instrument, however, is as widely accepted.

To summarize, it may be stated that the three discussed subdivisions of stereotactic neurosurgery are of a completely different background. The history of functional stereotactics is comparatively long and evaluation of the validity of the various functional procedures therefore relatively easy. Mass lesions stereotactics is strongly connected to oncology and diseases that might arise in patients with cancer. Stereotactic biopsy is a safe and reliable way to obtain information required to plan the best strategy of medical treatment. Finally, stereotactic localization, with or without combined open surgery, is the latest development. This localization often makes it possible to approach and expose small lesions with the help of the

CT scan and computer facilities, which have become available. However, most of the publications relating to this matter give preliminary results and the time for evaluation has not yet come. On the other hand, a discussion on the continuously expanding field should not exclude these promising results, because most certainly computer assistance in the operating room will be vital to neurosurgery in the near future.

# Chapter 4

# Modern Instrumentation

## I. Introduction

In chapter 2 we described the four most popular types of the many different stereotactic apparatus which have been developed: i.e. the instruments of Talairach, Riechert-Mundinger, Leksell and Todd-Wells. These instruments in their original construction are only suited to perform conventional stereotactic surgery, i.e. with the aid of standard X-ray equipment, such as is used in angiography and ventriculography. The break-through in radiologic imaging with computerized scanning techniques (CT, NMR, and PET scanning) has made visualization of normal as well as pathological anatomy of the brain feasible and has given the impetus to the development of new stereotactic instrumentation.

The already existing apparatus needed technical adaptation to make them suitable for computerized scanning methods. The construction needed to be adapted too, to give the least scanner artifacts, and special designs have been developed with carbon fiber fixation pins. With this adapted instrumentation it became possible to visualize targets of interest inside the brain with the stereotactic apparatus mounted to the skull during the scanning procedure (Fig. 46).

Stereotactic space (i.e. the brain in a fixed relation to the stereotactic instrument) could now be studied with the scanner computer facilities. Brown (1979) was the first to describe these possibilities and he presented a prototype stereotactic frame for use in the CT scanner, with a complete three-dimensional computer graphics approach to optimum stereotactic orientation. An overview of CT based stereotactic systems has been given by Alker (*et al.* 1984).

On the other hand, the development of these CT guided stereotactic methods does not imply that the conventional X-ray stereotactic principles are out of date. There are still situations in which the so-called conventional approach is essential for optimal target visualization, e.g. in the localization of small arteriovenous malformations (Fig. 47) which may not be visible on CT and thus need angiography (especially in the case of adjacent intracerebral hematoma). Sometimes angiotomography in stereotactic space is needed to acquire an exact target calculation. Moreover, at the

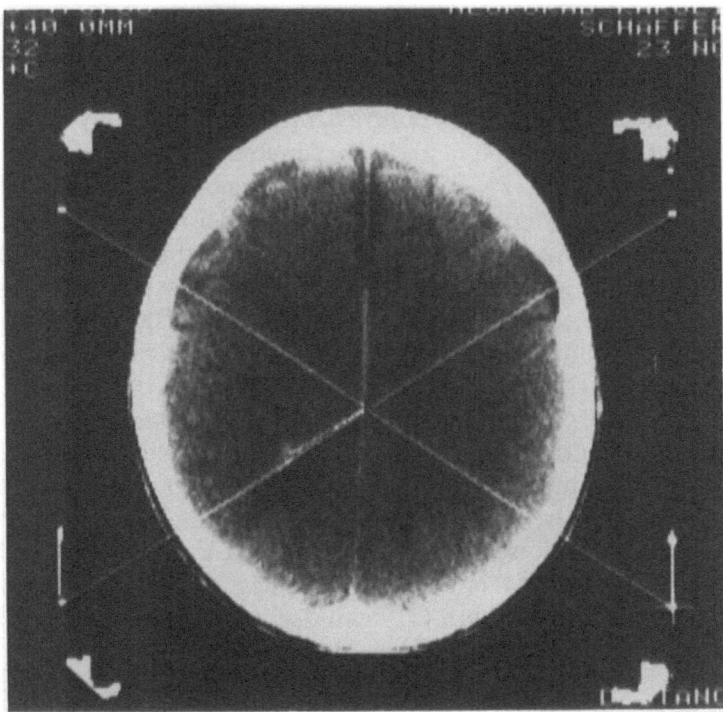

Fig. 46. CT scan picture of a deep seated small brain tumor, which is localized in stereotactic space with the instrument of Leksell

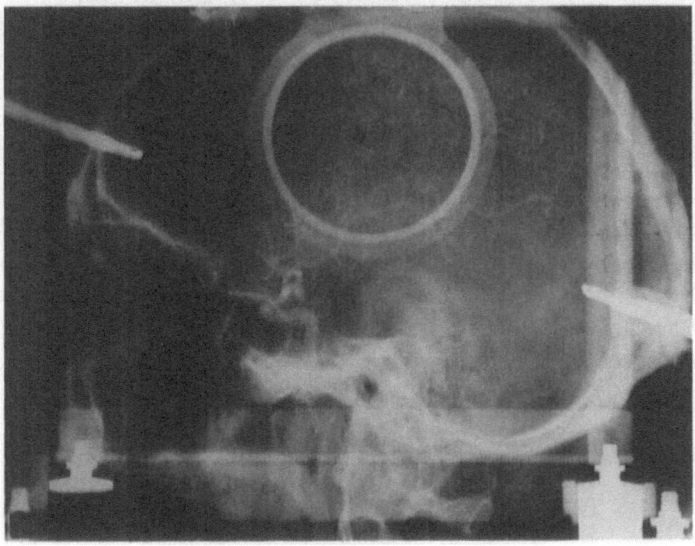

Fig. 47. Angiography in stereotactic space to visualize a tiny paraventricular arteriovenous malformation (arrow)

moment CT guided localization is often more time consuming and may need stereotactic CT studies prior to the day of surgery. In functional stereotactics CT guided stereotactic surgery is demanding highly sophisticated computer software, this being in contrast with the rather simple and reliable method of ventriculography. Indeed, functional surgery rests on the construction of the AC—PC-line, being at present the most safely achieved with stereotactic ventriculography as compared to computer techniques with sagittal plane imaging and computer graphical reconstruction of the intercommissural plane (Hardy *et al.* 1983). In the assessment of the lateral coordinate, however, CT and NMR scanning are of great value, as with these imaging techniques the thalamic width in the individual patient can be measured (Hitchcock and Cadavid 1984).

In cases which present moderately large deep seated mass lesions, diagnostic stereotactic surgery is obviously as easily performed with conventional techniques (chapter 2), using the angiographic films for target positioning. Moreover, to avoid the risk of damaging vessels in tumor biopsy an angiographic study is necessary, and the target should in our opinion always be chosen from these films, unless digitizing of angiographic data and combining these with CT scan derived target data is carried out prior to surgery.

The era of computerized stereotactic surgery with its new instrumentation is not only characterized by the introduction of scanning machines, but also by results attained in the—not completely on these machines dependent—evolution of computer technology (Bertrand 1982). The computer itself with its excellent facilities as to graphical reconstruction and calculation of three-dimensional objects, together with the possibility of computer simulation prior to the actual surgical performance, have provided the neurosurgeon with a tool to study the true volume and shape of any lesion plus the safest trajectory towards it. During the performance and the actual introduction of a probe, its position may be checked with the aid of a computer display of a digitized X-ray film. A major advance has been made with CT and NMR imaging in stereotactic space, which enables the neurosurgeon to continue after stereotactic localization with open surgery. Stereotactic resections of lesions or certain brain areas (e.g. the hippocampus in epileptics) may be carried out with computer monitored microsurgical techniques.

## II. CT Guided Stereotactic Apparatus; Technical Aspects

### A. Riechert-Mundinger System

The Riechert-Mundinger stereotactic instrument has been adapted for CT stereotaxy by Birg and Mundinger (1982) and Mundinger and Birg

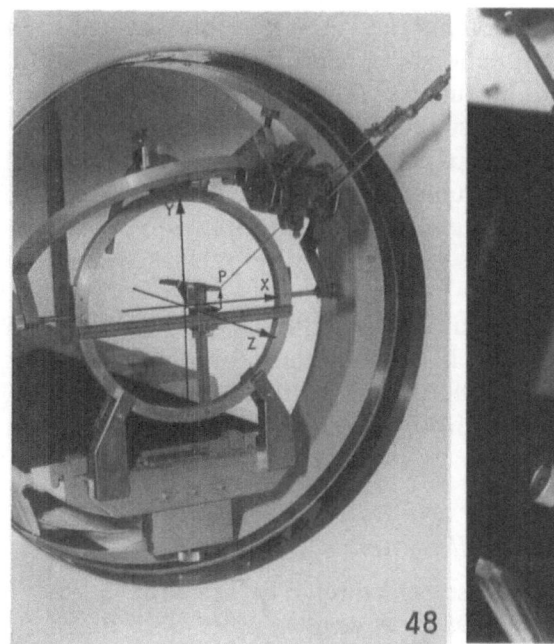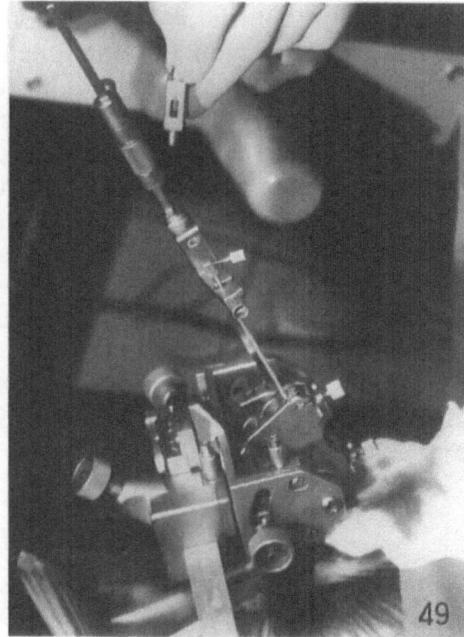

Fig. 48. The Riechert-Mundinger apparatus for CT guided stereotaxy (by courtesy of Prof. Mundinger)

Fig. 49. Close view of the instrument carrier and aiming device (by courtesy of Prof. Mundinger)

(1984). In fact, the value of CT information in interstitial irradiation (stereotactic curietherapy) is obvious, and the computerization of interstitial irradiation had already been started at an earlier stage by the Freiburg center of stereotactic surgery. CT makes exact positioning of the therapy probe possible as well as the exact determination of the volume/dosage relationship after input of CT data into a computer. Mundinger (*et al.* 1978 a, b) describes the value of computer calculations for therapeutic stereotactics and CT scanning under stereotactic conditions. Birg and Mundinger (1982) subsequently developed a system to attain the target coordinates directly from the scan pictures, obtained by scanning with their stereotactic apparatus fixed to the skull. The instrument only needed a special CT holder and low density fixation pins. Pictures are made at a gantry angle of 0 degrees, i.e. parallel to the stereotactic base ring. The computer accuracy in the determination of any target has been shown to have a maximum deviation of 0.6 mm. Both functional and diagnostic interventions have been carried out with satisfactory results with the aid of CT guided coordinates setting. CT reconstruction of the midsagittal plane makes measurement of the intercommissural line possible and thus the assessment of coordinates for functional targets. Even the trephination point can be determined prior to surgery. The set-up of the Riechert-Mundinger apparatus for CT guided stereotaxy is shown in Figs. 48 and 49. Gahbauer (*et al.* 1983) published a paper on the results with interstitial irradiation using this CT guided intrumentation with both intraoperative CT scanning and angiography. They transferred enlarged CT reconstructions to angiographic films and selected puncture tracks according to the orientation of the blood vessels.

Combined surgery with craniotomy in the stereotactic instrument can easily be performed with the Riechert-Mundinger-Birg system, as is beautifully shown by Jacques (*et al.* 1980) in a paper on stereotactic removal of small intracerebral lesions. Further information on this technique is given by Shelden (*et al.* 1980, 1982).

## B. Leksell System

The Leksell stereotactic system has been adapted to direct use in the CT scanner by Leksell and Jernberg (1980). A scan adapter with magnetic attachment has been constructed which can be used in all types of body CT scanners and secures a fixed position of the headframe to the scanner bed (Fig. 50). Fixation pins are made of carbon fiber, avoiding artifacts on the CT pictures. A localizing pair of plastic discs can be mounted on the headframe (Fig. 51), which allows rapid coordinates calculation of any intracranial target directly from the scan pictures. Fig. 52 shows in a drawing how these calculations can easily be made with the help of a standard CT ruler. During the last years further refinements have been designed, all of them for safe and reliable management in both CT and NMR scanners, and for rapid calculation of target coordinates with the scan computer (Lunsford and Nelson 1982, Lunsford and Martinez 1984). A probe holder for performing stereotactic surgery in the CT scanner has been developed by Lunsford (*et al.* 1983, 1984 a), who has a CT scan machine dedicated to surgery in the operating room (Fig. 53). Boëthius (*et al.* 1980) described a baseplate that is fixed to the skull to achieve a constant relationship between the Leksell headframe and the CT scanner, which enables the surgeon to localize and calculate the target position with the CT computer software only.

The newest type of Leksell instrument has been reconstructed for use in both CT and NMR imaging, including a coordinate system that is modified according to the standard terminology used in NMR and CT scanning. Specially designed coordinate indicators and rulers make coordinate calculation in both CT and NMR easy procedures (Fig. 54).

Mackay (*et al.* 1982) reports a group of patients who had biopsy and

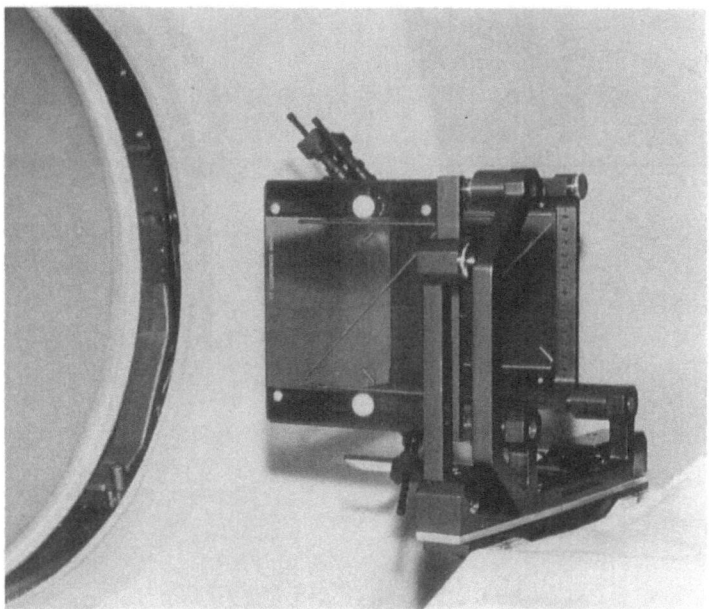

Fig. 50. The Leksell instrument for CT guided stereotaxy, with CT scan adapter securing a fixed position to the scanner bed (by courtesy of Prof. Leksell)

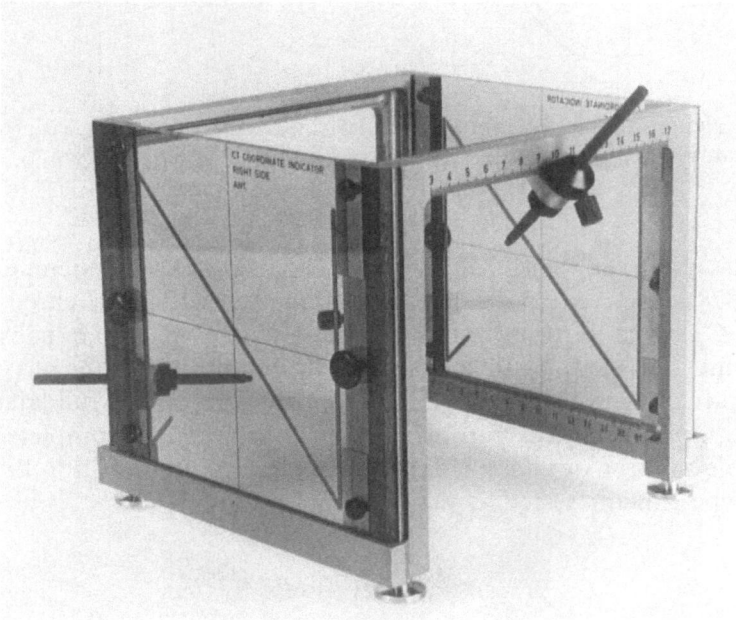

Fig. 51. The Leksell headframe with coordinate indicator discs for use in CT scanning (by courtesy of Prof. Leksell)

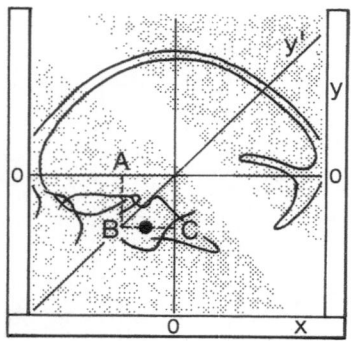

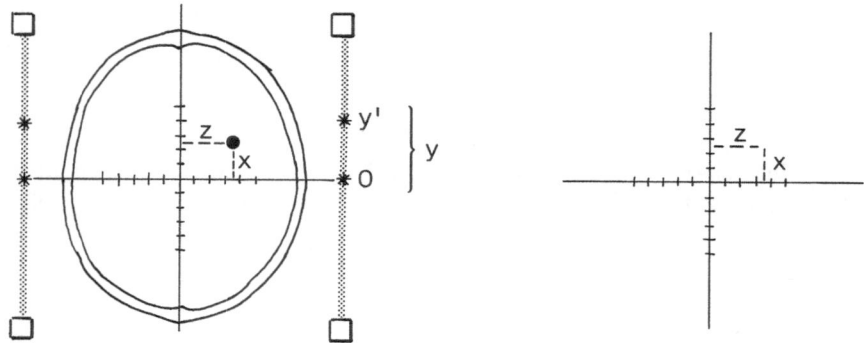

Fig. 52. Calculating the coordinates for a leftsided temporal tumor with the aid of the indicator discs. As AB = BC the distance OY′ = $y$, whereas $x$ and $z$ can be calculated directly from the scan picture

interstitial irradiation with help of the CT guided Leksell system. Gleason (*et al.* 1978) described coordinates determination with the Leksell system and the CT scan. For craniotomy in stereotactic space (i.e. subsequent craniotomy after stereotactic localization) the cubic headframe has certainly its disadvantages, because of its side-bars which prevent full lateral and temporal approach. To permit combined surgery a completely new headframe has been developed (Leksell, personal communication 1985) and a prototype is being tested at the moment.

## C. Brown-Roberts-Wells System

The Brown-Roberts-Wells system is a new stereotactic instrument that enables accurate localization of CT scan determined targets. It is a modern version of the original Todd-Wells apparatus discussed in chapter 2 (sub D,

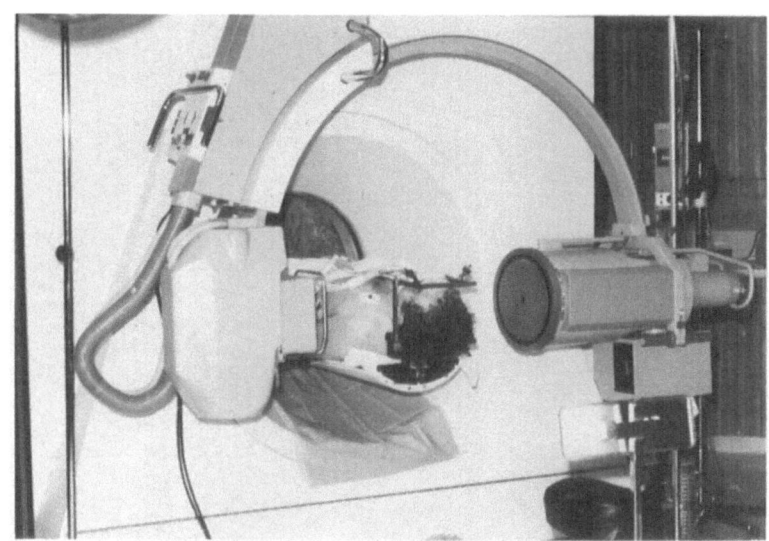

Fig. 53. The combined set up allowing intraoperative angiography with a ceiling mounted fluoroscope that may be used over the intraoperative CT scanner; Pittsburgh (by courtesy of Dr. Lunsford; published in Surg. Neurol. *22*, 222—230; 1984)

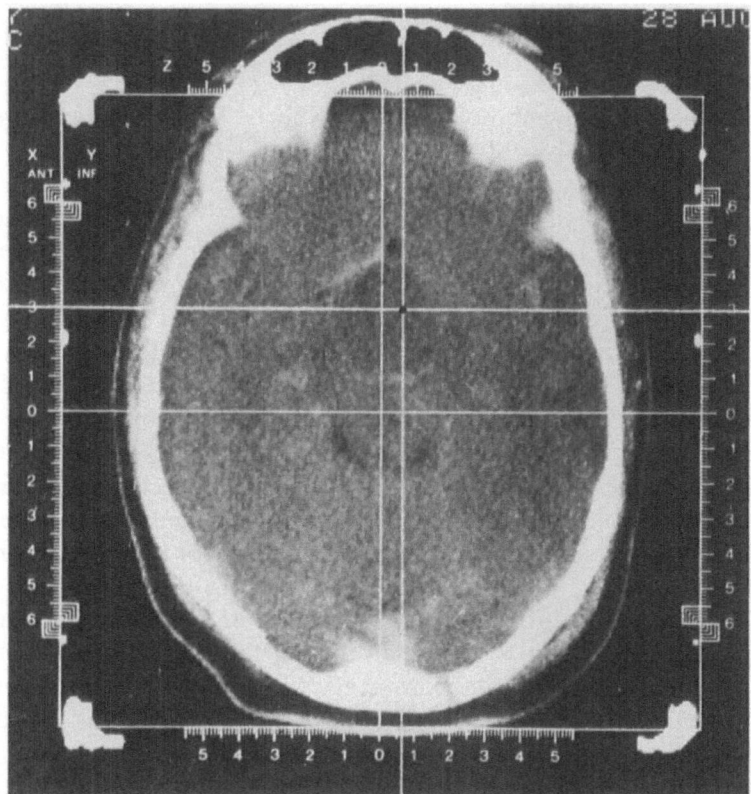

Fig. 54. Coordinate ruler over stereotactic CT scan picture with the Leksell instrument. The target point (black dot) is easily defined in stereotactic space: $x = 30$ mm ant.; $y = 20$ mm inf.; $z = 7$ mm lateral (by courtesy of Prof. Leksell)

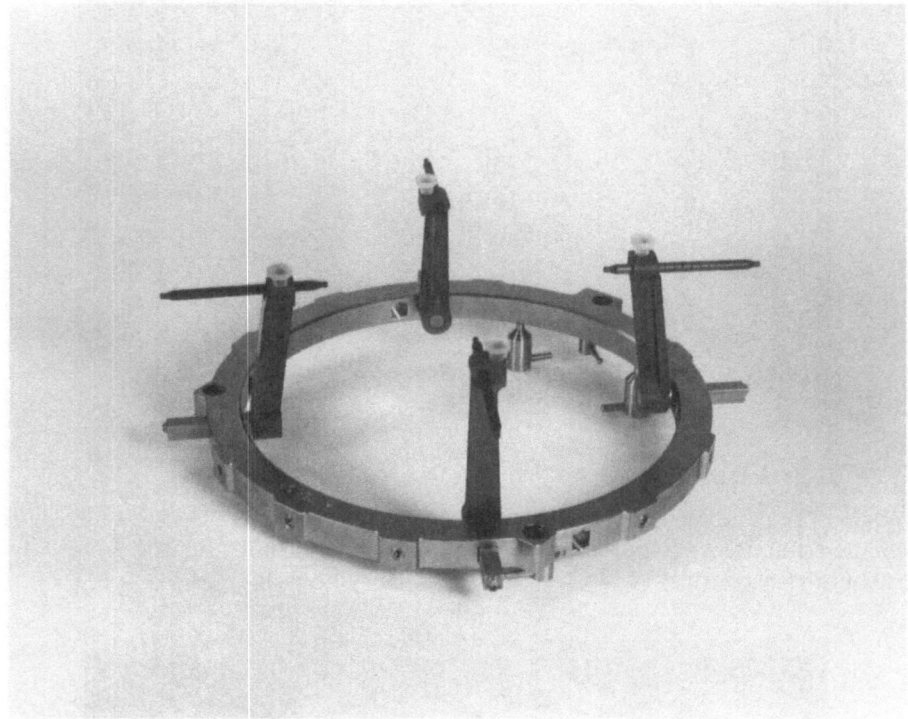

Fig. 55. The head ring assembly of the Brown-Roberts-Wells stereotactic system for
CT guided surgery (by courtesy of Dr. Cosman)

4), and is available as the **B-R-W** CT stereotactic system from Radionics
(Instruction Manual 1983). The computerized approach to stereotactic
localization has been tested and published by Brown (1979) and clinical
experience with a prototype instrument was presented by Heilbrun (*et al.*
1983), Apuzzo and Sabshin (1983), and Thomas (*et al.* 1984). The system is
designed in such a way, that all coordinates are referenced to a ring fixed to
the skull (the so-called head ring assembly with 4 fixation screws, Fig. 55),
which eliminates the necessity of a fixed relationship between the base ring
and the CT scanner gantry (this in contrast with the Leksell and Riechert-
Mundinger systems). This makes, however, the calculation of the target
coordinates more elaborate, and therefore a calculator is needed to program
the position as to the reference points on the base ring.

The **B-R-W** system is dependent on the scanner only for identification of
the target and localizing rods (which during the scanning procedure are
temporarily mounted on the base ring, Fig. 56). All subsequent data
processing can be performed away from the CT scan area with a hand-held
programmable calculator. As has been described by Heilbrun (*et al.* 1983),
the target's coordinates are derived from the localizing rods coordinates on

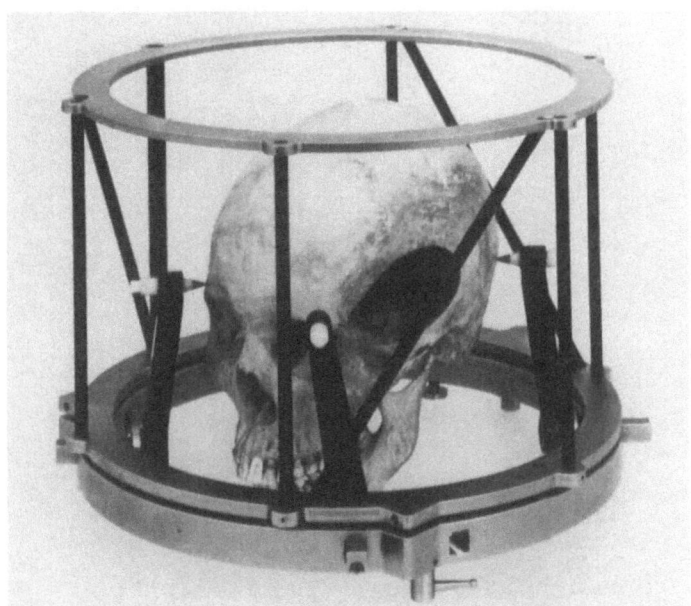

Fig. 56. System of localizing rods mounted on the head ring for stereotactic CT scanning and calculation of the target's coordinates (by courtesy of Dr. Cosman)

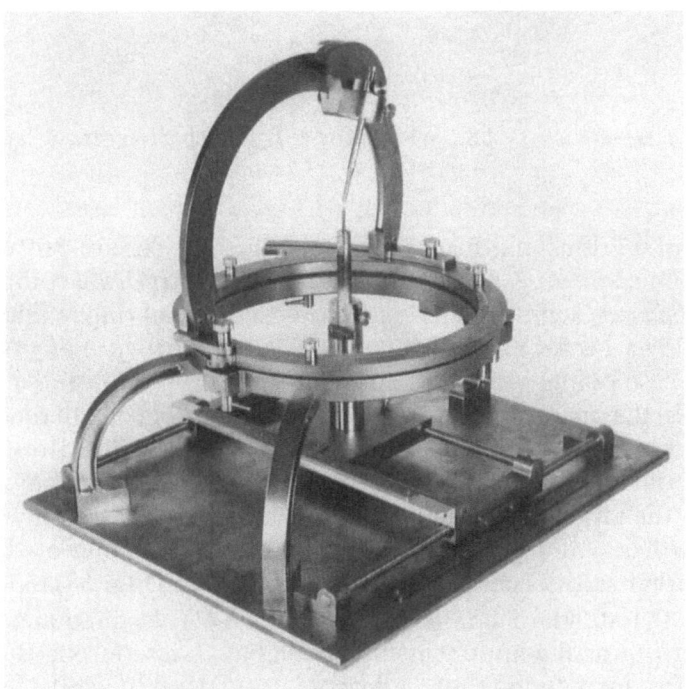

Fig. 57. Simulation of stereotactic performance on the phantom base assembly (B—R—W-system; by courtesy of Dr. Cosman)

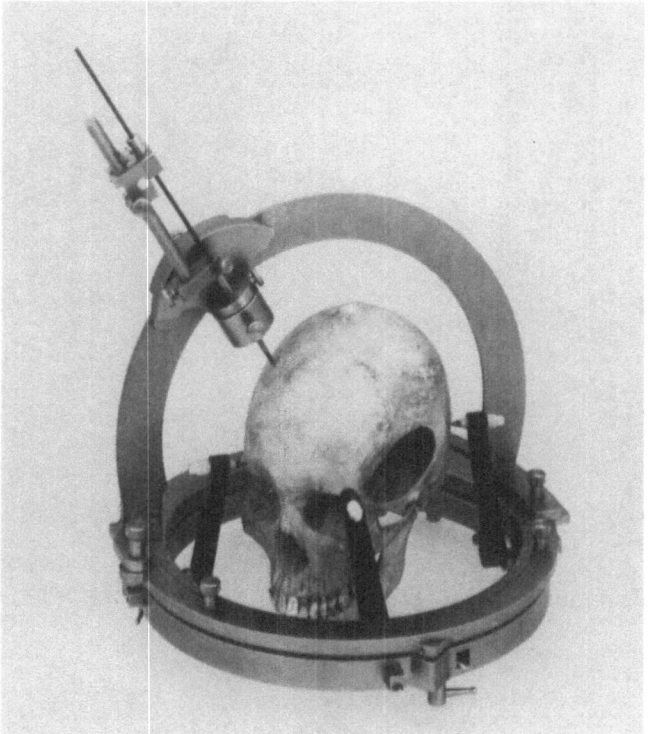

Fig. 58. The B—R—W-system set up for CT guided stereotactic surgery (by courtesy of Dr. Cosman)

the basis of various mathematical formulae, which are stored in the computer. Once the x, y, and z coordinates of the target are computed, the design of the arc system (which is mounted on the head ring to allow guided surgery) allows a course and distance to be plotted between any two points in space. These points generally represent the entry point on the skull and the target. In the operating room the patient is positioned with the head ring attached to a special floor stand or to the Mayfield head-rest. Having performed data processing with the calculator, the arc settings and the distance to the target are simulated on a phantom base assembly (Fig. 57). The system has five degrees of freedom in the positioning of the guided probe. Thereafter the operation can be carried out (Fig. 58).

Besides the standard components of the B-R-W stereotactic system, many other optional components are available for use in NMR and PET scanning, for introduction of endoscopic and laser devices, as well as various biopsy instruments and RF lesion electrodes. Also the original Talairach grids for parallel introduction of electrodes (see chapter 2, sub D, 1) are available in adapted form for use with this system (Fig. 59), and a NIH

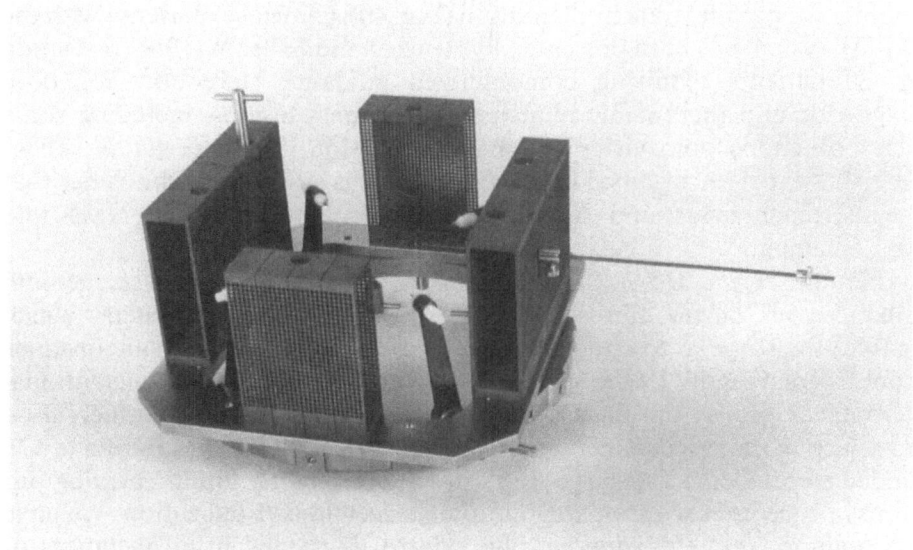

Fig. 59. The Talairach grids for parallel introduction of electrodes in adapted form for use with the B—R—W-system (by courtesy of Dr. Cosman)

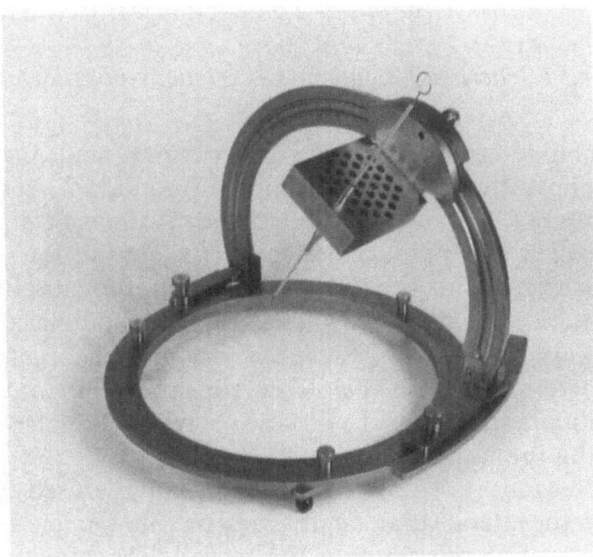

Fig. 60. The NIH adapter for parallel tract implantation (B—R—W-system; by courtesy of Dr. Cosman)

adapter for parallel tract implantation (Fig. 60). Clinical experience with the B-R-W system has been presented by Apuzzo and Sabshin (1983) in a study on 80 patients requiring computerized guidance stereotaxy for both diagnostic and therapeutic management of mass lesions, including some cases of endoscopic visualization and excision. Thomas (*et al.* 1984) describes experience gained in London with this system and concludes that the instrument is safe and easy in use and is also applicable with NMR and PET imaging.

Nauta (*et al.* 1984) discusses the arterial bolus contrast medium enhancement during stereotactic CT scanning with this system, which enables the surgeon to choose a target inside the tumor at a safe distance from major vessels. This paper is of importance, because in conventional stereotactic biopsy the arterial and venous angiograms are routinely used for selecting the target and avoiding injury to these vessels. In the era of CT guided stereotactics the surgeon is apt to think lightly about carrying out biopsy procedures without angiographic target area visualization. We have the opinion, that this angiographic control is needed in all instances of tumor biopsy, because fatal bleeding at the biopsy site is in fact almost the only real danger in stereotactic biopsy (about 1–2% ; see also chapter 8, sub C).

## D. Other Computed Tomography Based Systems

### 1. CT Based Intracranial Landmark Technique of Gildenberg (et al. 1982, 1983)

This technique comprises a lateral scout film made on the CT scanner, which demonstrates reproducible bony landmarks. A baseline through these landmarks is drawn and a first slice is done through this baseline, which is called the reference slice. After completion of the scanning procedure a zero point is calculated, which represents the point midway between anterior and posterior and lateral bony boundaries. The zero point is then displayed on all slices. Relationships for each target point to this zero point are determined with the CT cursor and yield two coordinates. The third coordinate stands for the distance between the reference slice and the slice showing the target.

Thereafter any stereotactic instrument may be used in the theatre for surgery. On the lateral stereotactic X-ray picture the reference line is drawn as well as the line representing the target slice (after appropriate mag-nification). The zero point is then marked on this line, and then the target itself can be marked on both the lateral and anteroposterior X-ray pictures. Calculations for the coordinates of the target regarding the stereotactic apparatus are then performed with the methods described in chapter 2 for conventional stereotactic target determination. This technique has the advantage that it is applicable to all types of instrumentation. The only drawback is, that there is no fixed relationship between the head of the patient and the scanner, leading to non-parallel slices in case of restlessness. Bullard (*et al.* 1984) presents a series of biopsy cases, in which this CT guided technique has been followed with satisfactory results. Gildenberg reviews (1982 b) various CT guided systems, including his own, in the chapter on "computerized tomography and stereotactic surgery" in Spiegel's monograph on guided brain operations (Spiegel 1982).

## 2. The Computerized, CT Guided, Stereotactic System with 3-D Reconstruction of Shelden (et al. 1980) and Jacques (et al. 1980)

This sophisticated system employs a modified Riechert-Mundinger head ring plus computer processing of CT scan data from the region of interest by filtering, magnifying, color-coding, and three-dimensional reconstruction (Shelden *et al.* 1980). Thus any lesion can be three-dimensionally reconstructed before stereotactic surgery to better define the exact volume, size, and shape. The system depends on transfer of CT scan data to magnetic tape, that is fed into a computer (a PDP 1145 type) for coordinate calculation and 3-D reconstruction.

After simulation of the procedure in a phantom ring, surgery can begin with the help of a micromanipulator and a type of stereotactic speculum that is introduced into the brain after appropriate trephination. The lesion of interest is reached using a series of dilators, whereafter the speculum ("tulip") is opened to expose the lesion at the calculated depth. Actual surgery is carried out with binocular vision afforded by a specially designed endoscope for use with this speculum. True removal of minute lesions has been achieved (Jacques *et al.* 1980) with the aid of this preoperative 3-D reconstruction in stereotactic space.

## 3. The Computer-monitored, CT Based, Stereotactic System with 3-D Reconstruction of Kelly and Alker (Kelly et al. 1982 a, b, 1983, 1984 a–c)

This completely computer-monitored system enables the surgeon to perform microsurgery in stereotactic space, with continuous computer information during actual surgery as to the position of the microsurgical instruments inside the area of interest (tumor, malformation, dysfunctional brain). Complete laser ablation of tumors and arteriovenous malformations has been presented by Kelly and his co-workers thanks to 3-D reconstruction of the target area and display in the operative field of the microscope and on a computer screen in the operating room (Kelly *et al.* 1984 b). The stereotactic apparatus used is a modified Todd-Wells head ring, with the target placed into the focal point of the sphere described by the arc-quadrant stereotactic frame. An operating microscope and a $CO_2$ laser

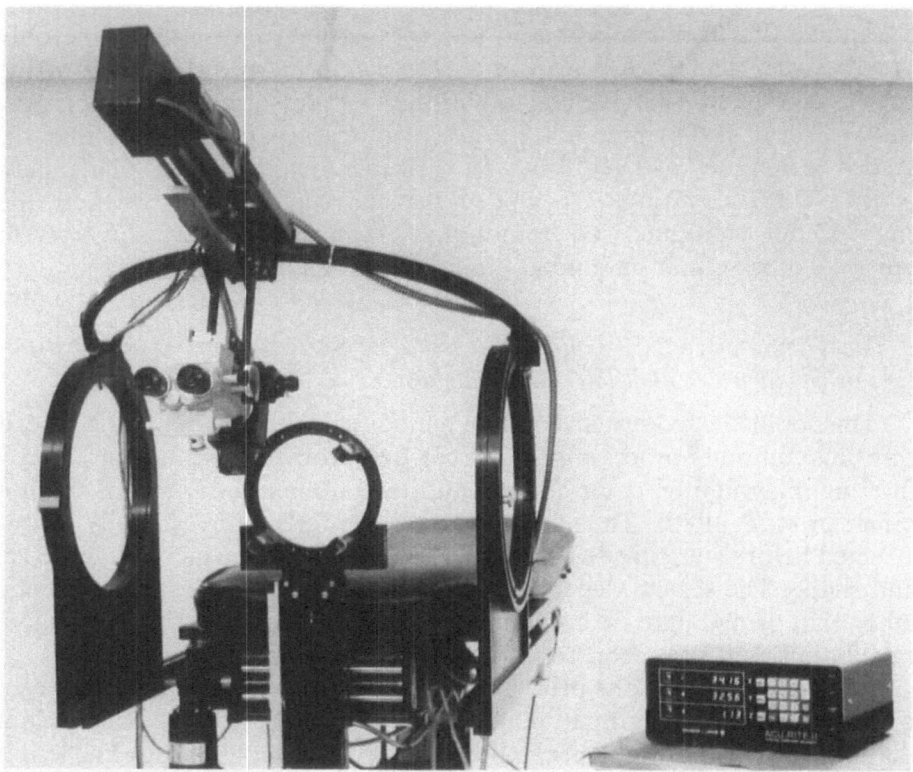

Fig. 61. The combined set up allowing computer-monitored, CT based, stereotactic resections with the aid of an operating microscope and a $CO_2$ laser; Mayo Clinic, Rochester (by courtesy of Dr. Kelly)

micromanipulator box run perpendicularly to a tangent to a 400 mm arc mounted on the stereotactic frame (Fig. 61), and after trephination these instruments automatically focus at the target point. The computer tape containing CT or NMR data derived from stereotactic scanning (which normally is performed a day prior to surgery) is transferred to the operating room computer system (IPDC type) and is displayed on a Ramtek raster display console. Programs written for 3-D reconstruction are available for display at any desired angle and depth of the volume of interest. In this way the actual boundaries of this volume in relation to the microsurgical instruments is secured during surgery. This enables the surgeon to resect a predetermined volume of tissue, whether a tumor or dysfunctional brain tissue (e.g. the hippocampus).

In this system arteriographic control during CT guided biopsy of tumors can be incorporated (Kelly *et al.* 1984a), using arteriography under stereotactic conditions and subsequent arteriographic data processing by digitizing a pair of stereoscopic angiograms.

The to this system inherent 3-D reconstruction of tumor volumes makes it particularly useful for tumor treatment with interstitial irradiation. Computer simulation, prior to the actual stereotactic placement of radio-nuclide sources, of various source positions in the reconstructed tumor volume may achieve the best fitting isodose configurations and offers a safer management of intracranial non-resectable mass lesions. This is of par-ticular importance in the treatment of the so-called low grade gliomas. For more information the reader is referred to Kelly (*et al.* 1984 c).

Whether this computer-monitored way of tumor treatment will bring complete recovery (this in contrast with biopsy alone plus external irradiation) remains to be proven and clearly depends on the extent to which the visualized tumor boundaries (on CT or NMR) match the histological boundaries. The borders of neuro-oncology, however, are by this system expanded into the computer age.

## III. CT Guided Stereotactic Surgery

### A. General Principles

"It was only natural that two techniques which involve accurate localization of neurological structures would marry to introduce new possibilities in the field of neurosurgery" (quoted from Gildenberg 1983). CT scanning allows visualization of the exact position of any target, whereas stereotactic surgery allows the introduction of any surgical tool into the target.

It is evident, however, that the visualization of lesions is a more convenient CT technique than the visualization of ventricular landmarks, such as the anterior and posterior commissures, which are necessary for the construction of the line AC—PC in functional stereotactics. Although it is difficult to transfer CT images to a stereotactic atlas of the standard brain in order to calculate stereotactic coordinates for determination of a functional (invisible) target, in the future computers may be able to generate the patient's individual stereotactic brain map, as is preluded to by Kelly in his special article on future possibilities (1983). In fact, stereotactic hippocam-pectomy has already been developed by Kelly (personal information 1985), based upon the transfer of stereotactic atlas plates to the patient's actual CT scan pictures. Hardy (*et al.* 1983) also presented a computer graphic technique for use in CT guided functional stereotactics, which simulates an otherwise blind surgical procedure on a graphics screen for use during surgery. Their system involves software which allows selective storage and display of electricophysiological data from stimulation and micro-electrode recordings in the individual patient. The brain maps stored in the system's memory are mainly those from the Schaltenbrand and Wahren atlas (1977).

The atlas maps can be expanded or contracted in different dimensions and overlayed on corresponding CT pictures.

On the other hand, the possibilities for CT guided and computer-monitored stereotactic surgery in the fields of diagnostic, therapeutic, and localizing performances have become more widely recognized, because in these fields the impressive technical advances have led to hitherto impossible operations.

After visualization of a lesion (visible target) with CT, NMR, or even PET scanning computer calculations of the wanted coordinates and the reconstruction of shape and volume may become a routine, resulting in easier performing of stereotactic surgery in common practice. A specialization in the field of stereotactics—as was usual in former days—will not be necessary any longer and the integration into clinical neurosurgery (chapter 13) is at least theoretically spoken a fact. The use of the computer as an indispensable instrument in surgical neurology will follow this integration.

## B. Advantages over Conventional Stereotactic Surgery

Apart from the main advantage over conventional stereotactics, i.e. converting essentially blind surgical procedures to visualized and computer-monitored performances (Figs. 62 and 63), including the continuous possibility to check target and instrument position during surgery (Fig. 64), there are also less pitfalls. Firstly, the standard deviation in computerized target determination is less than 1 mm (as compared with a 2–3 mm deviation in conventional systems). Secondly, the position of the entrance point (i.e. the burrhole or trephination) may also be computed, including the proposed trajectory towards the target area. This opportunity lessens the problems presented by blind angles of stereotactic instruments and skull openings to a minimum. Finally, a major advance is presented by the feasibility to proceed with any type of craniotomy in stereotactic space, as the modern instrumentation offers both sufficient room for performing craniotomies and is accompanied by computer software which enables the surgeon to resect calculated, and predetermined volumes of tissue. Adjustments for mounting the stereotactic frame on a Mayfield head-rest still

Fig. 62. Visualization of rightsided brainstem tumor by stereotactic CT, with positive contrast in the aqueduct and lateral ventricles as well as around the brainstem

Fig. 63. The area of interest (brainstem) is enlarged; the tumor shows some contrast enhancement as well as a hypodense zone inside it. Marked shift of midline to the left

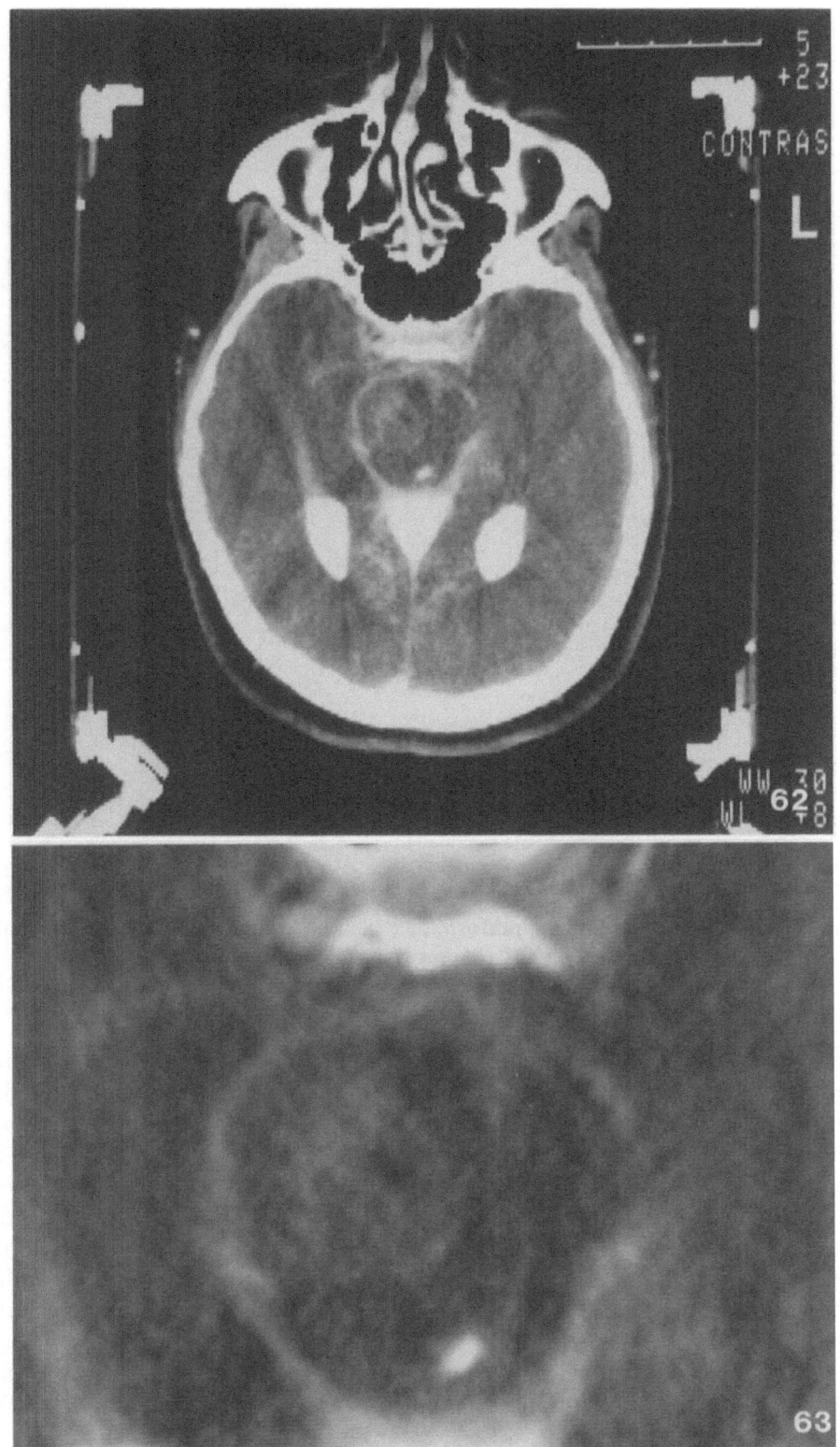

Figs. 62 and 63

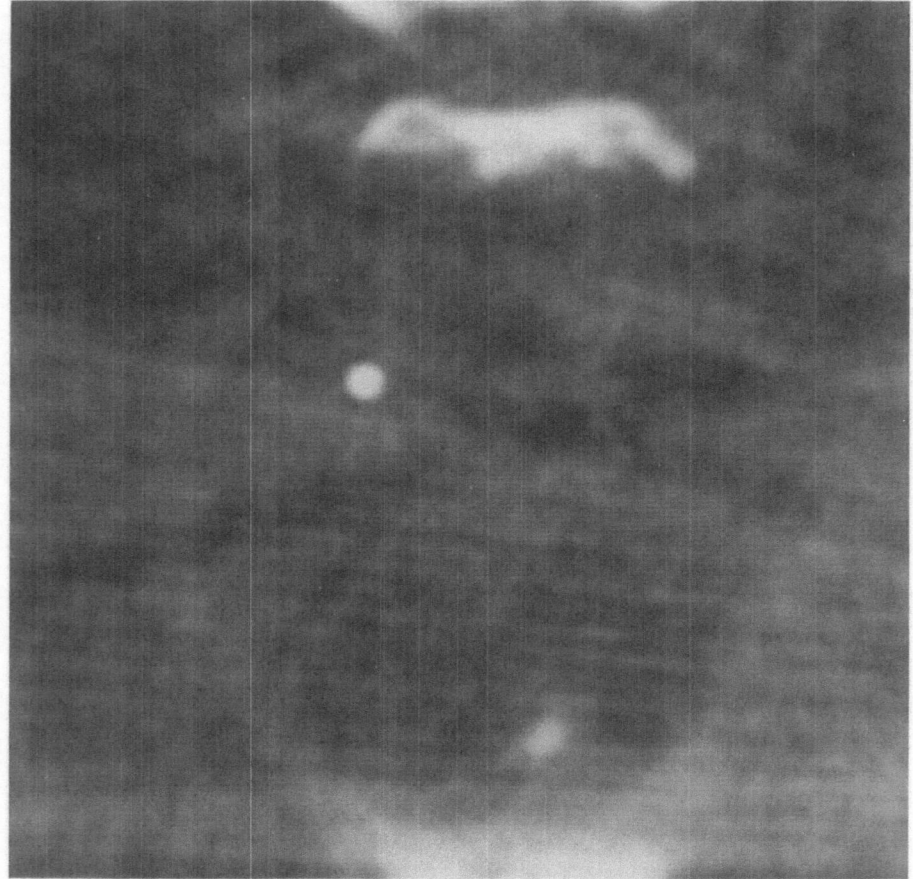

Fig. 64. During the stereotactic performance the position of the biopsy instrument
is checked with CT (diagnosis: astrocytoma grade 2)

amplify the versatility of the patient's head for optimal positioning during
surgery. In therapeutic performances the obvious advantages include
simulation of surgical performances prior to actual surgery, i.e. probe
insertion and placement of radionuclide sources at various targets inside a
tumor to achieve optimal isodose configurations (Kelly *et al.* 1984c).

Pre-operative computer studies of stereotactic space may be carried out
prior to the day of surgery, because repositioning of the stereotactic
instrument is easily done with micrometer control as to the depth of pin
insertion. In this field progress in the near future is to be expected,
particularly with the use of local hyperthermia, coagulation, freezing,
irradiation and intracavitary drug delivery, all of them being results of
ongoing research in the treatment of intracranial malignancies (chapter 14).

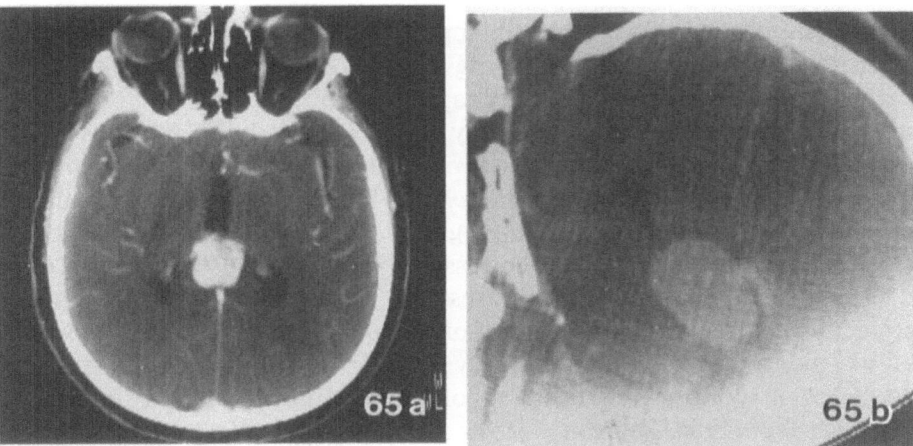

Fig. 65. Axial CT scanning (a) shows a pineal region tumor (after contrastenhancement). Because scanning without contrast already showed a hyperdense lesion, a sagittal scan was performed, revealing a vascular lesion (b)

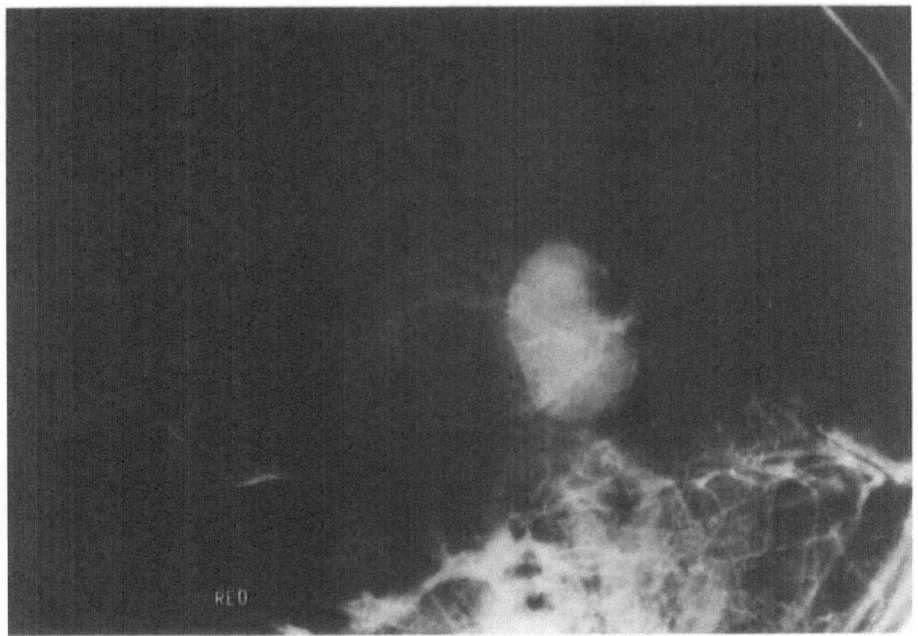

Fig. 66. Angiography confirmed the presence of an arteriovenous malformation (venous phase)

## C. Pitfall

On the other hand, the most important complication in stereotactic surgery will always be (fatal) bleeding at the target site, due to manipulation with stereotactic instruments (see chapter 8, sub I, C). This complication is not expected to be met less frequently with CT guided interventions (about 1–2%). With CT scan images [even with arterial bolus injection of contrast medium, as described by Nauta (et al. 1984)] as well as with digital information from stereoscopic angiograms (Kelly et al. 1984 a) the surgeon can never visualize small caliber vessels, which may also cause bleeding. Therefore, we would like to stress in this age of computer guided stereotactic surgery the importance of angiographic examinations prior to all but functional stereotactic surgery (Figs. 65 and 66). Although technical advances in computer processing of angiographic data are impressive (Suetens et al. 1984, Kelly et al. 1984 a), biopsy of a rather vascular tumor using conventional methods, and thus with angiographic visualization of the target on both lateral and anteroposterior X-ray pictures, will in our opinion remain the procedure of choice.

In conclusion the computer as surgical instrument in the operating room, together with the display of CT or NMR data with 3-D imaging in stereotactic space, will bring stereotaxy close to the general neurosurgeon. The computer will prove its particular value in the proper management of small and deep seated intracerebral lesions and the stereotactic approach to these will become common practice. Moreover, neuro-oncology may become a more sophisticated field of research and may at last bring some true results in the treatment of the various intracerebral malignancies.

# Chapter 5

# Indications for Stereotactic Interventions

Having discussed stereotactic principles in general and the nowadays available stereotactic instrumentation we will proceed with the established benefits of stereotactic neurosurgery. These include indications, contra-indications and the available techniques, which will be discussed in the following chapters. Ample information will be given regarding the implications of different techniques.

Indications for stereotactic interventions are in our opinion only those applications that have been proved to be of great value as to the treatment of the underlying disease. Therefore, the more rare applications of functional stereotactics will not be described here and the reader is referred for these more specific cases (including questionable ones) to the textbook of Schaltenbrand and Walker (1982), various symposium proceedings (Gildenberg and Marino 1978, Gillingham *et al.* 1980, Gybels *et al.* 1984), and to the monography by Spiegel (1982).

It must be emphasized, that until recently almost all pertinent literature concerns functional stereotactics only. This is self-evident from a historical point of view, the other stereotactics being generally accepted only during the last years. On the other hand, established indications in all groups of stereotactics form a rather heterogenous body that for the sake of clarity must be divided in both absolute and relative, regarding both the underlying disease and the patient under consideration.

*Absolute* indications regarding the disease are interventions that can only be carried out by stereotactic techniques: coagulation of a specified thalamic nucleus and biopsy of mass lesions that can only be reached safely by stereotactics (e.g. deep seated small brain tumor).

*Relative* indications regarding the disease are interventions that can also be carried out with conventional neurosurgery: e.g. amygdalotomy versus hippocampectomy (in epileptics) and treatment of mass lesions that can be reached just as safely with craniotomy (e.g. colloid cyst of third ventricle).

*Absolute* indications regarding the patient are stereotactic interventions that form the only possible treatment left: e.g. anterior capsulotomy or cingulotomy on psychiatric patients suffering from compulsive neurosis, and biopsy in mass lesions in the elderly who can't sustain major surgery.

*Relative* indications regarding the patient are interventions that form only one of the treatment modalities available: e.g. dentatotomy versus medical treatment in spasticity and biopsy in mass lesions that apparently no longer need histological proof (e.g. multiple lesions of the brain in advanced systemic cancer).

Established indications for stereotactic interventions can be subdivided in the following groups:

I indications for functional, II indications for diagnostic, III indications for therapeutic, IV indications for localizing interventions.

## I. Indications for Functional Stereotactic Interventions

### A. Movement Disorders

In movement disorders the treatment of hyperkinesias has become predominantly pharmacological. However, in tremor and dystonia stereotactic lesioning is often of great benefit (Walker 1982 a).

#### 1. Parkinsonian Tremor

Tremor of Parkinson's disease (4 to 6 Hz tremor of rest with typical alternating contractions of agonist and antagonist muscles) is normally treated with anticholinergic drugs, levodopa preparations, and direct dopamin agents. However, sometimes tremor is the only symptom of the disease or it is more resistant than the other symptoms to medical treatment. In these cases stereotactic thalamotomy (see chapter 9) with lesioning of the ventrolateral thalamic nucleus is indicated. A relative indication is present in bilateral symptomatology to relieve tremor at the most disabling side (usually the dominant one) or even to relieve—in stages—tremor by bilateral surgery. Long-term follow-up was reviewed by Matsumoto (et al. 1984) both for unilateral and bilateral thalamotomy in Japanese patients. Their results were slightly better than those reported on Caucasian patients with parkinsonism (Kelly and Gillingham 1980, our own results) and amounted to an 80% chance of almost complete relief of tremor.

#### 2. Essential Tremor

Hereditary or essential tremor (8 to 12 Hz action tremor of the upper limbs) may sometimes benefit by stereotactic surgery. It is advisable, however, to treat it with a $\beta$-blocking agent such as propanolol (40–80 mg, 3–4 times a day) prior to surgery. Contra-indications for medical treatment are asthma, cardiac failure and a heart block. Care is required in diabetics, in whom a $\beta$-blocker may conceal the symptoms of hypoglycaemia. Sometimes primidone has been found to be of help for some patients (O'Brien et al. 1981). In severe cases a stereotactic thalamotomy (nucleus Vl) is indicated (Van Manen 1974).

### 3. Cerebellar Tremor

Cerebellar or intention tremor (increasing in frequency as the goal of a voluntary movement is reached) cannot be treated effectively by pharmacological means. This target-seeking intention tremor is commonly found in patients with multiple sclerosis and only rarely responds to choline chloride or isoniazide. This condition may, at times, be so severe that stereotactic (Vl) thalamotomy should be applied, although disabling ataxia may sometimes follow surgery.

### 4. Posttraumatic Movement Disorders

Posttraumatic movement disorders following severe closed head injury have been described to improve considerably after stereotactic thalamotomy (Vl nucleus) by both Andrew (*et al.* 1982) and Bullard and Nashold (1984). In this clinical syndrome almost always more than one type of movement disorder is present as a result of significant brainstem dysfunction. The most frequent disorder is a type of action tremor in combination with hemiballistic or choreoathetoid movements, or with truncal ataxia. This posttraumatic syndrome responds badly to medical treatment, such as propanolol or clonazepam, and may therefore be an indication for stereotactic surgery. In all cases long-term results show some pertinent improvement with, in most patients only transient postoperative dysarthria.

### 5. Torsion Dystonia

Torsion dystonia in its generalized form is usually treated with high doses of anticholinergic drugs, but in the majority of cases little benefit is gained. Occasionally, bilateral thalamotomy (stereotactic lesioning of Vl, Vpl and Vpm nuclei) may provide effective relief, as Cooper (1965 b, 1982) described: 70% gained longstanding relief of dystonia in the young age of onset group (which is 50% jewish).

### 6. Torticollis Spastica

Spasmodic torticollis (one of the so-called focal dystonias) sometimes requires stereotactic intervention with a lesion placed in the contralateral Voi nucleus of the thalamus. As Hassler and Dieckmann (1970) pointed out, a head turned to the one side needs a lesion on the other side. On the other hand, torticollis due to neurovascular compression should be treated with the appropriate means.

### 7. Hemi-Dystonia

Hemi-dystonia forms one of the best indications for stereotactic surgery and an unilateral thalamotomy may be of considerable value. In fact, many of these cases show an acquired form of dystonia, after traumatic or vascular lesioning of the midbrain (Cooper 1982).


## B. Intractable Pain

In intractable pain syndromes, indications for stereotactic interventions are largely dependent on the nature of the syndrome itself and the life expectancy of the patient. Therapeutic lesions should only be performed on patients, who will not survive longer than one year, as after this period pain tends to recur, with concomitant postoperative central dysesthesias.

### 1. Cancer Pain

In cancer pain with only short time survival, stereotactic ablative surgery is of the utmost value. A mesencephalotomy or pontine tractotomy should be performed in all cases with pain above the C 5 level. Below this level one may choose a percutaneous cordotomy, when pain only has a unilateral distribution. Whenever there is pain bilaterally, however, a bilateral mesencephalotomy is to be preferred above a bilateral percutaneous cordotomy, because after bilateral cordotomy serious complications may occur. Ischia (*et al.* 1984) reviews bilateral cordotomy in 36 patients with neoplastic disease and reports a 10% mortality rate and a 30–40% permanent bladder dysfunction. Bilateral mesencephalotomy is much safer, particularly because of the absence of respiratory complications and the greater distance between the target and the pyramidal tracts [in cordotomy a 5–8% incidence of paresis is met (Fig. 67)]. Lesions are made in the neospinothalamic system (lateral spinothalamic tract).

In midline cancer pain a stereotactic extralemniscal myelotomy, as originally described by Hitchcock (1970b), may be indicated. It will lead to less loss of functions (almost no sensory loss), than the already discussed interventions. It has been suggested that its beneficial effect may be due to the interruption of an ascending paleospinothalamic system (central spinoreticular fibers).

In diffuse bone metastasis pain a stereotactic (or free-hand) chemical hypophysectomy may be indicated with the instillation of absolute ethanol (5 cc at 3 different targets inside the pituitary gland), as described by Katz and Levin (1977), Tindall (*et al.* 1979) and Levin (*et al.* 1980).


### 2. Chronic Intractable Pain

Chronic "benign" intractable pain syndromes include the thalamic syndrome, the phantom limb and other denervation pain syndromes, postherpetic neuralgia and various postoperative neuralgias, such as the "failed disc" pseudoradicular pains. Therapeutic lesions should be

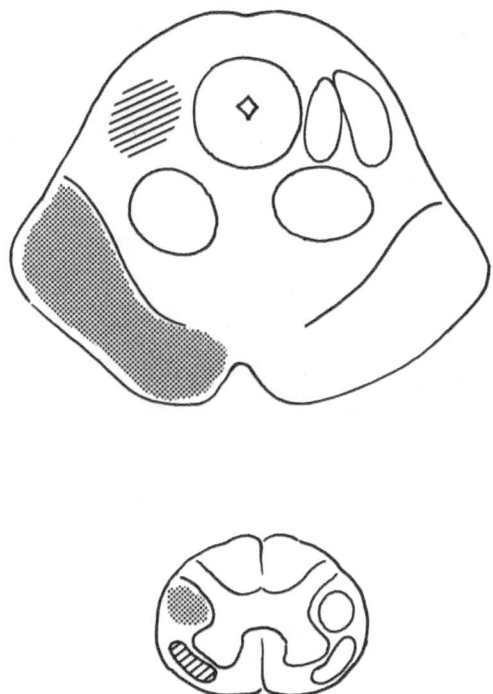

Fig. 67. Schematic representation of targets in stereotactic mesencephalotomy (above), and in cervical cordotomy (below); hatched areas. Pointed areas represent the pyramidal tracts. Note the different distances between target and motor system in these proportional drawings

abandoned here, as life is not limited by the disease and the mentioned patients will have no lasting benefit from these procedures. Too often pain surgery is carried out in these cases (including stereotactic interventions, posterior rhizotomies, peripheral nerve sectioning or blocking with ethanol) with a positively harmful effect in the long run, the short-term effect having worn away. Pain often recurs with a troubling anesthesia dolorosa as a complicating component. These de-afferentiation pains, referred to as burning and numbness are more stressing to the patient than the original pains. Therefore, there is only a relative indication for stereotactic interventions in the chronic intractable pain syndromes and all surgery should be non-ablative (i.e. therapeutic stimulation with electrodes). The effect of intracerebral stimulation with electrodes is highly unpredictable and therefore often produces unreliable results (Meyerson 1980, Kelly 1983). However, good results are described by Hosobuchi (1980) and Young (et al. 1985) in chronic pain syndromes with stereotactic placement of electrodes in the peri-aqueductal grey matter (PAG) (see chapters 3 and

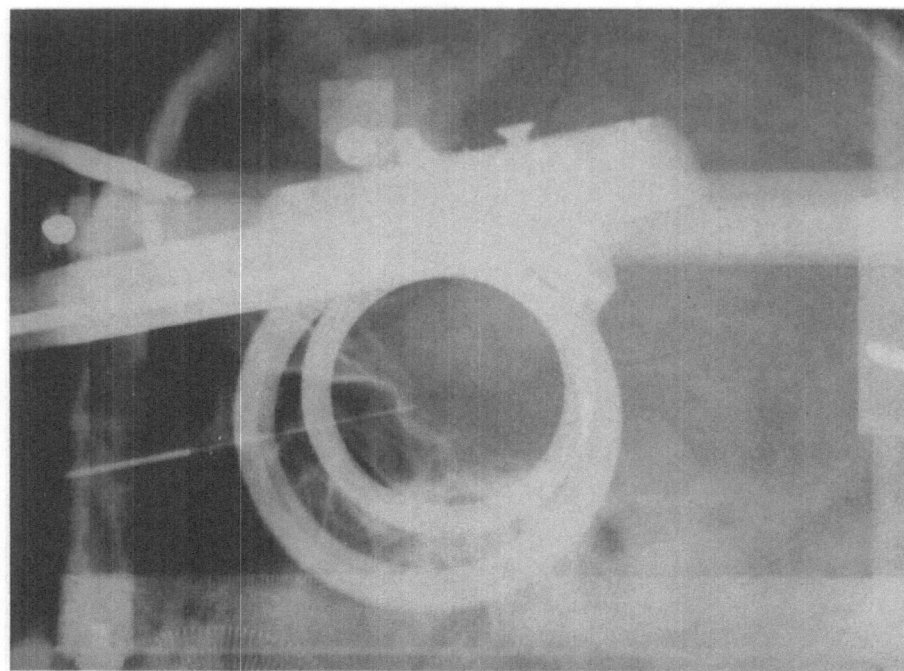

Fig. 68. Stereotactic chemical hypophysectomy with Leksell's system; patient suffering from thalamic syndrome pains

14). Seldom is a relative indication for ablative surgery present in the elderly, who suffer from intractable benign pain. Finally, in the thalamic pain syndrome, a stereotactic chemical hypophysectomy (Fig. 68) might be considered helpful for hitherto unknown reasons (Levin *et al.* 1983). Further research is needed to evaluate the benefits of this approach to the chronic de-afferentiation pain syndromes.

For further extensive information the reader is referred to Spiegel's monography (1982, pp. 46–59).

## C. Otherwise Intractable Epilepsy

Stereotactic lesioning may be performed in otherwise intractable epilepsy with interruption of the conduction pathways of focal epileptic discharge. The indication is present in cases in which the epileptic focus cannot be defined and resected by surgical means. PET scanning may alter indications (see chapter 14). According to Gillingham (*et al.* 1980) stereotactic lesions in the ipsilateral pallidum will lead to a 50–75% reduction in seizure frequency. On the other hand, cortical resection(s) of the epileptogenic area will also produce substantial reduction in the

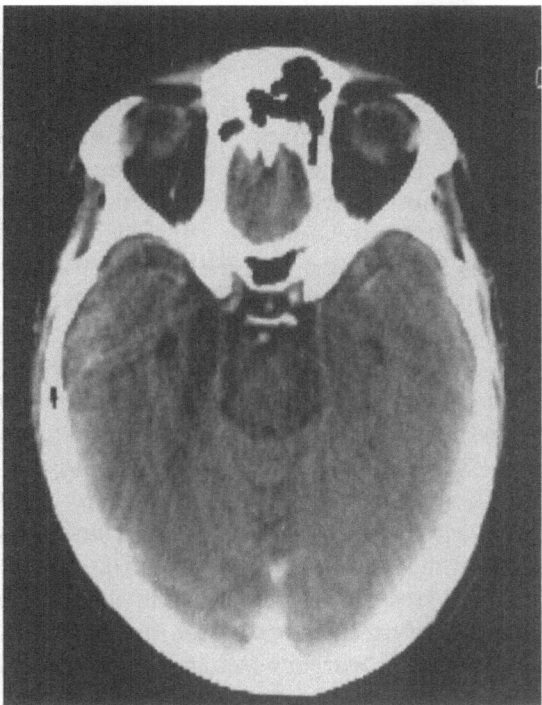

Fig. 69. Case of medically refractory epilepsy with rightsided temporal enhancing lesion and relatively widened right temporal horn. Biopsy revealed gliotic scarring due to anoxia (boy aged 16 years)

patient's seizure tendency (Rasmussen 1979), and therefore resection should be considered a good alternative whenever such an area can be defined.

Much experience was booked at the Montreal Neurological Institute dating back to Dr. Wilder Penfield's studies and first seizure operations (1928). Their studies include the results on about 1,500 patients with nontumoral epileptogenic lesions and on about 400 cases with epilepsy caused by tumors or vascular malformations. Particularly in recent years, CT scanning has proved to be essential in the differentiation between medically refractory epilepsy due to tumors and epilepsy due to non-tumoral lesions (trauma, anoxia, post-inflammatory scarring) (Fig. 69). Nowadays the tumor cases will no longer be of interest to functional but to diagnostic stereotactics (see sub II). For further reading regarding the various sites of lesioning in convulsive disorders (including amygdalotomy and hippocampectotomy) Spiegel's monography (1982, pp. 78–85) is recommended.

## D. Psychiatric Disease

Otherwise intractable psychiatric disease may be influenced effectively by stereotactic interventions. Particularly before the introduction of potent neuroleptic drugs surgical treatment was frequently employed. Today, indications for surgery are only relative according to psychiatrists and in many countries (stereotactic) surgery is no longer accepted in the treatment of psychiatric diseases. However, cases of severe obsessive-compulsive neurosis and phobias, which have proved to be refractory to all kinds of psychiatric and medical treatment, may successfully be treated this way (Wycis 1972). The targets of choice are always bilateral and are located in the anterior cingulum (Ballantine et al. 1967) or in the anterior part of the internal capsule (Bingley et al. 1973). The selection of patients for surgery is a much debated issue everywhere. Careful follow-up by psychologists (Teuber et al. 1977) revealed no serious neurological or psychiatric complications, making stereotactic psychosurgery—though sometimes politicized—a comparatively safe procedure. In a survey of psychosurgery, Rylander (1973) pointed out that the standard lobotomy has become unpopular due to unforeseen and undesirable personality changes, but nevertheless renewed interest developed with the introduction of restricted operations as in stereotactic surgery (see also: Spiegel 1982: pp. 34–45).

## II. Indications for Diagnostic Stereotactic Interventions

Any mass lesion inside the skull needs histological diagnosis for rational and adequate treatment, whether tumoral or non-tumoral in origin. The neurosurgeon or radiotherapist requires tissue identification in order to decide upon the most suitable treatment for the patient. Years ago certain mass lesions were treated by external irradiation following only a presumptive diagnosis based on the clinical picture plus neuroradiological studies. At that time conservatism in operative exposure of deep seated tumors was justified (Conway 1977), because of the relative inaccessibility of deep brain areas and a high incidence of tumors not amenable to surgery. Today, microsurgical techniques allow the direct surgical "attack" of tumors in or about the sella turcica, and intraventricular tumors without an unacceptable morbidity and mortality rate. *Mass lesions in the thalamus, basal ganglia and brainstem, however, will never benefit from direct surgical approach without stereotactic and computer monitored guidance.* A stereotactic biopsy will then form the first step towards rational treatment (Figs. 70 and 71). Histological diagnosis (Scarabin et al. 1978) is the key to further planning of CT guided surgery or—in selected cases—non-surgical treatment (radiotherapy and chemotherapy).

Stereotactic biopsy is indicated in all lesions of the brain, in which open surgery is not preferable or is inadvisable to perform for a variety of reasons.

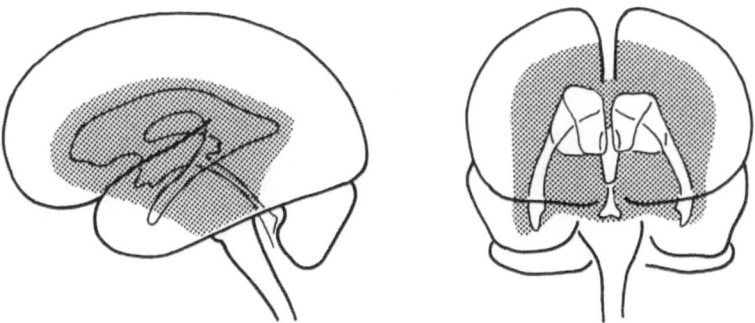

Fig. 70. Schematic representation of brain areas, where open surgery without stereotactic techniques is not recommended (hatched areas)

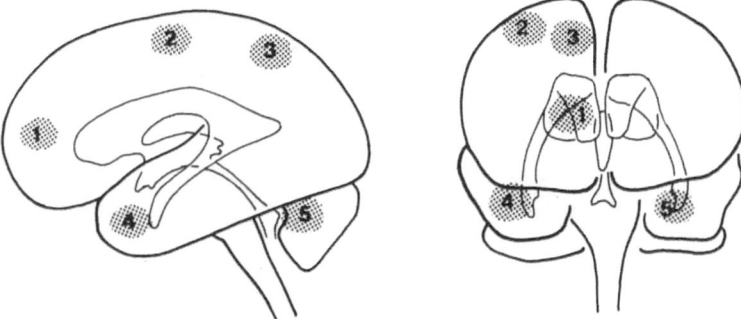

Fig. 71. Drawing showing the more common regions of the brain, where conventional open surgery may be carried out

Mass lesions not amenable to open surgery present an absolute indication for stereotactic biopsy (Bosch 1980). Computer-guided stereotactic resection may sometimes follow biopsy (see chapters 4, 13 and 14). Therefore a stereotactic intervention is indicated in all the following circumstances:
— mass lesions that are deep seated
— mass lesions that lie bilaterally (butterfly growth)
— mass lesions that present multiple, and vital locations
— mass lesions that grow diffusely without true demarcation on CT
— mass lesions that are of suspected infectious origin (herpes, AIDS)
— mass lesions that are of suspected systemic origin (Hodgkin, leukemia)
— mass lesions that have invaded the skull base considerably.
    In all of the mentioned instances it can be stated that conventional open surgery with bulk resection is not feasible, whereas a histological diagnosis may lead to other treatment modalities and sometimes to a complete cure.

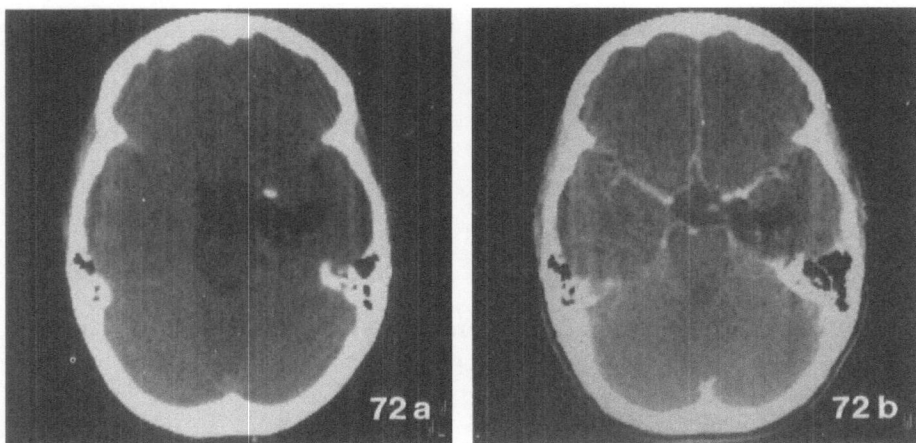

Fig. 72. CT scan pictures (b: after contrast) showing a leftsided, deep seated temporal lesion (boy aged 12 years). Biopsy revealed an epidermoid, which was subsequently removed with craniotomy

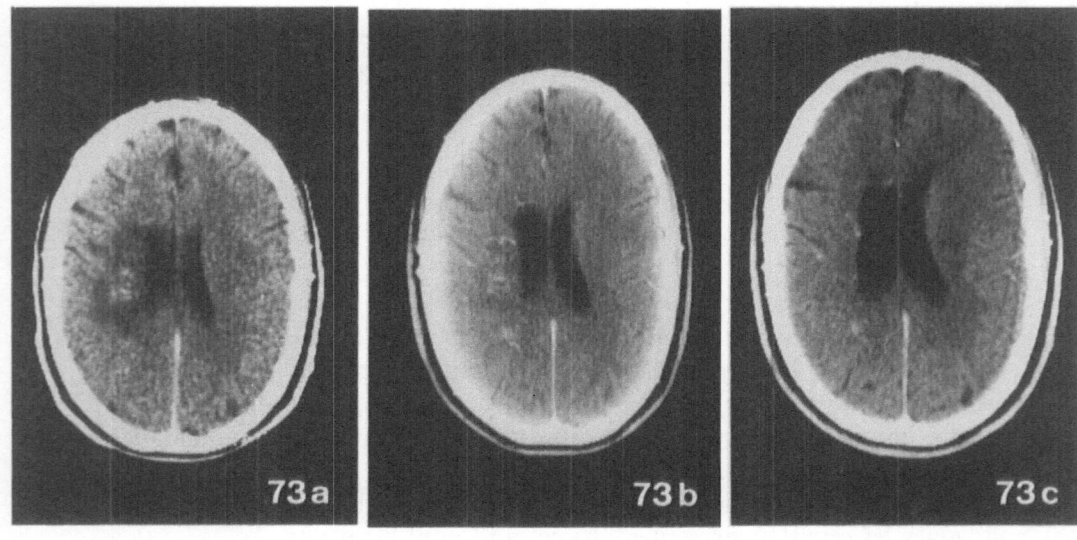

Fig. 73. CT scan pictures (after contrast enhancement); case with subacute leftsided hemiparesis (man aged 35 years). At intake (a) angiography showed no abnormalities and a biopsy was carried out to rule out the possibility of a tumor (see Fig. 74). Follow-up scanning (b, c: 3 months and 1 year) showed resolution of the lesion and finally some widening of the right lateral ventricle (c). Presumptive diagnosis: cryptic vascular malformation

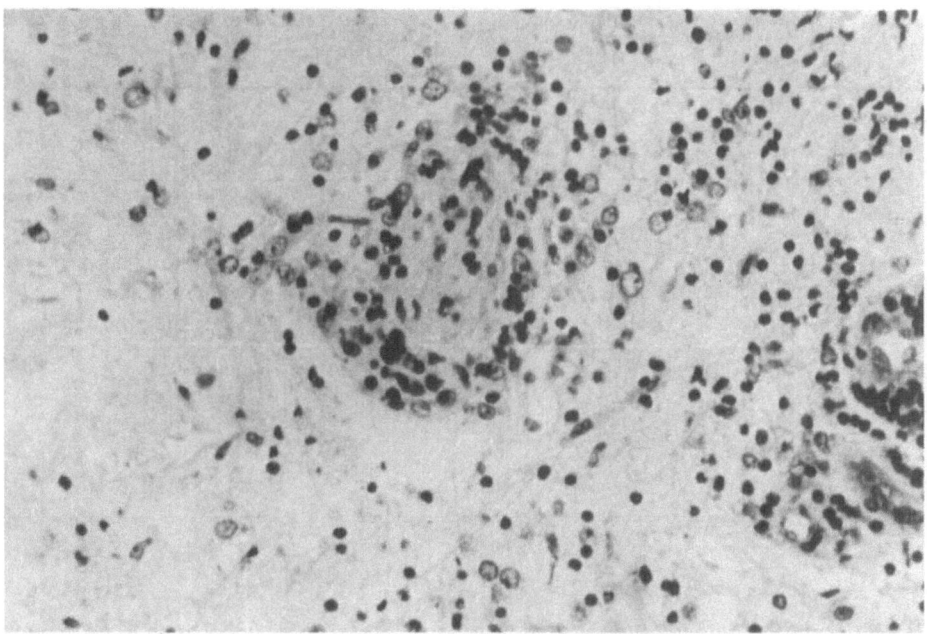

Fig. 74. Biopsy specimen of case presented in Fig. 73. Reactive picture with infiltration of brain tissue by lymphocytes (H & E staining)

An example of the obtainable cure is presented by a case of dysgerminoma of the pineal gland region. This tumor is highly radiosensitive and is preferably treated with radiotherapy after histological proof (illustrative case 2; chapter 12). A relative indication for stereotactic biopsy is given by mass lesions in which a differential diagnosis between a resectable and a non-resectable process exists. The following examples may be given: a medial temporal lobe oligodendroglioma versus an epidermoid of the temporal fossa (Fig. 72), a small white matter glioma versus a small and cryptic arteriovenous malformation (Figs. 73 and 74), or a deep seated glioma versus a toxoplasmosis deposit (Handler *et al.* 1983). Another relative indication exists in patients, who otherwise require a high risk craniotomy or cerebral transit (Apuzzo and Sabshin 1983). By obtaining a tissue diagnosis preoperative strategic planning may be brought into sharper focus and sometimes the relatively simple and safe biopsy performance can take the place of open surgery (e.g. in glioblastoma), leading to a much less invasive treatment and furthermore a considerable reduction in the hospitalization period.

In discussing the indications for stereotactic diagnostic biopsy in mass lesions of the brain, four different groups of patients can be distinguished (Bosch 1980):

Table 1. *Indications for Stereotactic Biopsy in Brain Tumors in Cases Without Known Primary Tumor Elsewhere*

| Mass lesion number | Surgical technique | Histology |
|---|---|---|
| 1 | removable: craniotomy | glioma<br>lymphoma |
|  | not removable: biopsy, if further treatment is justified | metastasis<br>miscellaneous |
| ≧ 2 | biopsies, if further treatment is justified | metastases<br>multiple<br>primaries<br>miscellaneous |

Table 2. *Indications for Stereotactic Biopsy in Brain Tumors in Cases With Known Primary Tumor Elsewhere, but Without Other Metastatic Spread*

| Mass lesion number | Surgical technique | Histology |
|---|---|---|
| 1 | removable: craniotomy | metastasis<br>second tumor |
|  | not removable: biopsy, if further treatment is justified | non-neoplastic<br>disease<br>miscellaneous |
| ≧ 2 | biopsies, if further treatment is justified | metastases<br>non-neoplastic<br>disease<br>miscellaneous |

## A. Patients Without Previous History of Tumor Who Present a Single Mass Lesion

In general this is the case in primary tumors of the brain, but sometimes a secondary (still solitary) tumor will be encountered in a patient with an unknown primary malignancy elsewhere. Open craniotomy should be carried out whenever the possibility exists of removing the lesion, as even bulk resection of a glioma is preferable to biopsy if radiotherapy is to be given afterwards. As Sheline (1975) pointed out, after partial resection in low grade gliomas irradiation influences the survival rate favorably. The only exception is the cystic cerebellar astrocytoma (commonly named: juvenile pilocytic), which can often be controlled by surgery alone (Geissinger and Bucy 1971).

## B. Patients Without Previous History of Tumor Who Present Multiple Mass Lesions

These patients are, of course, suspected of having a malignancy elsewhere in the body and should therefore be investigated thoroughly. However, screening is time consuming, and it is not uncommon that a primary tumor cannot be found. Also, previous immunosuppressive treatment (as in transplant recipients) or immunodeficiency syndromes (as in AIDS) may lead to opportunistic infections inside the brain (Aspergillus, Toxoplasma among other) or even *de novo* developing brain tumors (e.g. malignant lymphoma). As in these cases the lesions only occasionally permit open surgery because of their multiplicity and often are preferably not treated by surgical means, we perform a stereotactic biopsy of one or two of the lesions in order to assist the oncologist in providing him with the histological characteristics of the process (e.g. squamous cell carcinoma, adenocarcinoma, lymphoma). At the same time bacteriological studies are started to detect possible infectious disease. Finally, the possibility of two independent primaries of the brain has to be ruled out (2.5% in all glioma cases according to Fewer (*et al.* 1976).

## C. Patients with a Known Primary Tumor Elsewhere, Who Present a Single Mass Lesion, but Having no Signs of Metastasis Elsewhere in the Body

Their management is dependent on site and size of the lesion. If at all possible, an open craniotomy should be performed to resect the lesion in toto. If not, stereotactic biopsy is indicated to ascertain the pathology of the lesion, since it is not always a metastasis of the primary tumor. With the improvement in tumor therapy, survival tends to increase so that, at the same time, the incidence of a second tumor increases. Moreover, the frequency of non-neoplastic disease in the brain is higher in patients treated for malignancies elsewhere. Of course, one should also be aware of the higher incidence of meningiomas in breast cancer patients (Schoenberg *et al.* 1975) and perform open surgery whenever this suspicion arises.

## D. Patients with a Known Primary Tumor Elsewhere, Who Present Multiple Mass Lesions in the Brain Without Other Metastatic Spread

A decision should be made as to the desirability of any further treatment on the basis of the patient's condition and the characteristics of the primary tumor. If irradiation or chemotherapy, or both, are considered helpful, histological proof of metastasis should be obtained because of the weight of the decision for both patient and doctor. As already pointed out, the mass lesions detected could be of a non-tumoral nature. The differentiation between metastatic and non-neoplastic tissue is most easily obtained by stereotactic biopsy, leading to a relative indication in these instances.

A survey of these groups is presented in Tables 1 and 2 (Bosch 1980). To summarize, open surgery is performed far more often than stereotactic biopsy. Especially in cases where metastasis is suspected, complete removal is the only option. Stereotactic diagnostic interventions are on the other hand the required procedure in patients who cannot be treated by open surgical techniques. Sometimes patients present a very small subcortical lesion, detected only with CT scanning, that could be resected totally if it were found at craniotomy. This special group benefits from stereotactic *localization* and subsequent open surgery in stereotactic space, and is discussed seperately under IV.

## III. Indications for Therapeutic Stereotactic Interventions

As many results in the pertinent literature are still preliminary (see chapter 3 sub II, B for details), the indications which are established are by now quite few. Indications fall apart in three groups, being:
— aspiration and evacuation of fluids
— interstitial radioisotope application
— stereotactic radiosurgery.

## A. Evacuation of Fluids

Stereotactic evacuation of fluids may be indicated in the following circumstances:

### 1. Cystic Craniopharyngioma

Cystic craniopharyngioma may be punctured stereotactically and—after calculation of its total volume—treated by the application of a sufficiently high dose of $^{90}$Yttrium to let it shrink. This mode of treatment is indicated in cases of unresectable craniopharyngioma and may be followed by external irradiation of the solid tumor parts (Georgi *et al.* 1980, Huk and Mahlstedt 1983). In Stockholm all craniopharyngiomas are treated stereotactically according to the studies of Backlund (1972, *et al.* 1972, 1973, 1979). Their strategy is twofold: the cystic component is treated with the application of radioisotopes and the solid part is treated with radiosurgery (see sub C).

### 2. Cystic Glioma

Deep seated cystic gliomas are—besides biopsy and irradiation (in many centers interstitial radioisotope application; Szikla 1979 a)—often candidates for stereotactic evacuation of the cyst contents (Fig. 75) and insertion of an indwelling catheter (Fig. 76) which allows repeated puncture at the subcutaneously placed reservoir (Rickham or Ommaya-type).

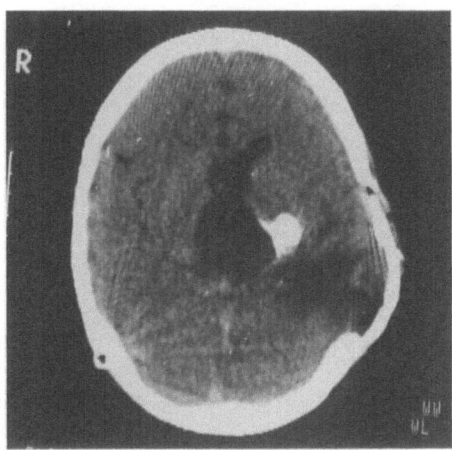

Fig. 75. Boy, 12 years old, with recurrent oligodendroglioma many years after open surgery and radiotherapy. CT shows cystic recurrence: Previously inserted CSF shunt showed dysfunction, due to the tumor cyst compressing the third ventricle and ventricular catheter

### 3. Subependymal or Leptomeningeal Cysts

Deep seated subependymal or leptomeningeal cysts. Biopsy of the cyst wall and evacuation of fluid is sometimes sufficient, but in other cases a permanent indwelling catheter has to be introduced stereotactically (Fig. 77) to be sure that refilling can be managed easily.

### 4. Colloid Cyst of Third Ventricle

Colloid cysts of the third ventricle form a relative indication, open surgery with microsurgical techniques being a good alternative. However, stereotactic aspiration of the colloid contents has been proved to be sufficient (Bosch *et al.* 1978, Lunsford *et al.* 1982). Hydrocephalus will

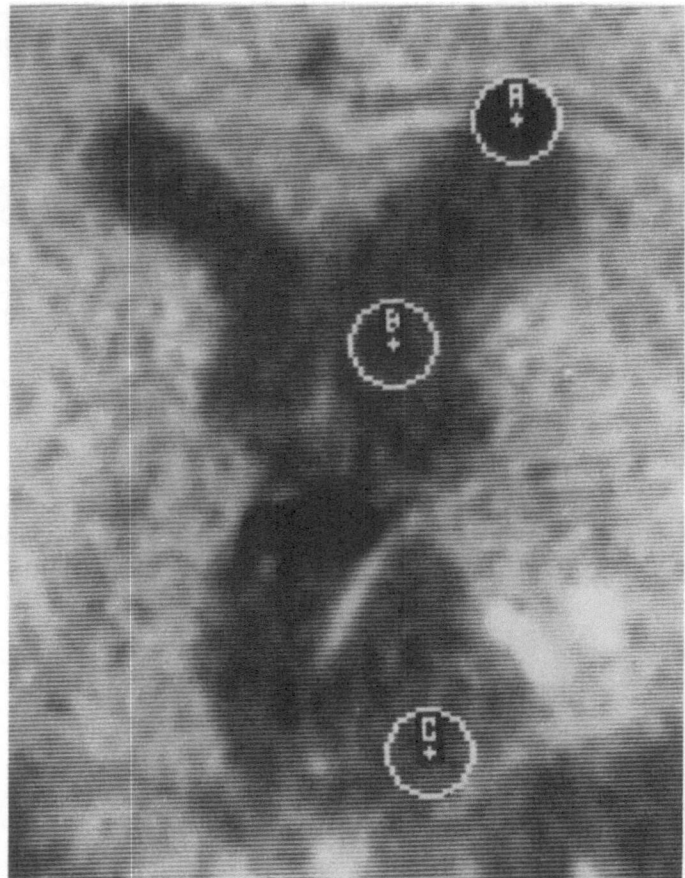

Fig. 76. Stereotactic drainage of the tumor cyst (case presented in Fig. 75). At *A* some air is seen in the left frontal horn; at *B* normal CSF density is measured; at *C* cyst fluid is present. Note that there is also some air entrapped inside the cyst at the point of entrance of the draining catheter

subside and until now follow-up has not shown signs of refilling. Due to the viscosity of the cyst's contents the inner diameter of the aspiration cannula should not be less than 1.5 mm and aspiration should be performed with fairly high negative pressure (see chapter 11, sub II).

## 5. Brain Abscess

Deep seated brain abscess should be treated stereotactically. This way of treatment is most rewarding since the lesion is critical and evacuation plus the application of the proper antibiotic drugs may cure the patient. For this mode of treatment the reader is referred to the papers by Wise and Gleason (1979) and Lunsford and Nelson (1982).

### 6. Primary Hematoma

Deep seated primary hematoma offers an absolute indication for stereotactic evacuation whenever the lesion gives rise to progressive impairment of consciousness, as pointed out by Higgins (*et al.* 1982). Particularly the primary hematoma of the brainstem, that has no known

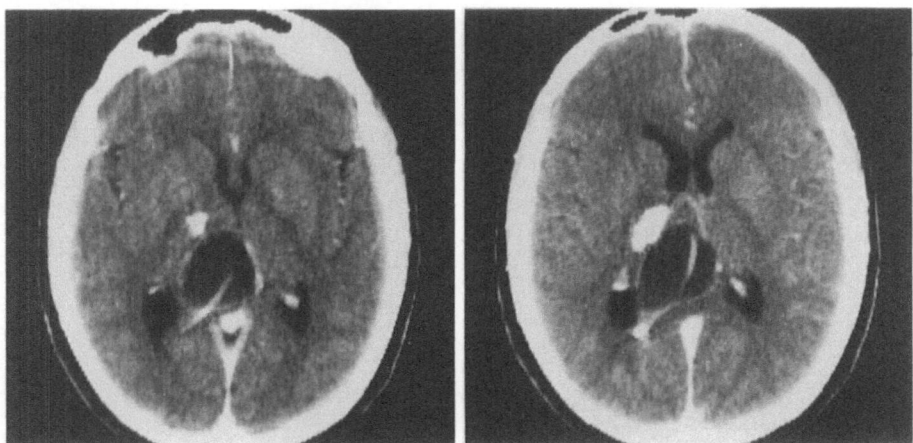

Fig. 77. Case of subependymal cyst, without ventricular enlargement, in a female, 18 years old. CT scan with contrast showing the stereotactically inserted catheter at two scanning levels. Biopsy of the cyst wall showed abnormalities compatible with a prenatally contracted bleeding of the subependymal cellular matrix (see Fig. 197)

connection with hypertension but is mostly due to cryptic vascular malformation, may be evacuated to cure the patient (Beatty and Zervas 1983, Bosch and Beute 1985). It should be emphasized, that the indication does not exist in cases of traumatic hematoma. In primary lobar hematoma the indication is only relative as microsurgical techniques have proved to give similar results. For further discussion see chapter 11, sub III.

## B. Interstitial Radioisotope Application

This so-called curie-therapy is used on patients with primary tumors of the brain, which are not removable or can only be partially resected. The Freiburg Center for Stereotactic Neurosurgery (Mundinger and collaborators) started this way of treating brain tumors back in 1958 and published the techniques and results in many papers (Mundinger 1966, 1970,

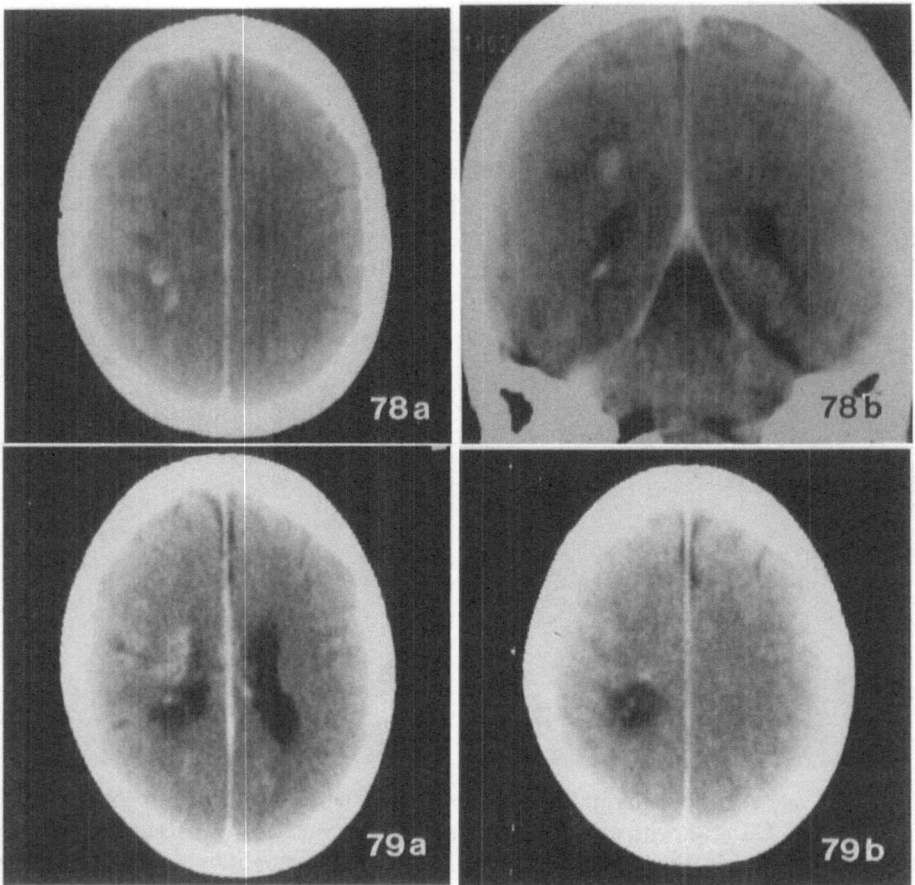

Fig. 78. CT scan pictures with contrast showing a deep seated small tumor. Biopsy revealed a highly malignant glioma and because of the very small diameter the patient (female 35 years) was sent for stereotactic irradiation in Stockholm

Fig. 79. Follow-up scanning (with contrast) after one year showed: recurrence of the tumor (a), and a necrotic target area of the irradiation treatment (b)

Mundinger *et al.* 1979). A review is available in the textbook of Schaltenbrand and Walker (Mundinger 1982 a). The following radioisotopes have among others been used: $^{32}$Phosphor, $^{192}$Iridium, $^{60}$Cobalt, $^{198}$Aurum and $^{90}$Yttrium. They can be delivered as pellets or as a suspension. With the information from CT studies concerning tumor boundaries and its exact position in relation to the stereotactic apparatus much progress has been achieved in dosimetry and exact localization of the radioactive implants. During the last years CT guided interstitial curie-therapy has become an established treatment modality, which offers the advantage of high radiation doses inside the tumor (up till 15,000 rads in one week) without undue exposure of the surrounding brain (Kelly *et al.* 1978, Gutin *et al.* 1981). One should make a distinction between permanent implantations and various types of temporary implantation (so-called brachy-curietherapy of Mundinger; 1982 a). This latter form is delivered with help of a contact radiation device and is reserved for the treatment of clearly malignant (anaplastic) tumors. Very large tumors cannot be treated successfully with interstitial irradiation. The low grade malignant glioma, which is well demarcated from surrounding brain on CT—in fact a rare finding—, forms the best indication.

## C. Stereotactic Radiosurgery

As only very few centers in the world have a stereotactic irradiation unit at their disposal (Stockholm and Boston being the first; chapter 3, sub II, B, 3) just some words will be mentioned on the indications. Leksell was the first in publishing experiments on stereotactic irradiation with Röntgen rays and proton beams (1951). In his book (Leksell 1971) a complete description is given of the stereotactic irradiation unit he constructed. Today, in Los Angeles and in Sheffield similar units are operational. Generally spoken, all non-malignant targets with a diameter less than 25 mm can be irradiated and destroyed, depending on careful dosimetry. Indications are vascular malformations which cannot be handled by microsurgery, solid parts of craniopharyngioma, hypersecreting pituitary adenomas and some small acoustic and pineal tumors (Backlund 1979, Rähn 1980, Steiner *et al.* 1974). Although malignant tumors of sufficiently small diameter would also be destroyed, our own experience with two cases (one survived) has proved (Figs. 78 and 79) that malignancy almost always infiltrates the surrounding tissue even further than the most sophisticated scanner or NMR-unit will show. The irradiation unit with its quality of destroying tissue is also effectively used in functional stereotactics, instead of thermal lesioning with electrodes.

## IV. Indications for Localizing Stereotactic Interventions

Localizing stereotactics is applying stereotactic methodology to remove a foreign body (e.g. a bullet) or to resect by subsequent open surgery in stereotactic space (e.g. vascular malformation, tumor) mass lesions, which are too small to localize by conventional means. Particularly, small subcortical, subependymal and brainstem lesions need this form of surgical approach to avoid damage to surrounding brain tissue. This group of stereotactic interventions will expand impressively in the near future thanks to computer facilities, becoming available to everybody and making three-dimensional reconstruction in stereotactic space feasible (see chapters 4 and 13 for detailed discussion). CT guided biopsy or localization with subsequent computer-directed removal has already been developed in some centers (Jacques *et al.* 1980, Kelly *et al.* 1983).

Absolute indications are the following:

## A. Small Tumors in the White Matter

Small tumors in the white matter, which could be removed if the exact position and extent is known. Stereotactic localizing is the first step, including a biopsy for histological diagnosis. Localization is done preferably by CT imaging and calculation of the coordinates with help of the computer. Nowadays most stereotactic apparatus have these CT facilities programmed (see chapter 4). In a second stage (during the same performance when frozen sections are used for histological examination or smear preparates for cytological investigation) a bone flap is made and the tumor is approached along the biopsy track that had been calculated to be safe beforehand. This methodological advance in neurosurgery will be employed successfully in an increasing number of centers over the world. The introduction of laser surgery will further develop this field of stereotactics.

## B. Small Subcortical Arteriovenous Malformations

Small subcortical arteriovenous malformations, which are known for their bleeding tendency and therefore have to be removed, can be resected microsurgically after exact localization. Intraoperative angiography is recommended for better target localization. The effectiveness of this approach is clearly shown by Kelly (*et al.* 1982 b), Garcia de Sola (*et al.* 1980) and our own results (chapter 11, sub IV).

## C. Small White Matter Abscesses

Small white matter brain abscess also calls for stereotactic localization. Evacuation of infectious material for bacteriological investigations is easily performed in this way and therefore further surgery is not needed.

## D. Lobar and Putaminal Hematomas

In primary lobar hematoma the indication is only relative, as many hematomas in this area tend to recover spontaneously (Kase *et al.* 1982). Medium sized (20–40 cc) lobar hematomas might benefit from surgery; stereotactic localization and evacuation (eventually with open surgery) offers the safest exploration. Matsumoto and Hondo (1984) recently discussed the stereotactic evacuation of hypertensive hematomas, which mostly lie in the putaminal region. Although their approach is not truly stereotactic, their results are encouraging.

## E. Subcortical Foreign Bodies

Subcortical foreign bodies—especially low velocity missiles—may lead to infection (Hagan 1971) and should be removed whenever possible.

Stereotactic removal is preferable, but stereotactic localization often mandatory, as reviewed by Hitchcock and Cowie (1983).

Reviewing the available textbooks on stereotactic neurosurgery (Riechert 1980, Schaltenbrand and Walker 1982, Spiegel 1982) one may conclude that only an oblique reference is made regarding the expanding field of neuro-oncology. Stereotactics in neuro-oncology is on the other hand extensively discussed in many papers mentioned in the text and listed under the references.

Chapter 6

# Contraindications for Stereotactic Interventions

With recent advances in surgical neurology some shifting from indication towards contraindication and vice versa is evident. Therefore, besides the contraindications in general for stereotactic surgery, those syndromes which no longer are treated by choice with stereotactic techniques will also be mentioned.

Contraindications *in general* are present under the following circumstances:

— Very young patients. It has been proved impossible to screw the pins of the stereotactic instrument into the skull in cases with a bone diameter of less than 3 mm. Moreover, whenever the skull bones have not yet grown together the placement of the apparatus is dangerous because of possible squeezing by the pins. This applies to children younger than 18–24 months and those who have hydrocephalic skulls. To circumvent this problem, the author once used a hard plastic cap made by the mouldroom staff (Fig. 80), which was moulded on the patient's skull some days beforehand. Although the cap itself can slide some millimeters over the skull, the stereotactic instrument can be fixed onto it firmly and in the usual way (Fig. 81), and with the use of general anaesthesia no real problem will be met. X-ray pictures (Fig. 82) are still readable.

— Patients with skull defects (whether congenital or posttraumatic) in the frontal or occipital area. At least three pins are needed in fixed position, to get a firm construction, allowing stereotactic surgery.

— Patients with disturbed blood cotting. Because one of the real dangers in stereotactics is a deep seated bleeding caused by the intervention, care should be taken to investigate bleeding and clotting times thoroughly beforehand. On the other hand, in patients with a normal clotting prophylactic heparin treatment is to be given before surgery as is usual in all other surgery with general anesthesia.

— Extremely rich vascularity of the target area may be a contraindication per se (Fig. 83). This is of course much depending on the intervention which is planned: a biopsy may be contraindicated, but the insertion of cannulas or catheters in localizing is tolerated without problems.

— All patients who are no longer suitable candidates for surgery due to hypertension, cardiac failure or other internal disease.

— In our opinion there is a contraindication to performing any stereotactic intervention without an up to date angiography, although much debated by others. Some pitfalls have been met (see chapter 8) which warrant angiography of the target area in every case, with the exception of functional surgery. Even after routine CT and angiography studies, we once came across a midbrain hemangioma that was almost totally sclerotized. The patient died suddenly due to rupture of a feeding vessel during the biopsy performance (Figs. 84, 85, and 86).

Contraindications *in detail*, according to the subgroups I–IV (chapter 5).

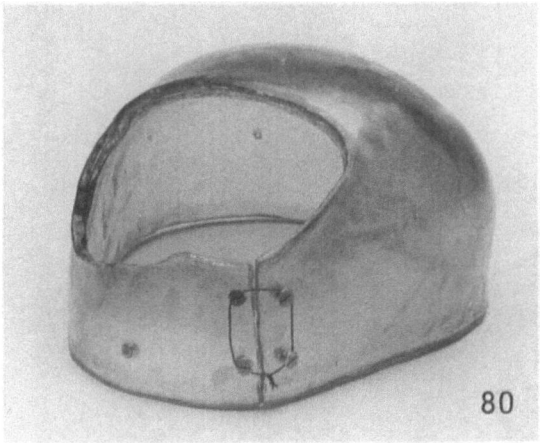

Fig. 80. Hard plastic cap, moulded on the skull, for use in the very young age group of patients

## I. Contraindications for Functional Stereotactic Interventions

### A. Movement Disorders

In movement disorders there is no established position for stereotactic treatment in cases of *chorea* and *athetosis*. Some benefit may, however, be achieved and the interested reader is referred to Narabayashi (1982) for more information. On the other hand, medical treatment is still developing, and Jankovic (1982) published promising results with tetrabenazine in the treatment of hyperkinetic movement disorders. Patients with *tardive dyskinesia* may also benefit by the administration of this drug. Stereotactic surgery is contraindicated in this syndrome, which is caused by chronic administration of major neuroleptic agents and closely resembles L-dopa—induced dyskinesias (Klawans *et al.* 1980, Narabayashi *et al.* 1984).

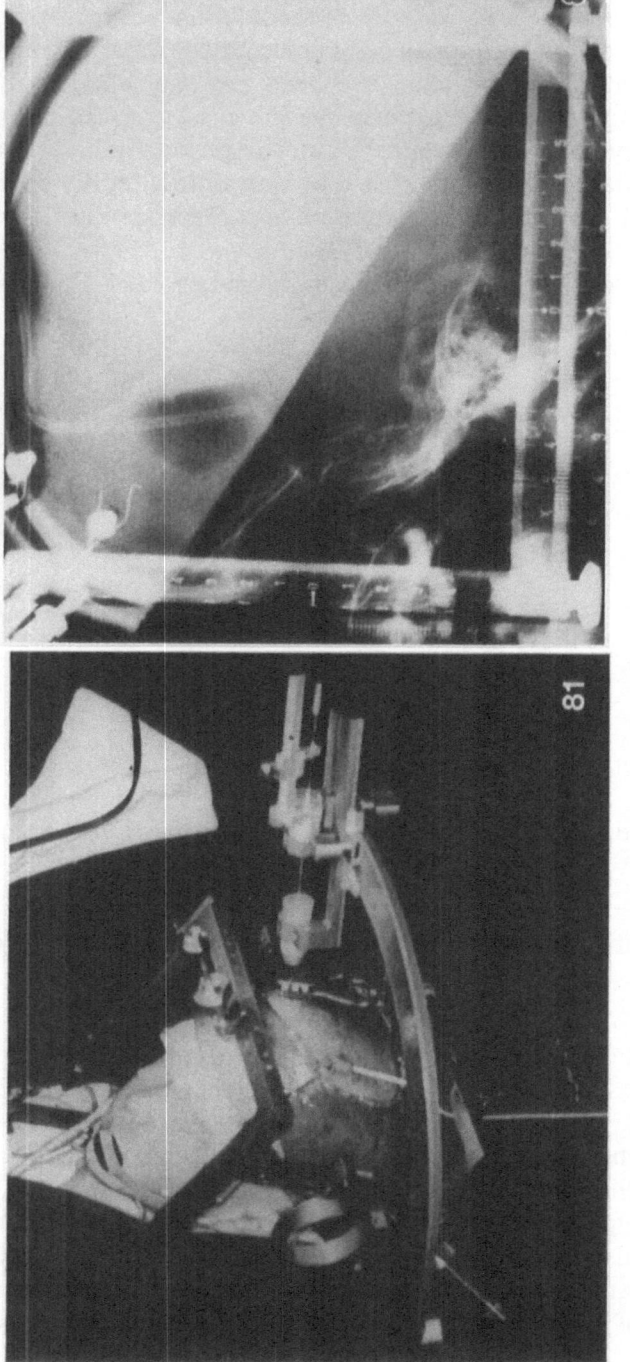

Fig. 81. The stereotactic apparatus fixed onto the plastic cap, which makes surgery possible in this hydrocephalic child

Fig. 82. Stereotactic X-ray pictures with the cap mounted on the skull are still readable. Note air and positive contrast in hydrocephalic lateral ventricles (tumor of the third ventricle)

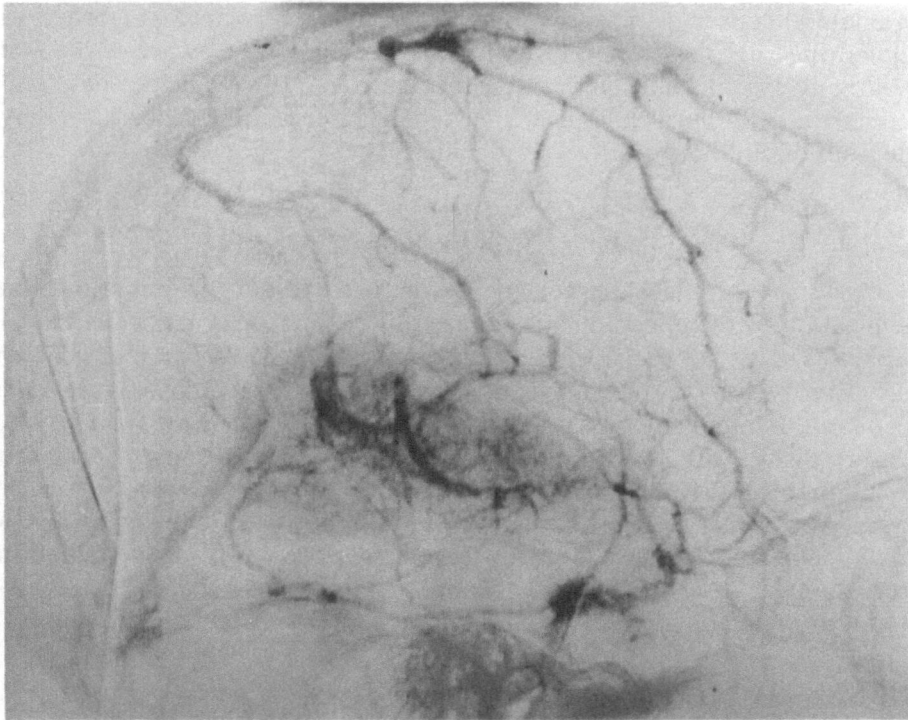

Fig. 83. Example of a vascular cerebral tumor (man, 65 years old), that showed to be an astrocytoma grade 3. Stereotactic biopsy (using the spiral needle) was carried out without bleeding problems

*Hemiballismus* will sometimes require a stereotactic intervention, in severe cases where no spontaneous regression appears. This experience is particularly relevant to the posttraumatic syndrome (Andrew *et al.* 1982, Bullard and Nashold 1984). A relative contraindication exists for performing *bilateral* thalamotomies, due to the unpredictable degree of dysarthria that will follow.

## B. Chronic Pain Syndromes

Stereotactic lesions to relieve pain states are absolutely contraindicated in patients who survive for more than 1–2 years after surgery, because a central type of de-afferentiation pain (dysesthesia) occurs by that time. For many patients this pain is even more troublesome than the original pains.

Bilateral lesions at the C 1–C 2 level (stereotactically or with free-hand percutaneous cordotomy) are contraindicated because of high morbidity and possible induction of sleep apnea (Ischia *et al.* 1984, Mooij *et al.* 1984).

In bilateral cancer pain at least one lesion should be placed at a lower or higher (mesencephalotomy) level. In fact, one should be aware of the fact that many chronic pain syndromes still lack effective treatment modes and often require both psychological and somatic intervention, such as given by the multidisciplinary staff of pain clinics.

## C. Medically Refractory Epilepsy

Resection of the epileptogenic focus after careful examination and delineation of the epileptogenic area with depth or stereotactic electroencephalography (stereo-EEG introduced by Talairach; Pecker *et al.* 1979 a) has proved to be very effective (Rasmussen 1979) and should be performed prior to stereotactic lesioning (Gillingham and Campbell 1980, Narabayashi 1980). Recent studies with PET scanning showed that this technique may demonstrate epileptic brain regions more precisely (Meyerson *et al.* 1984), leading to the possibility to localize those regions in stereotactic space with subsequent computer-guided stereotactic resection (see chapter 14). On the other hand, epilepsy is not often medically refractory nowadays, which makes surgical intervention less frequent.

## D. Psychiatric Disabling Disease

In the field of psychosurgery stereotactic interventions are performed less and less over the years, thanks to the continuous development of new and potent neuroleptic and thymoleptic drugs. By the time psychosurgery changed from open and often mutilating surgery to stereotactic and therefore sparing operations (Rylander 1973), drugs became available, being at least as effective as surgery in many of the previous indications. One may hope, that in the near future no indication will exist any longer for stereotactic interventions in psychiatric disease.

## E. Spasticity

The results of stereotactic dentatotomy for the treatment of spasticity are often disappointing, as symptoms frequently recur after some months

---

Fig. 84. CT scan pictures showing some enhancement after contrast in a mesencephalic tumor (man aged 28 years)

Fig. 85. Angiography showed a largely avascular tumor, and biopsy was performed revealing a sclerotized hemangioma!

Fig. 86. Histological specimen showing the large sclerotized vessels. Patient died due to rupture of a feeding vessel during biopsy

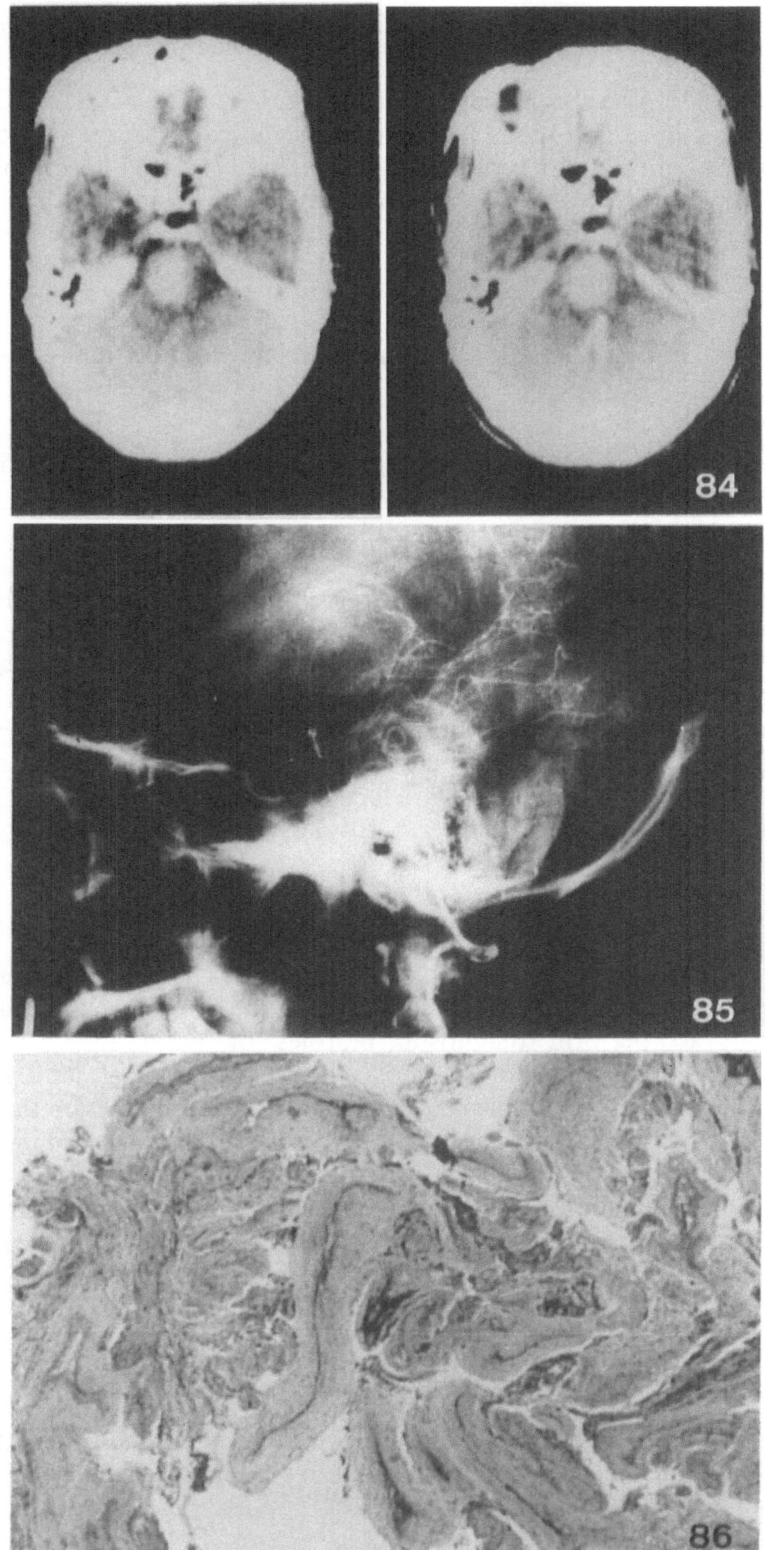

Figs. 84–86

(Spiegel 1982). Also chronic cerebellar stimulation, as advocated by Cooper (1978), does not lead to long standing and significant results. A review on stereotactic dentatotomy is presented by Siegfried (1982). Pharmacological treatment seems to become the treatment of choice together with intensive rehabilitation programs.

## II. Contraindications for Diagnostic Stereotactic Interventions

### A. Resectable Lesions

All those lesions, which can at least partially be resected by open surgical techniques should not be biopsied stereotactically. As discussed in chapter 5 (sub II) even bulk resection is preferable to performing a biopsy alone. Yet there are some important exceptions to this rule. Mass lesions in the basal ganglia, thalamus and pineal gland region should in the first place be explored stereotactically, even when they might seem to be resectable. Up to 10% of the tumors is very radiosensitive and thus cure can be achieved with irradiation. About 80% of the deep seated lesions will prove to be highly malignant gliomas or metastases and might only benefit from an attempt to stereotactic removal. Small subcortical resectable lesions should not be operated upon without stereotactic localization and calculation of a safe cerebral transit route (see chapter 5, sub IV).

### B. Normal Brain Tissue

In our opinion, the absence of any visible target after complete neuroradiological checkup is a contraindication. This means, that it is preferable to perform diagnostic biopsies of brain tissue using a craniotomy. Sometimes for diagnosis in child neurology and genetic counseling a biopsy of "normal" brain tissue is required. For thorough laboratory investigation about $1 \, cm^3$ of fresh brain tissue (including cortex and white matter) is necessary. Because cortical matter bleeds easily, microsurgical resection is mandatory in these cases. A similar situation is present for the diagnosis of a slow virus infection, in which even more problems may arise. Also the use of disposable instruments or at least very scrutinous desinfection (Gajdusek et al. 1977) is obligatory in this case.

### C. Intraventricular Tumors

Clearly intraventricularly exfoliating tumors should be treated with microsurgical techniques, as at least bulk resection can be achieved (Fig. 87). Paraventricular tumors, however, form an excellent target since they cannot be exposed by transventricular exploration. Exceptions to this rule are intraventricular cysts, which may be treated as safely stereotactically (eventually with the aid of fiberoptic instrumentation).

## D. Lower Brainstem Lesions

Diffuse mass lesions in the lower brainstem (pons and medulla oblongata) should not be treated with instruments designed for stereotactic biopsy (forceps, spiral needle). Stereotactic puncture, however, is relatively

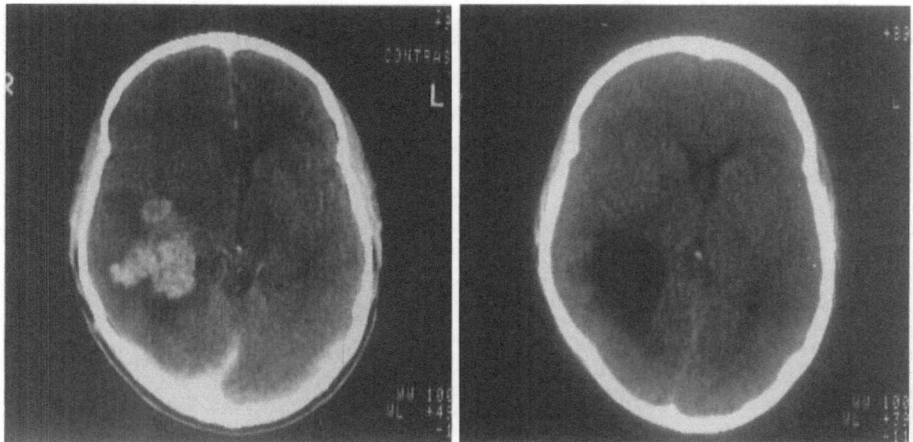

Fig. 87. Intraventricular tumor, clearly enhancing after contrast (left). Open microsurgical resection revealed a hemangioma that could be removed totally (right). Contraindication for biopsy

safe and aspiration can be tried to attain material for cytological and/or smear preparations. In our opinion, in well demarcated lesions (such as malignant tumors and abscesses—see Figs. 88 and 89) a biopsy instrument may be used. Otherwise, open biopsy via the posterior fossa is to be recommended, though it is more time consuming.

## E. Vascular Lesions

Mass lesions with very rich vascularity should not be treated with a stereotactic biopsy, because of the real danger of a bleeding, that is often fatal if it occurs. Particularly arterial bleeding is dangerous, as coagulation via the instrument or inserted electrode is ineffective. Some venous bleeding at the target is not uncommon, however, and is easy to handle when the cannula is left a little longer at the target until the bleeding has stopped. In

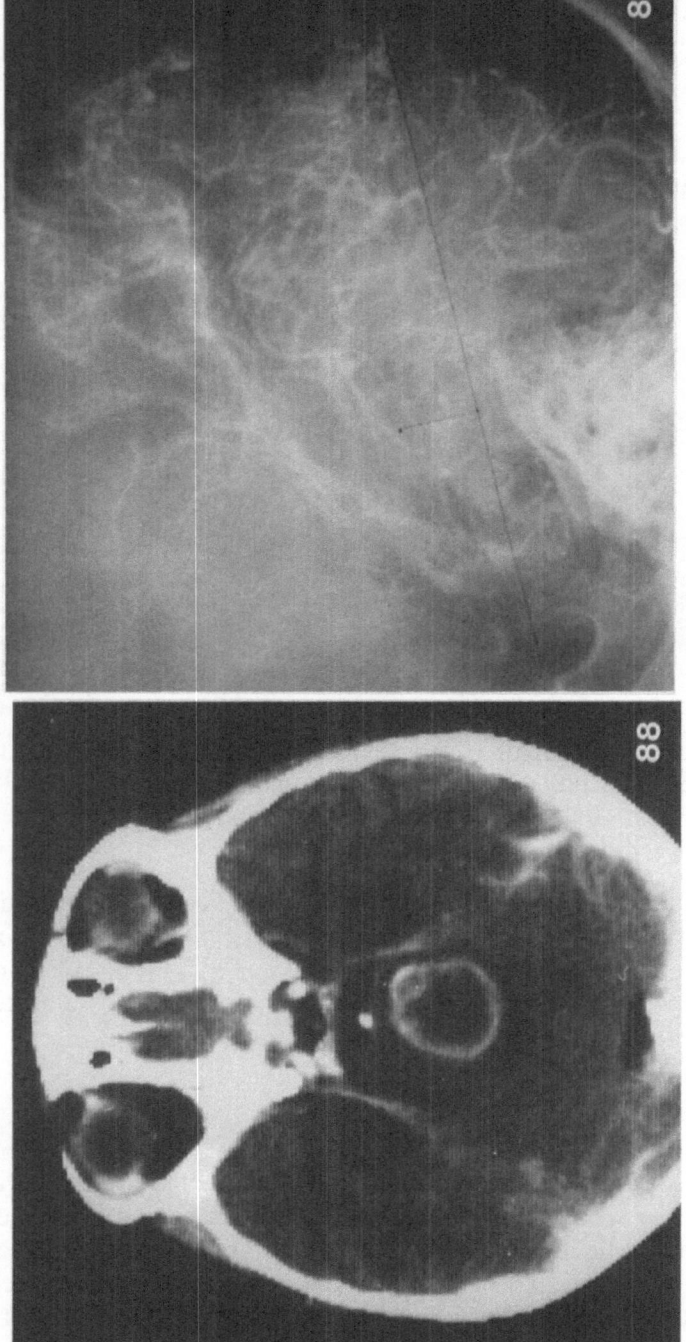

Fig. 88. Leftsided mesencephalic mass lesion in 15 years old boy. Almost no brainstem distortion is seen

Fig. 89. Angiography showed some vessel displacement and a target point was chosen for stereotactic biopsy; black dot. Histological examination revealed an astrocytoma grade 3

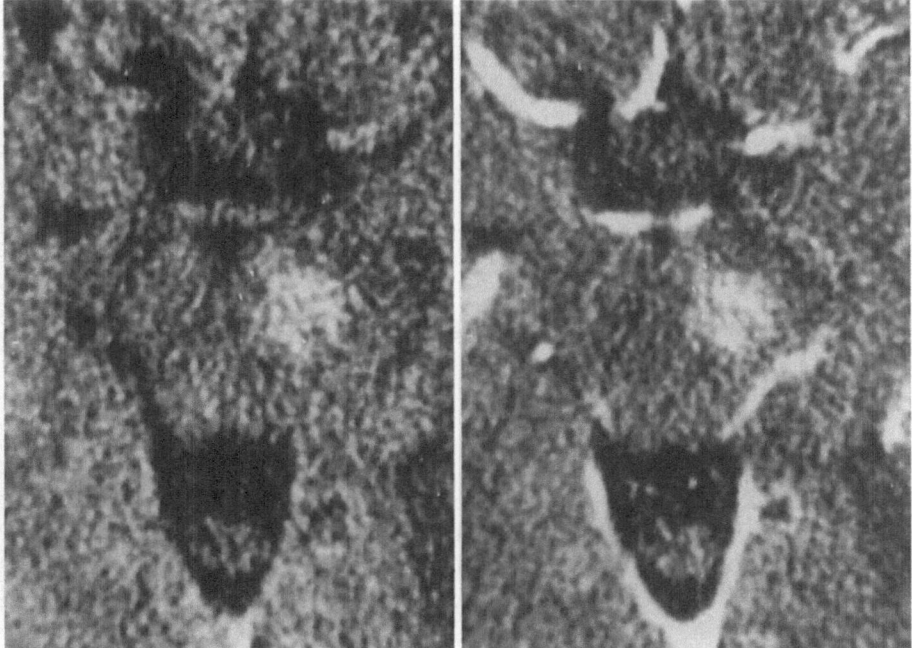

Fig. 90. CT scan pictures with and without contrast enhancement of a venous malformation in the left side of the mesencephalon. Lesion shows marked enhancement (right). Angiography demonstrated the venous malformation (see Fig. 121)

conclusion, a stereotactic biopsy is not acceptable without having done angiography beforehand. The overall mortality rate in large biopsy studies (Bosch 1980, *et al.* 1982, Ostertag *et al.* 1980, Edner 1981) amounts to about 2%, almost exclusively due to fatal bleeding at the target site.

Vascular malformations, particularly the venous malformations described by Huang (*et al.* 1984), may sometimes resemble tumors. On postcontrast CT scan pictures venous malformations may show marked enhancement, whilst angiography is not always positive. It is clear, that a stereotactic biopsy is contraindicated whenever the case history and the CT findings lead to the possibility of a venous malformation. Stereotactic localization and subsequent microsurgical resection is then the procedure of choice in the deep seated and small cases (Fig. 90).

### F. In or Near the Subarachnoid Space

Extreme care is demanded in stereotactic biopsy of small mass lesions, which lie in or around the subarachnoid spaces (the inner sylvian fissure, basal cisterns). The biopsy instrument (particularly the spiral needle of Backlund) can hook onto the arachnoid structures, and therewith tear minor arterial vessels. This applies especially to tumors located in the medial temporal region and parasellar area. It is advisable in this circumstance to make use of a side-window biopsy needle, such as the instrument constructed by Sedan.

## III. Contraindications for Therapeutic Stereotactic Interventions

### A. Aspiration and Evacuation of Fluids

#### 1. Cystic Craniopharyngioma

Stereotactic treatment of a hitherto untreated cystic craniopharyngioma with evacuation of fluid and the introduction of $^{90}$Yttrium has also its opponents among neurosurgeons. In particular, when the possibility for stereotactic radiosurgery of the solid tumor part is absent (as in most centers), open surgery is recommended. However, some craniopharyngiomas lie above the suprasellar cisterns and behind the optic chiasm and may offer an indication for stereotactic treatment (Fig. 91). External radiotherapy should always be given afterwards to stop the progress of the tumor rests. As Huk and Mahlstedt (1983) pointed out, the Backlund (1973) method of stereotactic treatment has much value in the chronic course of this disease (recurrent growth by cystic enlargement). Leakage of the radioisotope outside the cystic compartment should be avoided at any cost, because morbidity from adjacent brain irradiation may be considerable (one personal unpublished case).

#### 2. Posttraumatic Hematoma

In posttraumatic hematoma and those primary hematomas, which only give rise to transient symptomatology, stereotactic aspiration is contraindicated. In hypertensive putaminal hematoma open surgery is advocated by Kaneko (et al. 1977, 1983) in the early stage, in which the bleeding vessel can also be coagulated. In stereotactic evacuation, clots that cannot be aspirated by way of a cannula may be removed with the help of an Archimedes screw (Backlund and Von Holst 1978, Higgins et al. 1982).

### B. Interstitial Irradiation of Tumors

In highly malignant tumors interstitial irradiation with stereotactically implanted radioisotopes is not indicated (Mundinger 1982a). Short term

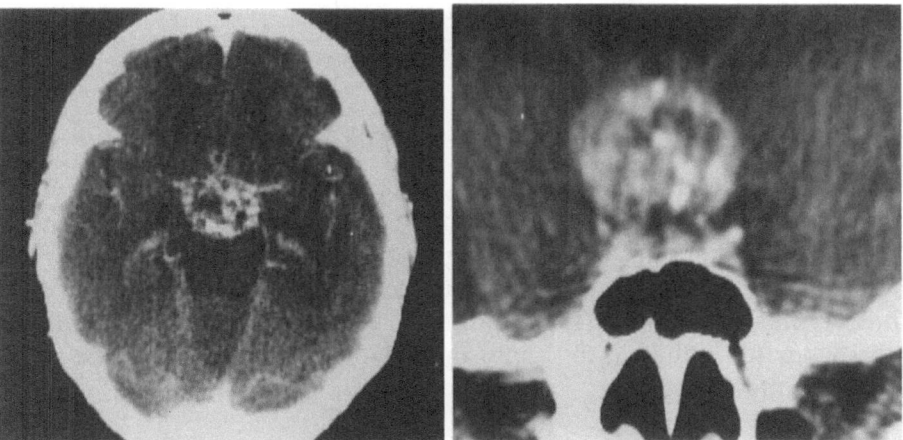

Fig. 91. CT scan pictures of a suprasellar craniopharyngioma, which extended markedly upwards. Indication for stereotactic treatment

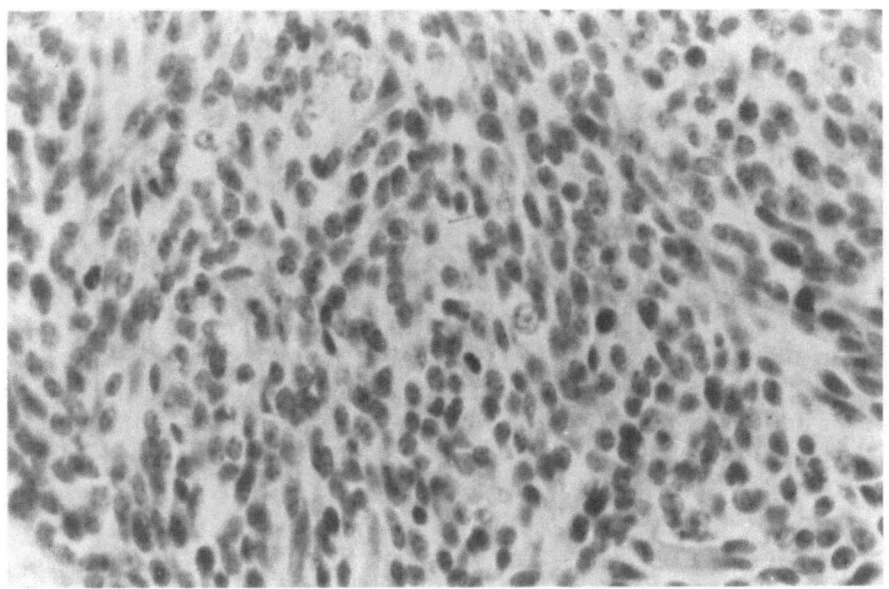

Fig. 92. Histological specimen of a pontine angle tumor, that invaded the pons (female, 25 years). Open biopsy revealed a fibrosarcoma. Stereotactic irradiation (Stockholm) cured the patient

palliative treatment with conventional external irradiation will have some effect, but in the already seriously ill one should perhaps refrain from any treatment except for dexamethasone.

## C. Stereotactic Radiosurgery

In malignant tumors, regardless grade of malignancy, radiosurgery is not indicated, as the target area is almost always more extensive than the irradiated volume. This is due to the growth characteristics (infiltrative) of these tumors. In only one case we succeeded in curing a patient with a fibrosarcoma of the pons (Fig. 92) that had given early clinical symptoms and was treated with Leksell's radiosurgical unit after open biopsy (survival 4 years; unpublished).

## IV. Contraindications for Localizing and Interventional Stereotactics

### A. Aneurysms

Although some publications are available on effective stereotactic treatment of otherwise inaccessible aneurysms (Mullan 1974, Kandel and Peresedov 1977, Smith and Alksne 1977, Sheptak et al. 1977), recent progress in both microsurgical and interventional neuroradiological techniques will lead to more reliable and effective aneurysm occlusion. See for further discussion chapter 3, sub III A.

### B. Deep Seated Arteriovenous Malformations

Arteriovenous malformations lying in the basal ganglia, thalamus or brainstem and bigger than about 25 mm in diameter are preferably treated nowadays with transvascular embolization techniques. Stereotactic radiosurgery can be performed in those less than about 25 mm in diameter.

### C. Foreign Bodies

High velocity missiles inside the brain will not lead to infection and are therefore preferably not extracted, whether stereotactically or with open surgery. Disconnected ventricular catheters may be extracted successfully, however (Blacklock and Maxwell 1985).

Foreign bodies, incidentally found on skull X-ray and lying inside the brain for an unknown period of time, should never be removed stereotactically because of adhesions which warrant open surgery in stereotactic space.

Apart from the contraindications mentioned, possibilities for stereotactic surgery depend largely on the technical details of the system used. Some are not built for use with the CT scanner or MR scanner and some have less degrees of freedom. In the following chapters the technical details of the Leksell system will be discussed at length and illustrative photographs will also show this system as it is in use in the author's department. In chapter 4 the various types of new instrumentation may be found.

# Chapter 7

# Stereotactic Techniques

With knowledge of the stereotactic principles and the various indications and contraindications, we may now proceed to the applications, technical details and pitfalls. Although the applicability differs a little from instrument to instrument, the commonly used and up to date systems of Riechert-Mundinger, Leksell and Brown-Roberts-Wells are all fully equipped for modern stereotactic surgery, including CT guidance. The stereotactic techniques will be described with the help of Leksell's apparatus, which is easy to understand because it lacks a phantom device and simply places the target in the center of the semicircular arc.

## I. Leksell's Apparatus

The stereotactic system constructed by Leksell (1971) consists of a cubical headframe, which is fixed to the skull with 3 or 4 pins (Fig. 25). It constitutes a threedimensional orthogonal coordinate system, with millimeter scales engraved on its edges. Conventional X-ray pictures are standardized to a 40% magnification at the zero plane by way of a mechanical X-ray coupling arm (Fig. 23). X-ray enlargement is corrected by the projection technique already discussed in chapter 2, with a geometric localizing diagram. The aiming device with instrument carrier consists of a semicircular arc that is fixed to the headframe according to the coordinates of the target in such a way that its center corresponds to the target point. Its construction permits both high quality X-ray pictures and CT scans, with the apparatus attached to the skull (see Figs. 46 and 47). For use with CT guidance the pins, after their fixation to the skull, are one by one exchanged for carbon fiber pins that allow scanning without artifact. A special CT ruler has been developed by Leksell and Jernberg (1980) to read off the coordinates of the target. This is done directly from the CT scan pictures (Figs. 52 and 54). Different instruments (electrode, needle, biopsy cannula, hematoma screw, etcetera) can be used by taking the appropriate guiding stops and placing them in the instrument carrier. The whole apparatus is easy to handle and a stereotactic intervention takes less than 2 hours, because the time needed for calculation of the target is relatively short. In the case of CT guided coordinate calculation the computer may be fed with a program that gives the coordinates directly.

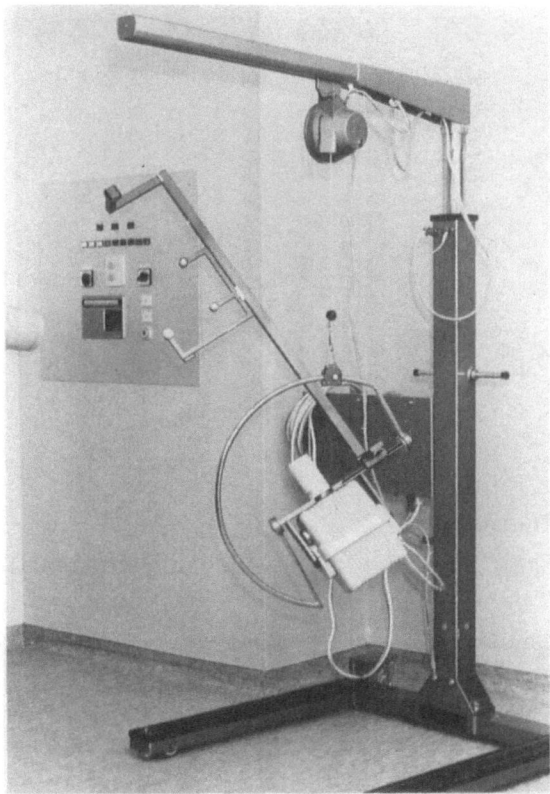

Fig. 93. X-ray tube with mechanical coupling arm and magnetic attachments for use with Leksell's stereotactic headframe

## II. Preparation of the Patient

In case of elective stereotactic surgery we perform only functional interventions under local anesthesia. Otherwise the normal procedure is followed for general anesthesia. 24 hours before the operation 4 × 5 mg dexamethasone is started, which after 4 days is lowered to zero. 2 hours prior to surgery medical treatment is started with fenytoin (2 × 100 mg), heparin calcium (2 × 5,000 U) and floxapen (2 × 1,000 mg). Antibiotics are only repeated twice (1,000 mg after 6 and 12 hrs) and anticoagulants will be continued until the patient is ambulatory again (third day). Antibiotics are only required, as we do not shave the hair, but only the area of transit (usually frontal). This means, that the instrument is no longer sterile after fixation onto the head (Fig. 95). After fixation, X-ray pictures in lateral and anteroposterior direction are made (Figs. 93 and 94), and the calculation is done in a dark room on the lightbox with the localizing diagram. During this time, the assistant cleans the skull and instrument once more and

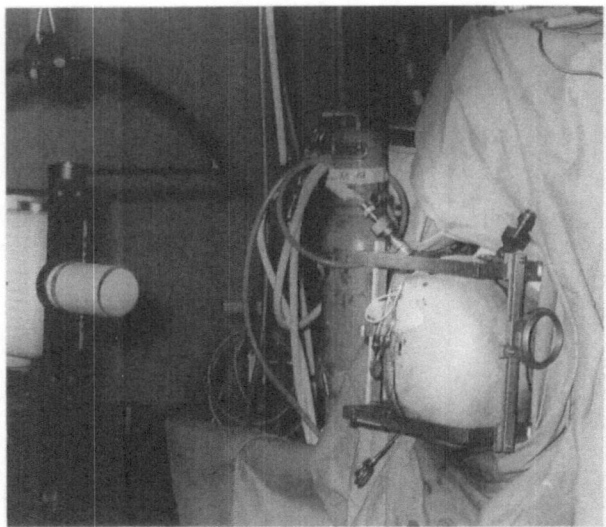

Fig. 94. Set-up for lateral X-ray picture during stereotactic surgery

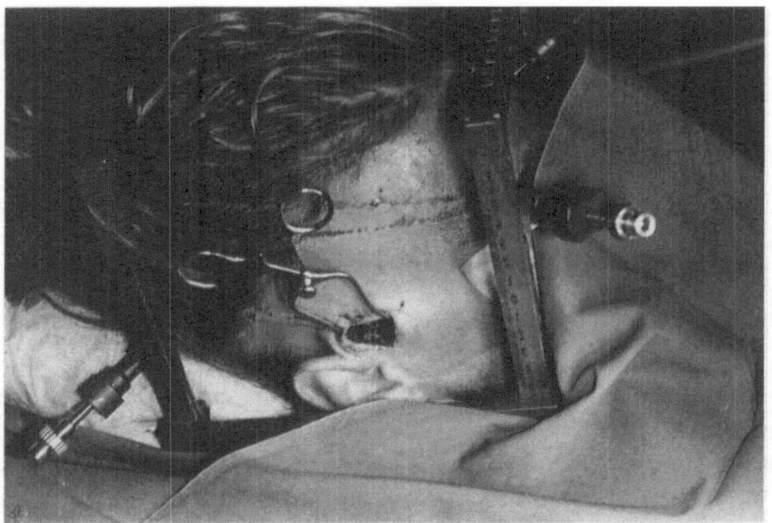

Fig. 95. Leksell's headframe after fixation onto the head. Preparation of a rightsided temporal skull opening

dresses the head of the patient as in conventional burrhole surgery. The surgeon, after washing and dressing himself, places the sidebars (Fig. 97) according to the coordinates x and y (i.e. y and z in the modern nomenclature). Thereafter the semicircular arc is placed in position on these sidebars (Fig. 98), after adjustment for the z (or x)-coordinate. Now a

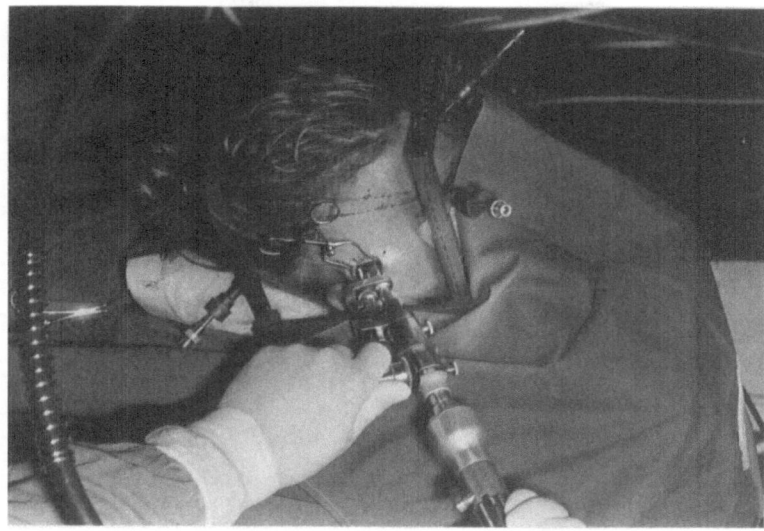

Fig. 96. The performing of the burrhole

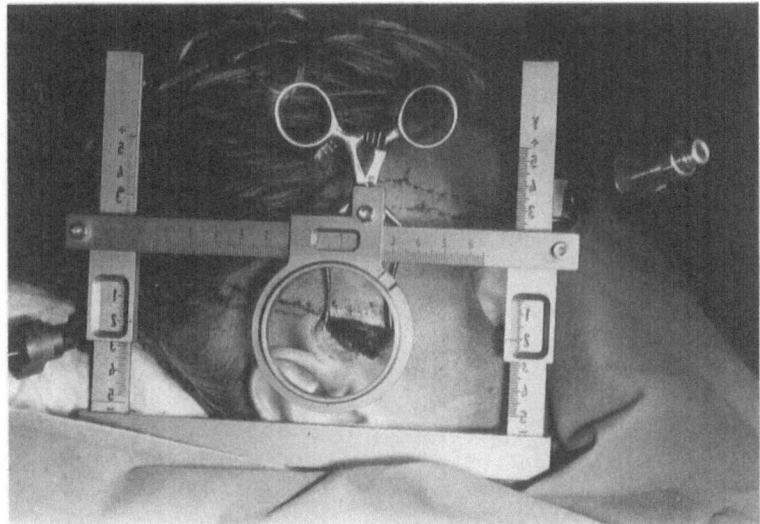

Fig. 97. The sidebars are mounted on the headframe

puncture needle is aimed through the instrument carrier and pointed to the site of entrance, which is marked. The semicircular arc is taken away or rotated in a way that leaves sufficient room for performing the burrhole (Fig. 96). By now the arc is properly positioned and the instrument needed is

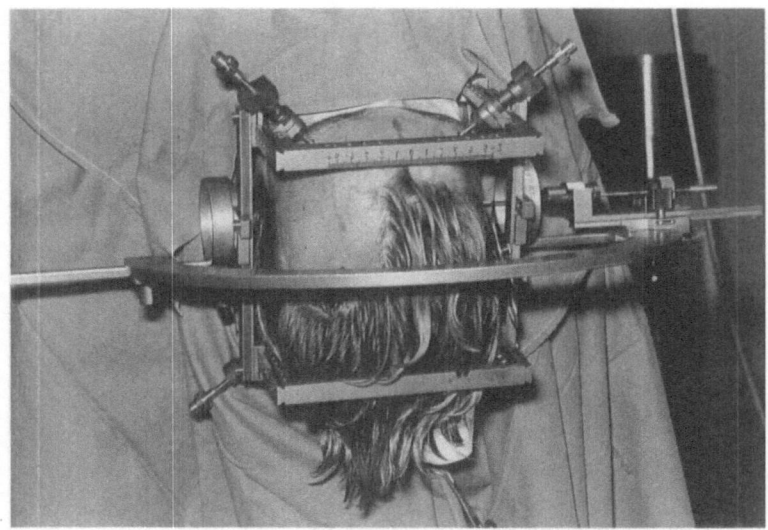

Fig. 98. The semicircular arc is placed in a proper position on the sidebars. Note that the center of the arc is in the right temporal area

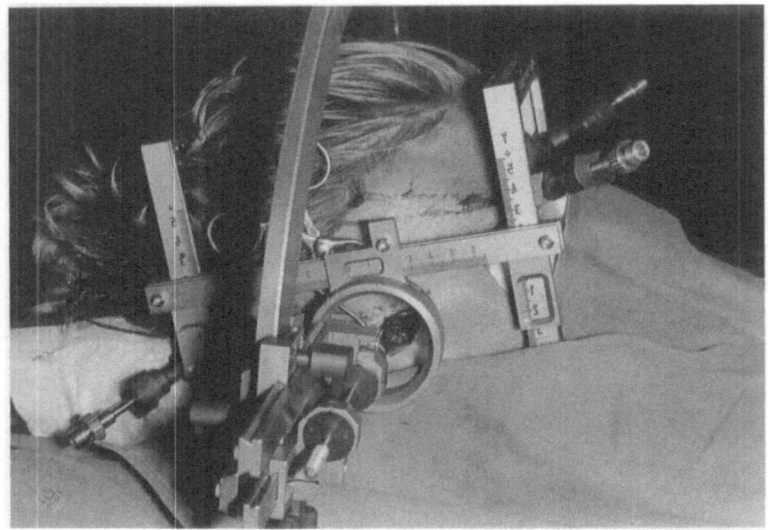

Fig. 99. The biopsy instrument is inserted through the instrument carrier

introduced through the instrument carrier and after depth adjustment advanced through the brain until the target is reached (Figs. 99 and 100). Resistance should not be met. True resistance can only be caused by the skull base, the falx and tentorium. Resistance can be checked by turning the instrument around a little whilst penetrating the tissue: vessels will give away to this turning. In functional and localizing stereotactics the target should be reached at once so as to perform the planned intervention.

## A. Diagnostic and Therapeutic Stereotactics

In diagnostic and therapeutic stereotactics, depending on the site and size of the target, one can start sampling biopsy tissue or fluid some distance in front of the target point (Fig. 101) and proceed with the sampling to some

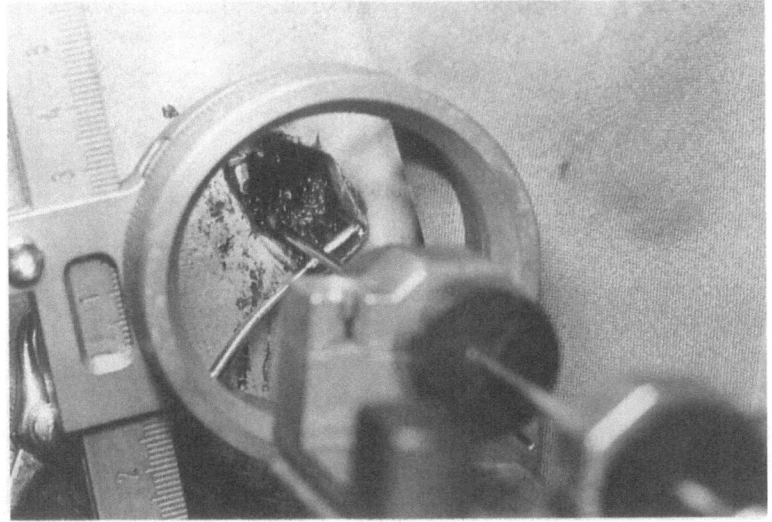

Fig. 100. Close-up view of biopsy instrument

distance behind it. As a standard procedure we take three samples along the puncture track if the location and size of the lesion permit this: one before reaching, one at, and one behind the calculated target point. If some more tissue is required by the pathologist, or if the biopsies produce too little material, another three samples are taken from a parallel track that is obtained by slightly altering the z-coordinate (Fig. 101). If the spiral needle (Backlund 1971) is used, the instrument is screwed into the target tissue after guided puncture, and by twisting the outer cannula the other way round, its sharp edge cuts away the material that is caught in the spiral (Fig. 102). As the spiral length is 12 mm and it has a 1.2 mm diameter, samples can be obtained of about 13 mm$^3$. The tissue samples are normally of excellent quality (Bosch 1980) for histological examination (no squeezing), and for this reason we prefer the spiral needle to the conventional aspiration needles (Fig. 103). It is sometimes necessary to puncture the tentorium to obtain

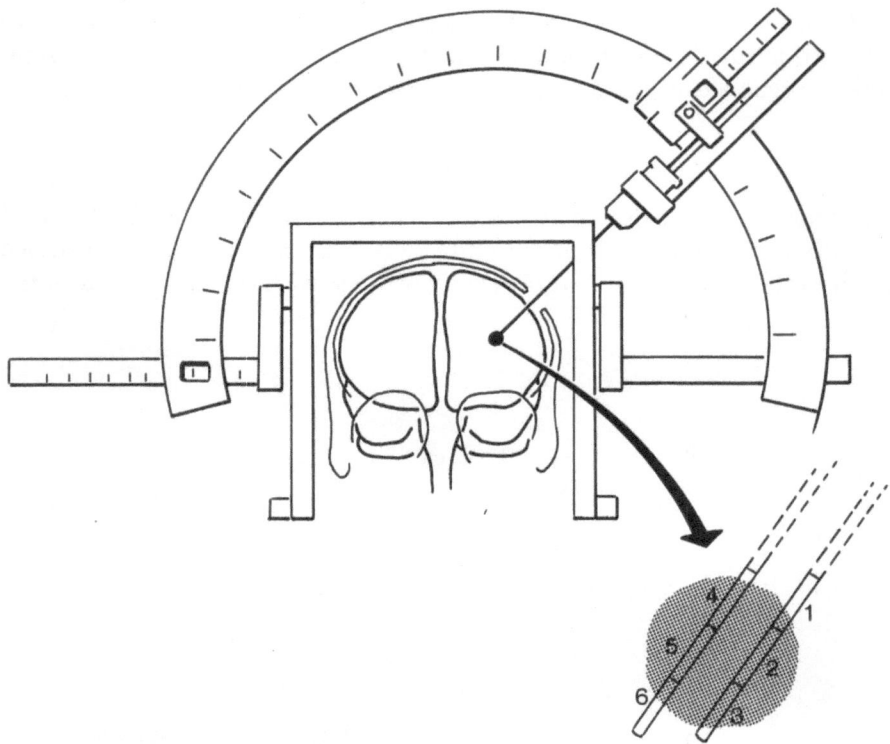

Fig. 101. Schematic drawing of the procedure of stereotactic tissue sampling. At the target site some consecutive biopsies are taken (*1–3*). After altering the lateral coordinate slightly, the biopsy needle is introduced once again and another series of biopsies (*4–6*) is taken

tissue at an infratentorial target. In that case, the inner, blunt, needle can be replaced by a sharp inner needle at the position on the tentorium, and after sharp puncture be directly replaced for the usual blunt inner needle. Tentorial puncture under local anesthesia may evoke a cough reflex by vagal stimulation. Usually, however, infratentorial interventions should be carried out with suboccipital trepanation, because cerebral transit is less.

## B. Functional Stereotactics

In functional stereotactics we use general anesthesia only in mesencephalotomies, because electrical stimulation at the target will cause strong emotional reactions (Nashold *et al.* 1969, 1982). In the treatment of movement disorders the patient should be awake and cooperative for neurological testing during stimulation and coagulation. Electrical stimulation is usually performed with a constant current with biphasic wave

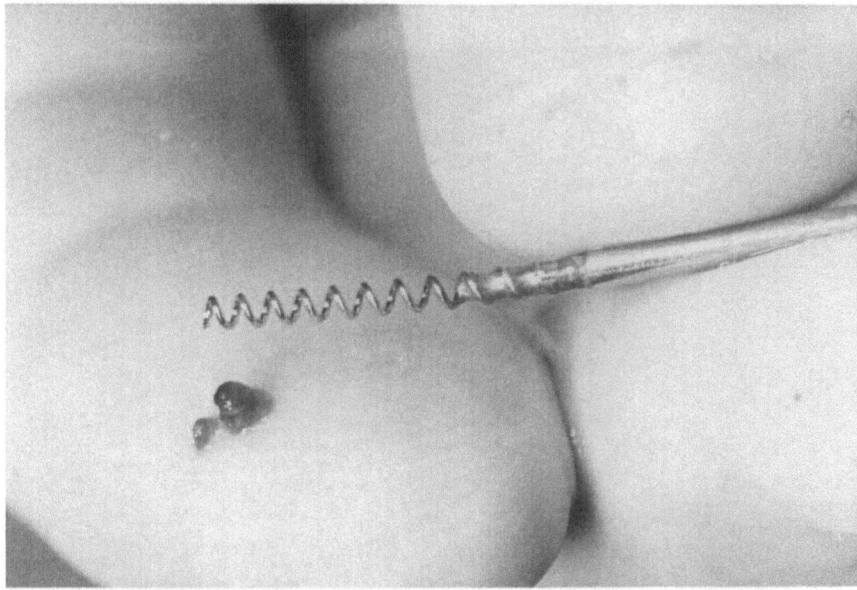

Fig. 102. Magnification picture of spiral needle of Backlund and a tissue specimen for histological investigation

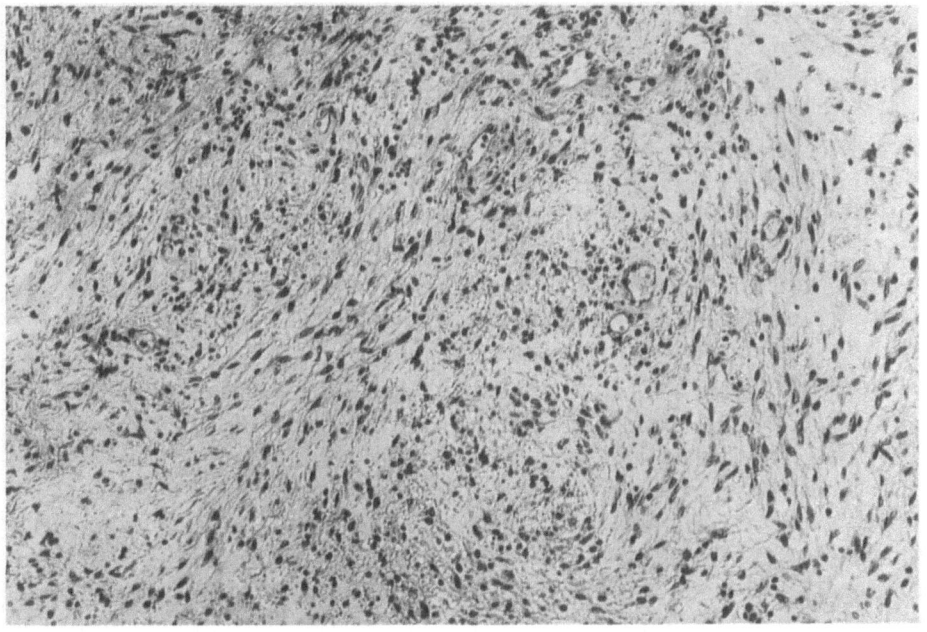

Fig. 103. Example of histological picture after a stereotactic biopsy with the spiral needle. No squeezing of the material and excellent quality for histological examination (astrocytoma grade 2; boy aged 6)

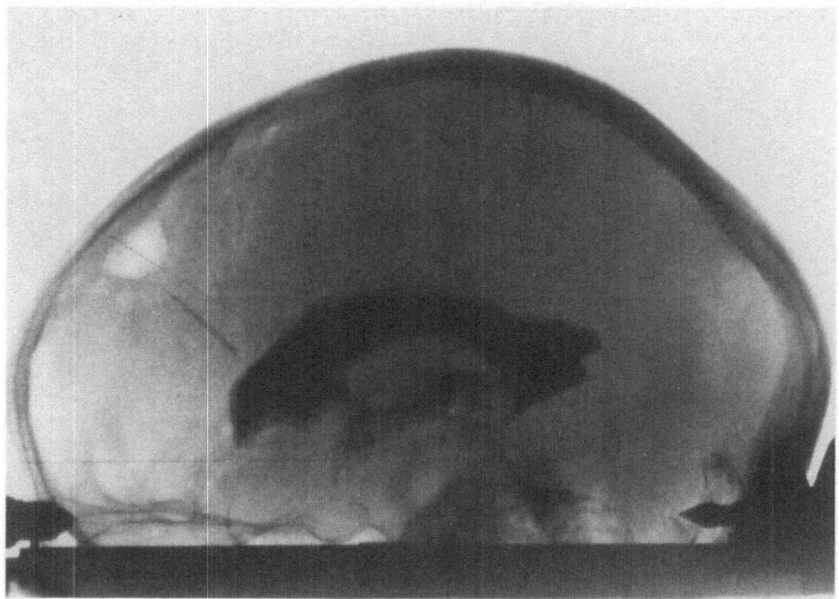

Fig. 104. Stereotactic ventriculography with positive contrast. Stereotactic apparatus of Van Manen; lateral view

forms and pulses of 1 ms duration. Frequencies range from 10–100 Hz. Motor responses are easiest observed with low frequency and indicate activity from the internal capsule (posterior limb). Normally motor responses are not seen with an electrode position within 10–12 mm from the midsagittal plane (Hardy *et al.* 1979). Sensory responses (tingling in the opposite side of the body) result from activity spreading towards the somatosensory thalamic nuclei, which lie posterior to the target. See for orientation Fig. 29 a and b. Micro-electrode introduction may register the fieldpotential of neurons at the target site, and help in localizing any thalamic nucleus by its firing pattern.

Discussing the details of stereotactic technique in functional surgery, we like to refer to the extensive description of the *invisible target* at which is aimed, as given in chapter 2. Because the target point represents a nucleus or fiber tract and cannot be visualized by neuro-radiological means, as in pathological conditions, the target point is called invisible and the stereotactic determination is done in two different steps with the use of two completely unrelated cartesian systems of axes. Although in magnetic resonance imaging white and grey matter are clearly differentiated, a special tract or nucleus cannot be visualized.

The first system of axes is erected in the cerebrum to determine the position of the target in relation to these axes with the help of a stereotactic

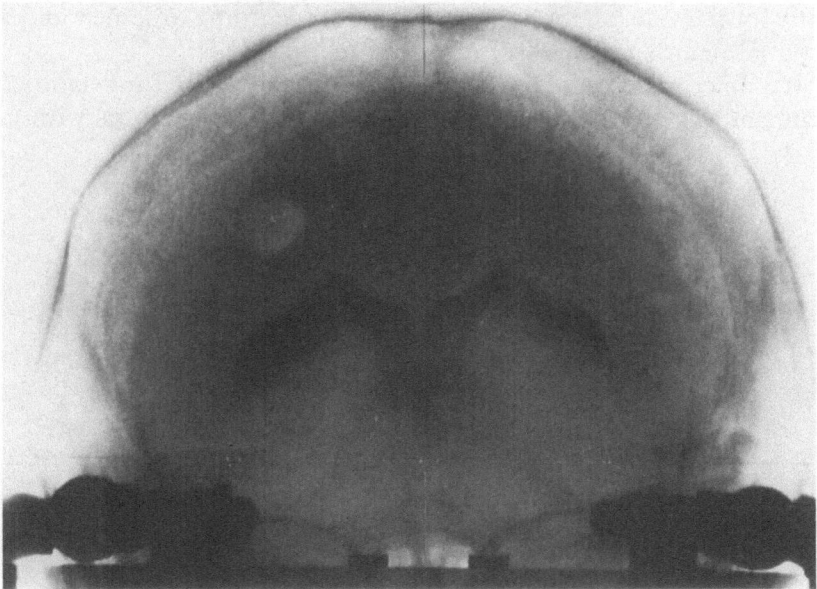

Fig. 105. Stereotactic ventriculography, anteroposterior view. Stereotactic apparatus of Van Manen

brain atlas (Fig. 7). The second system of axes is embodied by the stereotactic instrument that can be fixed to the skull in various positions. In practice, the erection of the (first) intracerebral system of axes (in the middle of the line AC—PC, according to Schaltenbrand and Bailey 1959) needs visualization of the anterior and posterior commissures.

There are two ways to visualize these reference points:

— CT scanning of the third ventricle in the sagittal plane with subsequent CT guided determination of the target point in relation to the second system of axes, namely that of the stereotactic instrument. This sophisticated method will require, however, extended computer facilities with the reconstruction of an axial tomogram running horizontally to the AC—PC line (Hardy et al. 1983, Kelly et al. 1984 d).

— intraoperative ventriculography with an isotonic contrast solution (Figs. 104 and 105), which will give the most reliable and easy way of target determination. This applies particularly to brainstem target points such as needed in mesencephalotomy and pontine tractotomy, in which visualization of the aqueduct and fourth ventricle are most helpful.

The position of the target point of choice in relation to the various ventricular reference points is extracted from the stereotactic atlas that is used by the surgeon. As is shown in Fig. 106 individual preferences may vary slightly for the ventrolateral thalamic target, according to some well-known functional neurosurgeons (see also: Laitinen 1985).

After determination of the target point, the coordinates in relation to the instrument system of axes are calculated in the same way as with visible targets.

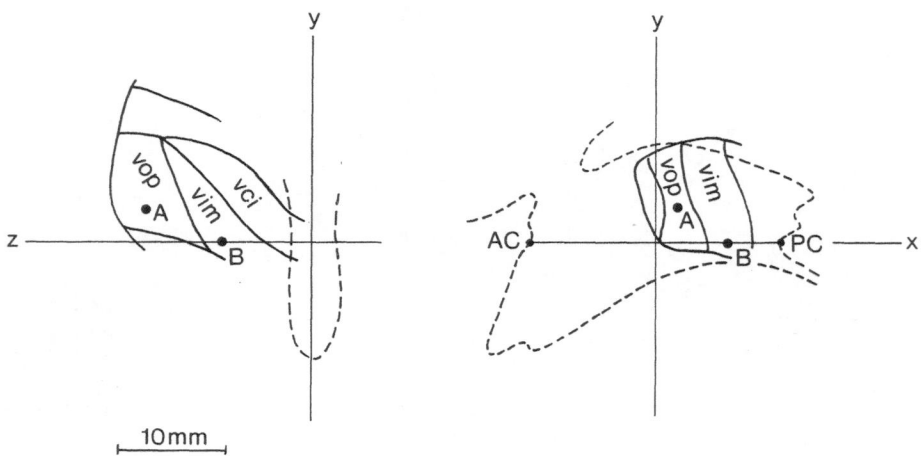

Fig. 106. Schematic drawing of the ventrolateral thalamic complex. Coronal and sagittal view, with 10 mm bar. Most frequently used target points are: nucleus *Vop* and nucleus *Vim* (*A* and *B*). For discussion see chapter 9, sub I A

## C. Localizing Stereotactics

In localization stereotactics followed by microsurgical exploration (as is advocated in small subcortical tumors and arteriovenous malformations) a careful planning should be made of the bone flap to secure the safest cerebral transit. In parietal lesions a more occipital approach may be considered the best, and the positioning of the apparatus on the skull should allow enough room to proceed with a craniotomy. Therefore, the surgeon should have sound judgement as to the possibilities and pitfalls of his stereotactic apparatus so as to overcome and anticipate problems during the second phase of open surgery.

Leksell's apparatus (as well as the other) offers many possibilities to place the headframe onto the skull. Graduated metal ear plugs are used for temporary fixation and alignment of the frame, and in this early phase the wanted position of the headframe must be tried out. As is shown in Fig. 107 b and c the earplug position can be changed to anterior and posterior by making appropriate extra holes in the headframe. This will allow for a relative shift to posterior or anterior of the headframe in relation to the

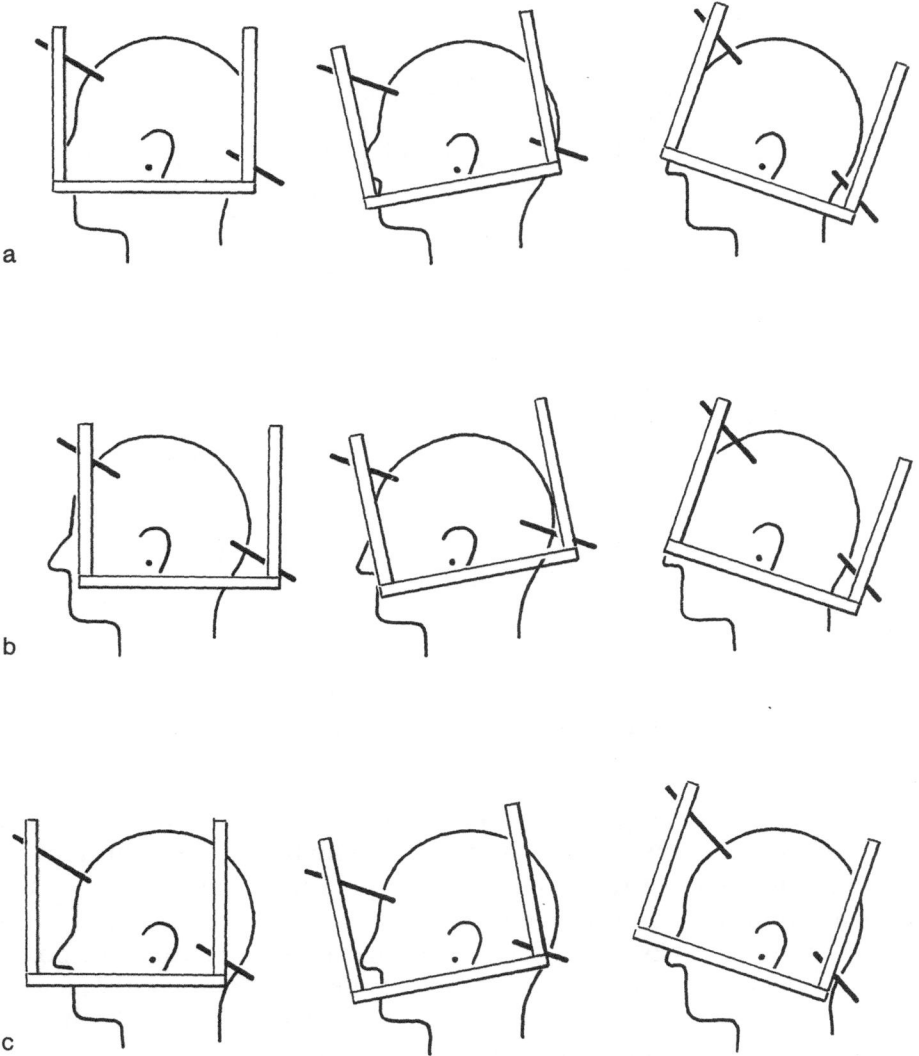

Fig. 107. Drawing of different frame positions. Ear plug axis as rotation point. In b) the ear plugs are placed more anterior, and in c) more posterior as compared with the normal position (a)

skull. The fixation pins should be available in standard and extra long sizes, enabling the surgeon to achieve every wanted frame position. Moreover, our own experience showed that the long size pins are often mandatory for stereotactics in children. A drawing may illustrate these different frame positions with the ear plug axis as a rotation point (Fig. 107). This rotation of the headframe may offer possibilities for more anterior or posterior

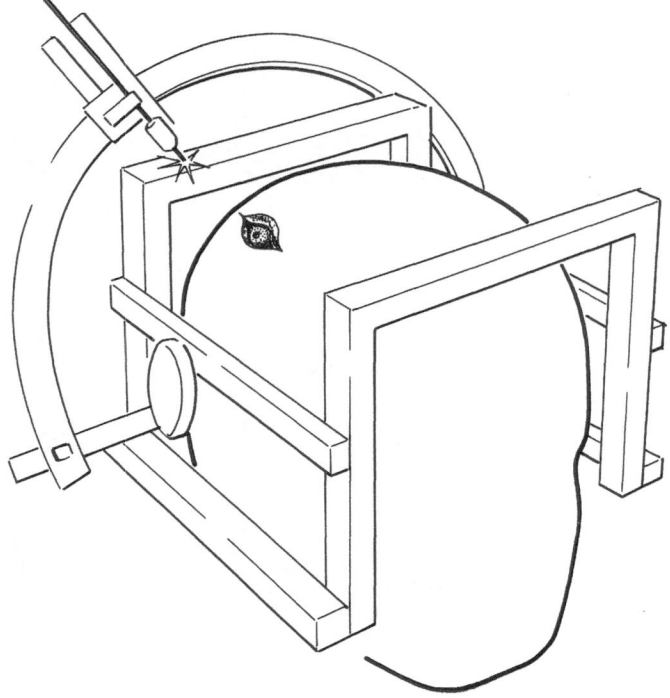

Fig. 108. Pitfall: blind angle of the stereotactic instrument

approaches. Even the carriers for the pins may be slided along the vertical edges of the headframe, if necessary. The standard Leksell headframe is, however, not suitable for a lateral approach with open surgery, as the sidebars allow no quarter turning. On the other hand a recently developed open headframe (Leksell, personal communication 1985) offers the possibility for all open surgery required. A stereotactic intervention without open surgery is, however, as easily performed using a lateral approach with the standard instrument (Figs. 99 and 100). Another pitfall is the so-called blind angle of any stereotactic instrument. As Fig. 108 illustrates, a part of the headframe may obstruct the passage of the aiming instrument. This is only prevented by insight of the surgeon in the planned approach. Moreover, any burrhole has a blind angle regarding the introduction of an aiming instrument towards a given target. This depends much on the thickness of the skull and the position of the target point (Fig. 109). To prevent the enlargement of the burrhole with bone tongs or even the making of a new burrhole, it is strongly recommended to postpone the opening of the skull until the exact position of the burrhole is known (e.g. after testing with arc and aiming instrument). The use of a gauging-rod instead of the aiming instrument is advisable for sake of sterility.

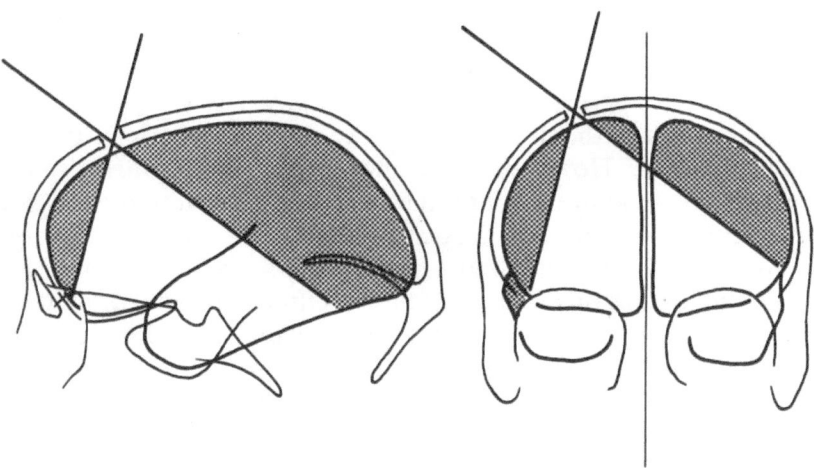

Fig. 109. Pitfall: blind angle of a burrhole. The pointed areas are inaccessible

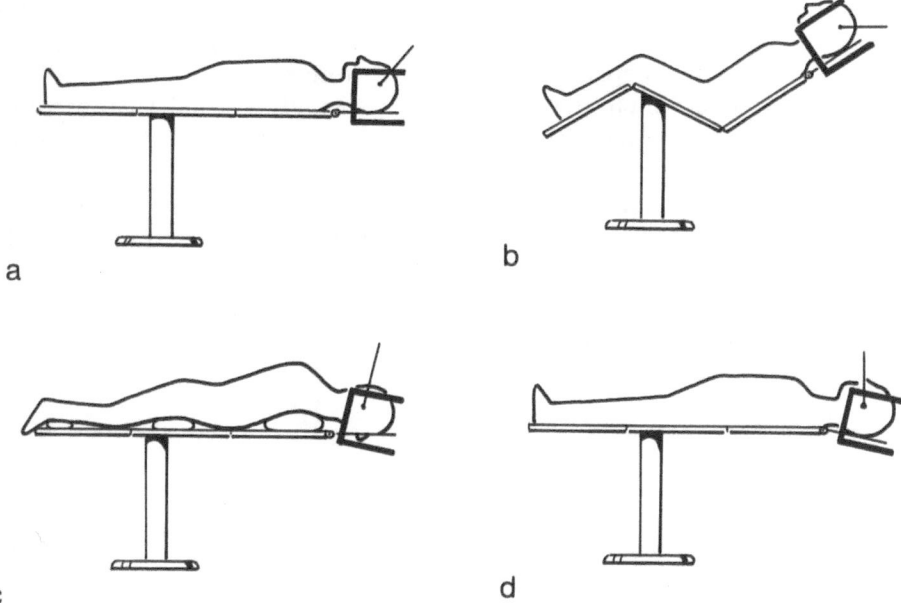

a

b

c

d

Fig. 110. Drawing of different patient positions. Recumbent (a), semi-recumbent or sitting (b), prone (c), and hyperextended position for transsphenoidal approach (d)

## III. The Positioning of the Patient (Fig. 110)

Normally the recumbent position is used. When the occipital approach is needed a patient may be placed in the semi-recumbent position. The suboccipital approach needs the prone position with use of a special headrest. The sitting position is often used in functional stereotactics, the patient being awake. The patient may sit in a type of dentist chair and lumbar puncture to perform air ventriculography may be used. To obtain reliable delineation of the third ventricle's commissures with air the sitting position is necessary. However, ventriculography with a contrast solution, after ventricular puncture through the burrhole, is preferred as it gives a complete ventriculogram in *one* X-ray picture. The disadvantage of air ventriculography is that it almost never shows both the anterior and posterior commissures on one lateral picture. Often two pictures are needed, which have to be superimposed to get a complete delineation of the third ventricle. To puncture the lateral ventricle, however, one needs some training as normally there is no ventricular enlargement. Ventricular CSF will have the normal clear appearance, whilst CSF evacuated from the interhemispheric fissure will be red stained, due to some contamination by blood after the burrhole surgery.

In conclusion, it is evident that some training is needed to become familiar with the different stereotactic techniques. However, when the principles are clear and calculations can be made quickly, the performance *per se* will present no special problems any longer.

The period in which stereotactics was strongly related to functional neurosurgery has become history. In the future any neurosurgeon will need help of stereotactic localization techniques in order to treat small lesions which can be detected nowadays. Computer software connected to CT and MR images of these lesions will bring stereotactic methods within his reach.

# Chapter 8

# Pitfalls

In this chapter some of the more usual pitfalls in stereotactic surgery will be mentioned. It is only possible to make a rough distinction between technical problems on the one hand and pitfalls presented by the underlying pathology on the other.

## I. Technical Problems

### A. The Superficial Target

In stereotactic surgery the superficially lying target is more difficult to reach than the deep seated one, the issue being that the intervention is carried out through a very small skull opening (a burrhole or even the opening made with a twist-drill). The central brain area can be reached by any hole, whereas the superficial target is only reached by an opening that is positioned exactly above it. This might be a technical reason to refrain from superficial interventions, unless required for exact localization of small lesions. Moreover, on the basis of proportional correction (chapter 2, sub V A 2) needed in conventional stereotactic X-ray studies, the small error in calculation that is thereoretically always present (about 1 mm) will be larger at the periphery. Thus, CT guided localization is preferable in superficial targets. Also, in lesions which are only detected on CT scan and have a completely normal angiography, a CT scannogram is required to reconstruct exactly the target position on the lateral stereotactic X-ray picture, unless there are CT-facilities for coordinate calculation. A well-known pitfall is the presumptive frontal position of a lesion that actually lies in the parietal region (Fig. 111), which is due to the commonly used canthomeatal plane of scanning in axial tomography. Whenever a reconstruction of the target on the lateral X-ray picture is not feasible a CT guided localization plus coordinate calculation is mandatory.

### B. Clinical Signs of Increased ICP

From a theoretical point of view there is no indication for stereotactic approach to a superficially lying large tumor. A craniotomy is a better surgical modality, because a bulk resection or even complete removal is the best option and leads to both diagnosis and therapy. In general practice, however, the question sometimes arises whether a stereotactic biopsy could be considered in case of large tumors, which have already led to a clinically significant rise in intracranial pressure. Reasons may be, that the patient is too ill to undergo open surgery or that the relatives and the patient himself like to know the histological diagnosis before deciding upon possible further treatment. Although this relative indication is sometimes considered

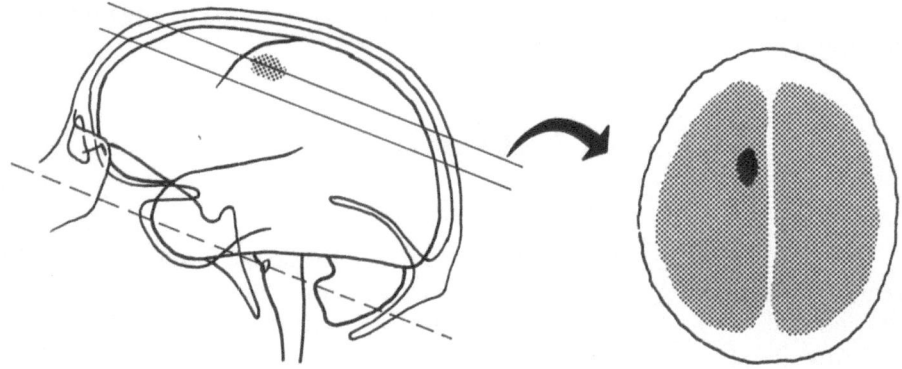

Fig. 111. Pitfall: presumptive frontal position of a lesion that actually lies in the parietal region (due to commonly used canthomeatal plane of scanning)

acceptable, the overall experience with such cases learns that operative morbidity will increase. The cause of clinical worsening is the induction of some reactive brain edema by the biopsy procedure: the biopsy site will always bleed a little, though undetected, and forms a focus for reactive signs to develop. Therefore, the wish to know the histological diagnosis must be strong enough to perform this type of biopsy and information should be given on the somewhat increased risk. We only accept this indication when strategic planning is justified because of the clinical picture and the suspicion that open surgery would not give a better outcome.

Increased intracranial pressure in centrally lying tumors may also be caused by obstruction of CSF pathways inside the brain. In these instances a CSF draining system should be inserted some days prior to the stereotactic procedure. Localization of the target should then be repeated on the day of surgery, because of possible changes in position of the target after normalization of the ICP.

During the pre-CT scan-period often large tumors were discovered, which after biopsy led to (not always transient) deterioration in consciousness and motor function. The progression of edema may ask for higher doses of dexamethasone with increased risk of complications (gastrointestinal bleeding and Cushing syndrome).

## C. Bleeding at the Target Site

If by accident a bleeding occurs at the target site, as sometimes happens with aspiration or biopsy techniques, it is extremely important to keep the instrument at the bleeding site. One should note the depth of the instrument tip by reading it off the scale on the instrument carrier, and should wait and at the same time repeatedly remove and replace the inner needle through the outer shaft. This allows spontaneous drainage without clotting inside the needle and may lead to spontaneous clotting at the target in the case of venous bleeding. After a 5–10 minutes waiting period, one should remove the instrument completely and introduce it once again down to the noted position of bleeding, withdraw the inner cannula and aspirate slowly to make sure the bleeding has stopped. Very seldom a depth coagulation is to be considered with the help of an electrode. Large vessels will never lead to bleeding, unless when ruptured by tearing; they give way to blunt instruments as used in stereotactics.

In only three instances (out of 250 biopsy cases) the author met bleeding problems that were fatal. All of these were arterial and due to the hooking of a vessel with the spiral needle at the biopsy site. The first case concerned a feeder vessel to a completely sclerotized hemangioma (therefore not seen on angiography), which was torn apart when taking the biopsy (Figs. 84, 85, and 86). The other two cases concerned mass lesions growing around the inner sylvian fissure. The spiral needle fastened itself in the arachnoid tissue and caused bleeding of one of the medial cerebral artery branches. Brain edema followed and emergency craniotomy within some hours in 1 case led only to a decerebrate state. These experiences led to the concept of more dangerous areas deep in the brain and to a strong belief that angiography is a obligatory preoperative investigation. The more dangerous areas comprise the major vessel trajectories such as the sylvian fissure, the epithalamic roof with deep cerebral veins, the parasellar and uncal areas and the superficial brainstem. With knowledge of these high risk regions it is almost always possible to select a safe target point inside the mass lesion. For this selection a careful analysis of the angiographic study is necessary and sometimes intraoperative angiography is to be recommended. With mass lesions that are very small (diameter of less than 15 mm) and furthermore lying in a high risk region the use of the spiral needle is to be avoided. Aspiration biopsy or the use of a specially designed biopsy forceps may be more safe (Apuzzo and Sabshin 1983).

## II. Pitfalls by Underlying Pathology

### A. Vascular Lesions

Vascular lesions sometimes offer a real pitfall to the neurosurgeon, especially when they are very large and closely resemble mass lesions on CT scan. The patient may be referred for stereotactic biopsy with the diagnosis "tumor of the pineal gland region" and accepted for this type of surgery (Fig. 112). We met such a case, in which routine preoperative angiography showed an extensive arteriovenous malformation (Figs. 113–116) that mimicked clinically a tumor (headache and hydrocephalus signs). More

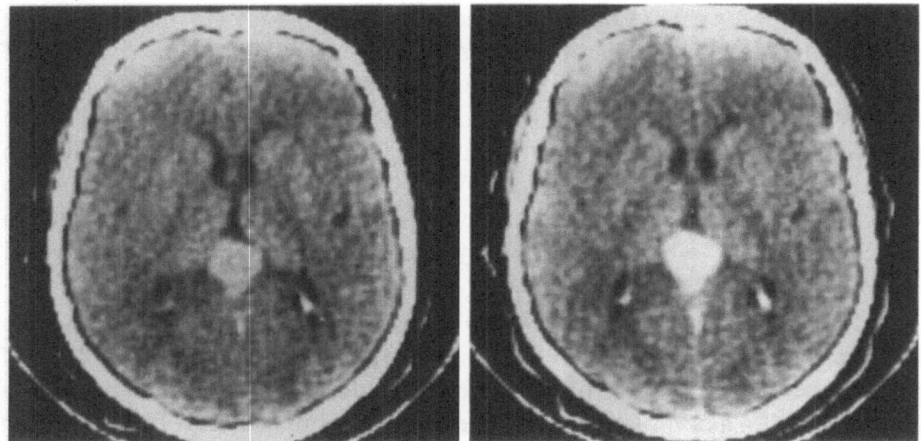

Fig. 112. Case presenting a "pineal region tumor" on CT scan. After contrast (right) there is clear enhancement of the lesion. After sagittal scanning (see Fig. 65 b) a vascular lesion was suspected

frequent are giant aneurysms, which did not bleed (yet) and may give rise to tumor symptoms. Particularly aneurysms lying at the top of the basilar artery may act as space occupying lesions, producing hydrocephalus by obstructing the third ventricle. CT scanning after contrast enhancement may show a variable filling, which may be so obscure that a presumptive diagnosis of tumor is made. Angiography, however, will then reveal the aneurysm, with sometimes a ring of calcification at the outer edge that, due to thrombosis, lies at some distance from the filling compartment. An example of a supraclinoidal tumor, which presented symptoms of headache and blurred vision on one eye, is presented in Figs. 117 and 118. After contrast enhancement some filling of the tumor can be detected, indicating the presence of an aneurysm as later on was shown with angiography (Fig. 119).

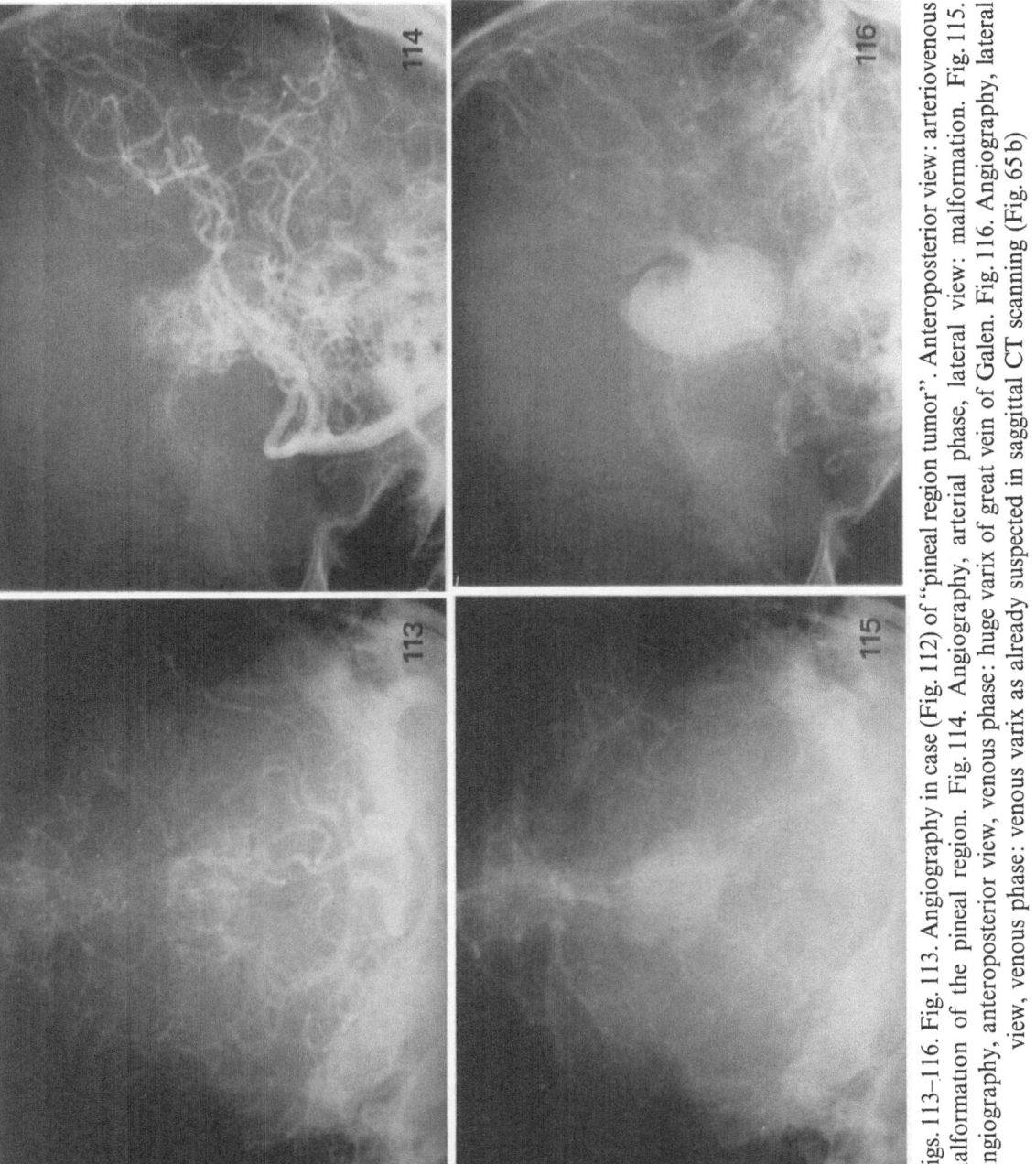

Figs. 113–116. Fig. 113. Angiography in case (Fig. 112) of "pineal region tumor". Anteroposterior view: arteriovenous malformation of the pineal region. Fig. 114. Angiography, arterial phase, lateral view: malformation. Fig. 115. Angiography, anteroposterior view, venous phase: huge varix of great vein of Galen. Fig. 116. Angiography, lateral view, venous phase: venous varix as already suspected in saggittal CT scanning (Fig. 65b)

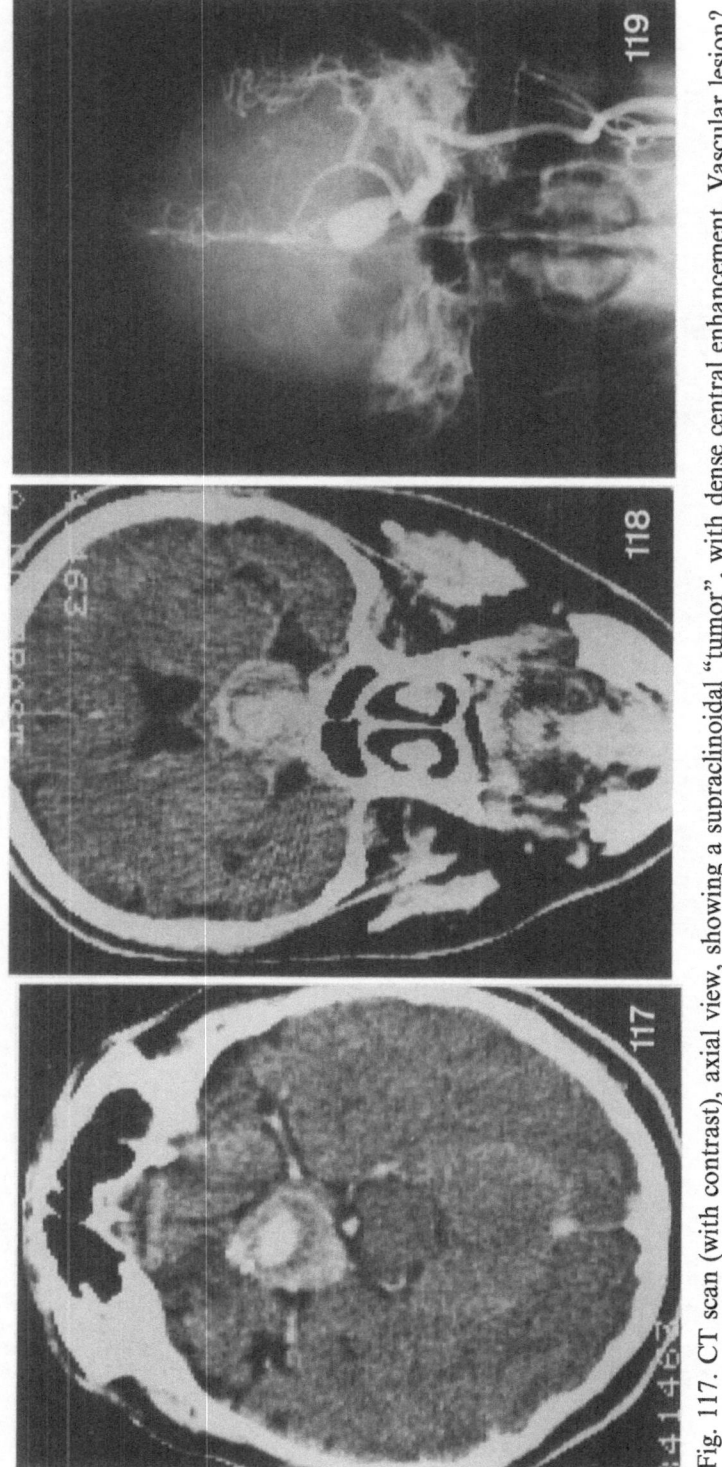

Fig. 117. CT scan (with contrast), axial view, showing a supraclinoidal "tumor", with dense central enhancement. Vascular lesion?

Fig. 118. CT scan (with contrast), coronal view, showing calcified outer edge and central accumulation of contrast medium

Fig. 119. Angiography (anteroposterior view, arterial phase) confirms the presence of a giant aneurysm of the carotid artery

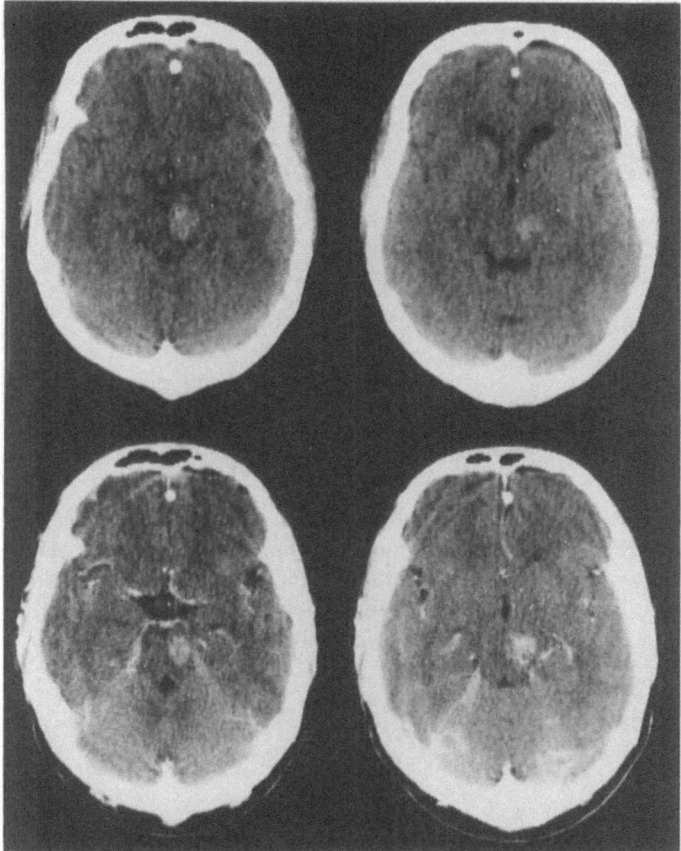

Fig. 120. Case of a cerebral venous malformation (according to Huang *et al.* 1984), lying in the left side of the mesencephalon. Upper pictures: without contrast medium injection; lower pictures: postcontrast CT scan pictures

A special problem is seen in the cerebral venous malformations, formerly called venous angiomas. Huang (*et al.* 1984) made a new classification and presented excellent pictures of cases, which resemble tumors. Medullary venous malformations may be multiple and mimick multiple metastases. The predilection site for these malformations is the paraventricular area (along the superior lateral corner of the lateral ventricle), and any enhancing lesion with no evidence of a mass effect at the ventricular corner should, according to Huang (*et al.* 1984), lead one to suspect a medullary venous malformation. Cavernous venous malformations are most frequently encountered in subcortical white matter and the pons. Angiograms are usually negative, and postcontrast CT scanning will show marked enhancement (particularly with delayed scanning). If there is one reason to perform angiography before carrying out a biopsy, it is this possibility of coming

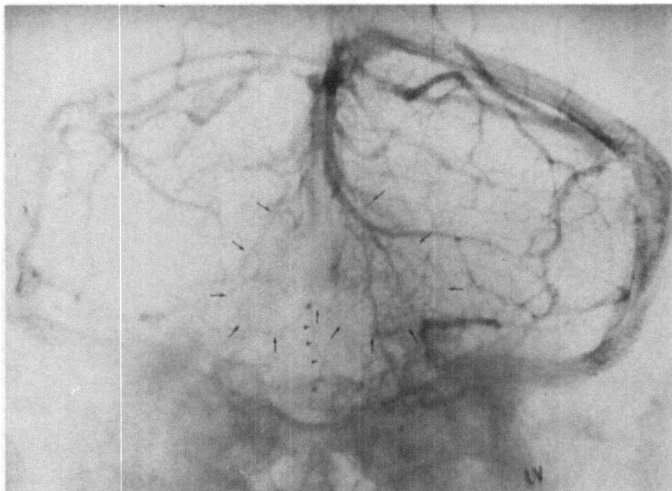

Fig. 121. Angiography (left vertebral, Towne position, venous phase) of case presented in Fig. 120: mesencephalic venous malformation. Arrows indicate contour of mesencephalon with lateral mesencephalic veins; arrow-heads indicate the anterior pontomesencephalic vein, which is slightly displaced. Note venous blush on left side

across some venous malformation, as is shown in one personal case (Figs. 120 and 121).

## B. False Positive and False Negative Results

In diagnostic stereotactics biopsy may sometimes lead to false positive and false negative results. These two problems will be discussed, because they—though infrequently—bother the surgeon when discovered as such, and may delude him when not discovered (see for review: Kleihues *et al.* 1984).

As *false positive* we define a histological diagnosis, revealing a pathological entity that is afterwards proved to be untrue. Edner (1981) defines false positive as misinterpretation. False positive results are very rare. In our own experience we have only 3 cases/250 biopsies (less than 1.5%), in which follow-up revealed other histological diagnoses. In 2 cases autopsy gave malignant lymphoma, whereas at biopsy a diagnosis of malignant astrocytoma was made. The other case was a pineal tumor, diagnosed as a pinealoma, that later on proved to be a dysgerminoma with multiple lesions by ventricular dissimination. In the other important biopsy studies the percentage was 0% in 35 cases (Broggi and Franzini 1981), 0% in 302 cases (Ostertag *et al.* 1980) and 2.7% in 345 cases (Edner 1981). Although these figures do not have much significance (in the series with 0% the possibility wasn't even considered), an overall percentage of about 2% seems to be false positive.

*False negative* results are encountered in those cases, where the pathological report states that normal or non-conclusive tissue has been found, whilst clinical picture, follow-up, or CT abnormalities disclose clear pathology. False negative results are obtained much more frequently in stereotactic biopsy as compared with false positive. Reasons for this are manyfold: technical failures; sampling errors; non-conclusive material and no material at all.

Technical failures are decreasing in frequency thanks to better CT localization facilities, although even minimal technical errors in calculation and positioning of the aiming device may lead to biopsy outside the target. In our own experience this has only once occurred; Edner (1981) mentioned 3/345. This possibility therefore is less than 1%. With the high resolution scanners nowadays available technical failures will become negligible.

The problem of sampling errors, however, is more important. Sampling errors may happen likewise in open surgery and lead to misinterpretation as the representative material is not taken. Sometimes these errors may even happen in the laboratory, when the pathologist does not examine all the given material. In as much as it is an accepted rule in histopathological diagnosis to grade malignancy according to the most malignant tumor part, the final diagnosis depends completely on the specimens obtained. Therefore, sometimes histological diagnosis may yield a grade 2 astrocytoma, although the surgeon suspects a truly malignant tumor on the basis of angiographic features and/or surrounding edema on CT. These cases should, however, not be listed as false negative but as positive with a dubious grading. A histological diagnosis of *normal* tissue, that is to be interpreted as false negative result, is obtained in cases of hamartomas (mostly lying in the floor of the third ventricle), and in cystic lesions, if the specimen of the cyst wall is normal. Often the cyst wall is abnormal, however, and the contents may be highly suggestive for a certain diagnosis (clear yellow and rapidly clotting in cystic astrocytoma; motoroil appearance in craniopharyngioma).

A nonconclusive diagnosis is found in highly malignant tumors when only necrotic material is obtained (metastasis and malignant glioma). As Apuzzo and Sabshin (1983) point out, this is due to obtaining biopsies from nonenhancing tumor regions (4/44 in their biopsy material).

To minimize this possibility we normally take three biopsies in one trajectory to make sure the whole mass lesion is penetrated. However, if only necrotic material is obtained, the differentiation between primary and metastatic malignancy is impossible.

Sometimes, massive gliosis is found without conclusive tissue.

"No material at all" is a possibility, that should also be kept in mind. The

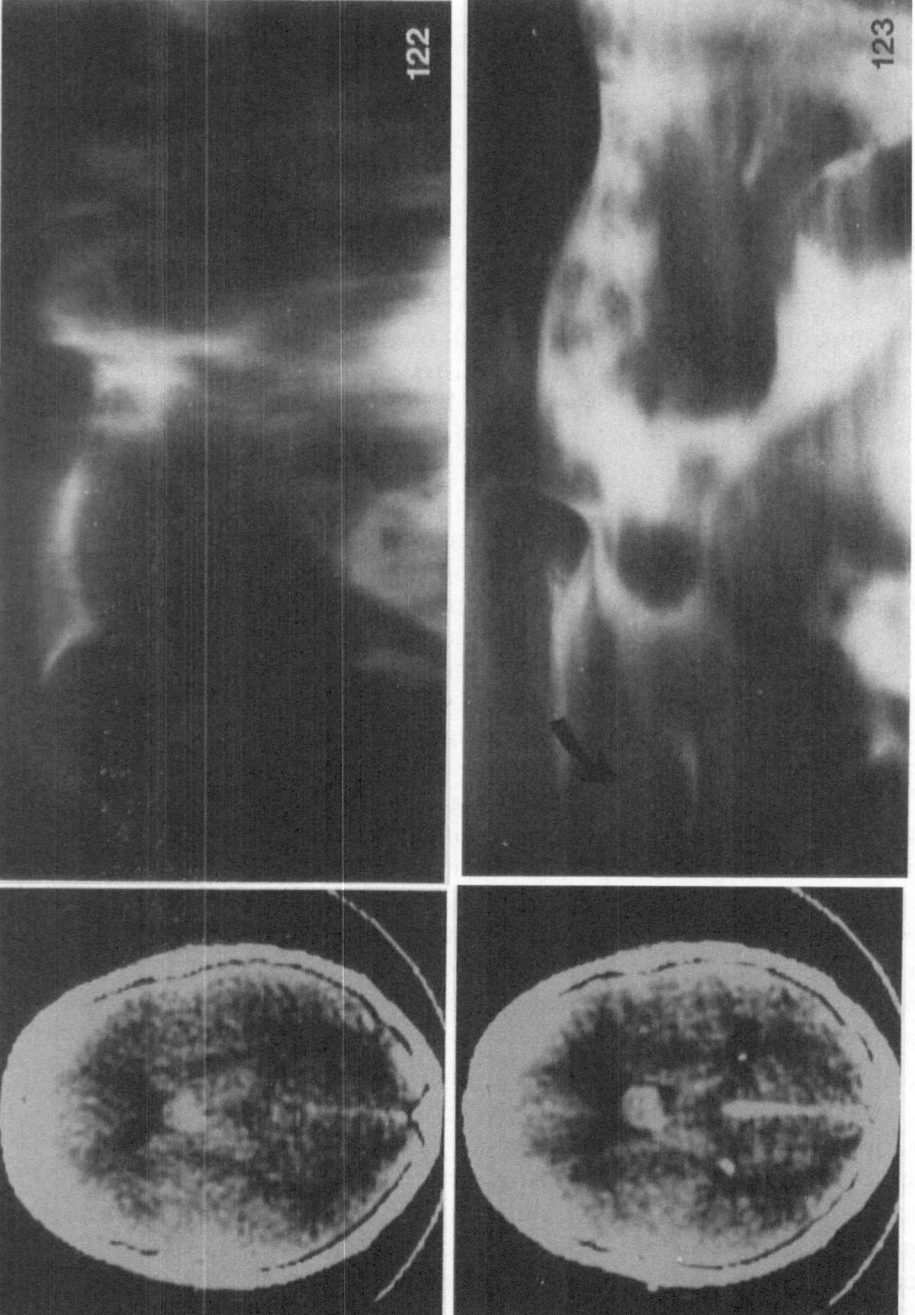

Fig. 122. CT scan (precontrast) and cisternography with positive contrast, showing a "tumor" in the anterior third ventricle (arrow)

Fig. 123. CT scan (postcontrast) and ventriculography with positive contrast of case presented in Fig. 122. Angiography showed no evident abnormalities. A stereotactic biopsy was carried out (arrow) and nonconclusive material was found at histological examination. A presumptive diagnosis of hematoma due to vascular malformation was made. Later on the lesion had simply disappeared

consistence of the target tissue may be so tough, that no specimen can be obtained with the spiral needle or aspiration techniques. ˞

A stereotactic forceps would be necessary, but tearing should be avoided. Ostertag (*et al.* 1980) used a specially designed forceps (Riechert *et al.* 1967) and published a percentage of non-conclusive results in 8.7% : in 26/302 biopsy cases they found only gliosis. Apuzzo and Sabshin (1983) used a 1 mm flexible cup bronchoscopy forceps through a cannula and

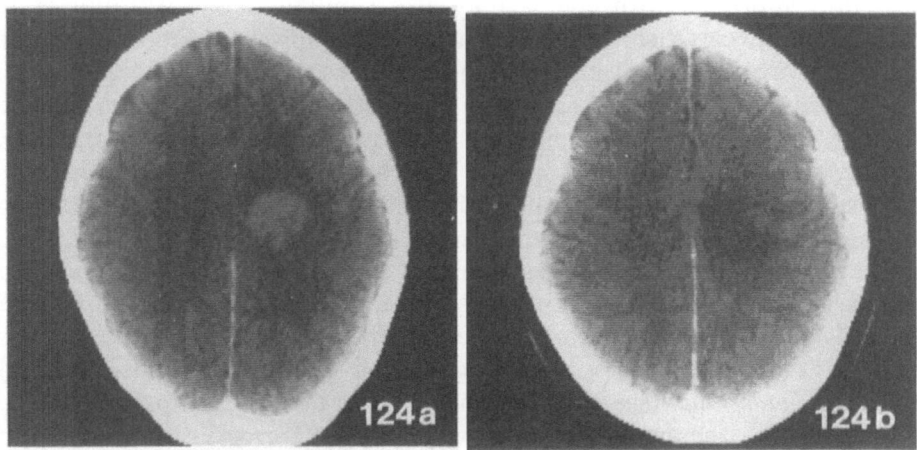

Fig. 124. CT scan pictures (postcontrast) showing a recent infarction (a), and after 2 weeks a disappearance of the hyperdense zone (b)

obtained nondiagnostic (necrotic) tissue in 11% (4/44). Edner (1981) noted a 9% of false negative results. Kleihues (*et al.* 1984) presented a percentage of 2.5% (15/600). In our own series we have 9 cases with "normal" tissue (of which 4 are believed to be third ventricle hamartomas and 5 tumors with non-conclusive material—some gliosis—), and 7 specimens that contained only necrotic tissue. Our percentage for false negative results is therefore 6.4% (16/250 cases). Moreover, we found 3 hematomas and 4 infarctions, which have been established by consecutive CT controls (Figs. 122 and 123). For detailed discussion the reader is referred to chapter 10, sub II.

## C. Unsuspected Mass Lesions

Besides unsuspected metastasis and infectious lesions, in *multiple sclerosis* plaques may present a pitfall, as they sometimes resemble cerebral tumors (Sagar *et al.* 1982, Wang *et al.* 1983). Although many reports on computed tomography in multiple sclerosis stress, that enhancing plaques are distinguishable from tumors by their lacking a mass effect, both Sagar (*et al.* 1982) and Wang (*et al.* 1983) present 3 histologically confirmed cases with acute demyelinating disease with enhancing lesions and mass effect on CT. From their photopresentation it is evident, that a diagnosis of tumor was made (eventually multiple cerebral metastases), whereas the clinical picture with headache, epileptic seizures and aphasia also suggested tumor growth. These authors performed both open and needle biopsy, and histological diagnosis of acute demyelinating disease was made (almost total lack of stainable myelin and perivascular cuffs of lymphocytes). Cerebral *infarction* with edema may also simulate cerebral tumor (Fig. 124 a). The development of signs and symptoms, however, is more explosive and therefore the clinical state will lead to the suspicion of a vascular lesion. In this case a follow-up CT scan may be expected before a decision is made to take a biopsy. The mass effect has disappeared after two weeks (Fig. 124 b), and the patient will improve. Very seldom intracerebral *hematoma* may simulate a neoplasm, as shown by Shinn-Zong Lin (*et al.* 1984). Ring formation on computerized tomography is often seen in the postoperative patient (Grand *et al.* 1978), particularly after clot evacuation, and also during the period of hematoma resolution. This picture should not be misjudged and held for a tumor, as stereotactic biopsy will only show gliosis indicating an active process of healing. Whenever a mass lesion is suspected to be an *epidermoid* (see Fig. 72), the samples taken at biopsy should be managed with the smear preparation technique to make the cholesterin visible; this is no longer possible after the chemical procedures of embedding for histological examination (Ostertag *et al.* 1980).

In conclusion, pitfalls regarding both the stereotactic technique and the underlying pathology are presented. To prevent the sampling of non-conclusive material and to avoid problems in localization, CT guided techniques have been developed (chapter 4). On the other hand, the surgeon himself should be aware of the various diagnostic entities that may lie behind the mass lesion the CT scanner shows. Moreover, enhancement after the administration of a contrast medium is also frequently seen in infectious disease (herpes simplex encephalitis: Lunsford *et al.* 1984 b; acute hemorrhagic leukoencephalitis: Valentine *et al.* 1982).

# Chapter 9

# Functional Stereotactics

In chapter 3 we discussed the five fields of functional stereotactics with the purpose to give a short review of the diseases, which may be treated with stereotactic techniques. It should be emphasized, however, that in the fields of epilepsy, psychiatric illness and spasticity only a limited number of stereotactic centers is involved. Partly because of the fact, that in these fields centralization is obligatory, and partly because the indications are less obvious and therefore depend on clinical experience, skill and to a lesser degree also on local habits.

Particularly in psychiatric disorders—such as compulsory neurosis and drug addiction (or even sexual offences)—in many countries stereotactic surgery is no longer an accepted way of treatment. Psychiatrists prefer pharmacological treatment and indeed this modality should be tried extensively before a diagnosis of *otherwise intractable* illness is made. The effect of ventromedial hypothalamotomy in these syndromes has been recently discussed by Spiegel (1982, pp. 37–40). Orthner (1982) published a report on a group of 34 patients with sexual disorders, treated by lesions in the ventromedial nucleus of the hypothalamus with good to excellent results.

In our description of the more usual indications for functional stereotactics (chapter 5, sub I) particularly patients with *extrapyramidal* and *cerebellar tremor* and with *intractable pain* syndromes proved to be good candidates for stereotactic surgery. First of all, because the incidence of these syndromes is fairly high (the incidence of Parkinson disease being 120–160/100,000 in Caucasians and 36–65/100,000 in Japanese), and therefore clinicians are familiar with these patients. Secondly, because the research and clinical experience with these entities are extensive and stereotactic interventions can offer reliable results.

In this chapter we like to present both our own experience and that of other authors on the two mentioned subjects. For technical details the reader is referred to chapter 7, sub II B.

## I. Extrapyramidal and Cerebellar Tremor

In 1963 Gybels has already published experimental data on the mechanism of parkinsonian tremor, in which he showed that a similar tremor can be induced experimentally in monkeys by a small lesion in the medio-ventral part of one side of the midbrain. He also pointed out the importance of the spinal reflex loop (the level of muscle tone) for the periodicity of the tremor. Recent experiences with stereotactic surgery in tremor led Narabayashi and Ohye (1978) to the conclusion that tremor-driving impulses almost certainly originate in the nucleus ventralis inter-medius (Vim) of the thalamus, whereas the spinal reflex loop is responsable for rhythm setting since it modulates the frequency. There is strong evidence that proprioceptive or kinesthetic sense, perhaps mainly muscle afferents, project to nucleus Vim of the thalamus.

When these two parts are in synchrony, according to these authors the tremor—whether postural or at rest—will be constant and rhythmic. Nucleus Vim lies slightly posterior to the ventrolateral nucleus (about 2 mm) and anterior to the ventroposterior nuclei, as is clearly outlined in the 3-dimensional diagram in their publication (Narabayashi and Ohye 1978). The coordinates for the nucleus Vim are: about 4/5 of the distance AC—PC behind AC, and 1–3 mm above the AC—PC line with a lateral coordinate of about 8 mm (Fig. 106). On the other hand, Hassler (et al. 1979) stresses, that the lesion should be placed slightly more anterior, namely in the nucleus Vop (ventralis oralis posterior = ventralis lateralis) to achieve abolishment of tremor without the danger of disturbing the speed and precision of hand and finger movements due to lesioning proprioceptive mechanisms. Also Van Manen (et al. 1984) prefers this more anterior target; the coordinates for the nucleus Vop are: about 3/5 of the distance AC—PC behind AC, and 3 mm above the AC—PC line with a lateral coordinate of about 13–15 mm (see Fig. 106). Recently Laitinen (1985) reviewed the various targets.

In Parkinson's disease the introduction of L-dopa has changed the indications for surgical interventions to a great extent. This drug is very effective in relieving most of the manifestations of the syndrome, but without altering the progression of the disease and with comparatively little effect on the tremor. Furthermore, in most patients, L-dopa becomes progressively ineffective after a few years, which warrants reservedness in starting L-dopa therapy (Kelly and Gillingham 1980). Long-term L-dopa therapy will also lead to serious side-effects, such as dyskinesia and psychosis. As L-dopa is particularly helpful in the treatment of bradyki-nesia, and as tremor and rigidity usually appear earlier in the course of the disease, it seems reasonable to re-introduce stereotactic surgery as an accepted way of treatment for patients, whose disability is due to tremor and rigidity. Later on in the course of the disease, when bradykinesia develops, L-dopa may be instituted, thus saving some years of active life for these Parkinson patients (Bosch et al. 1983, Gildenberg 1984, Kelly and Gillingham 1980, Matsumoto et al. 1984, Van Manen et al. 1984). Guiot (et al. 1976) also points out the complementary roles of stereotactic surgery and

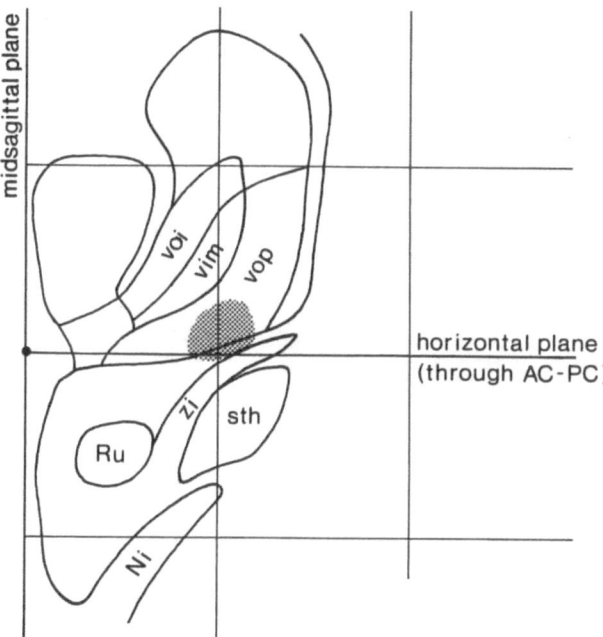

Fig. 125. Line drawing illustrating the topographical anatomy of the ventrolateral thalamus (after Schaltenbrand and Wahren 1977, Plate 27. With permission). Frontal section with 1 cm grid. The target area for thalamotomy in the treatment of tremor is indicated. For abbreviations see Fig. 29

pharmacological treatment, which issue has recently led more authors to recommend a protocol for a combined treatment. Because the efficacy of stereotactic thalamic surgery with lesioning of the Vop or Vim nucleus on the contralateral side is undoubtedly evident in the treatment of tremor and rigidity, Matsumoto (*et al.* 1984) advocates after 15 years' experience with L-dopa therapy and over 1,400 cases of Vl (= Vop) thalamotomies, to postpone drug institution as long as possible. This strategy leads to treatment with anticholinergic drugs prior to surgery and L-dopa institution only after surgery. It is self-evident, that delay of L-dopa treatment, until the patient shows marked bradykinesia, will also postpone the "long-term levodopa syndrome" of hyperkinesia and on-off phenomena, including mental changes and hallucinations which are often irreversible (Kelly 1983). Moreover, the response to L-dopa is no better in patients who did not undergo thalamic surgery (Hughes *et al.* 1971), while on the other hand dopa-induced hyperkinesia seems to occur less frequently at the operated side (Kelly and Gillingham 1980, Van Manen *et al.* 1984). Both conclusions being reasons to favour the proposed protocol of combined treatment (Gildenberg 1984, Narabayashi *et al.* 1984).

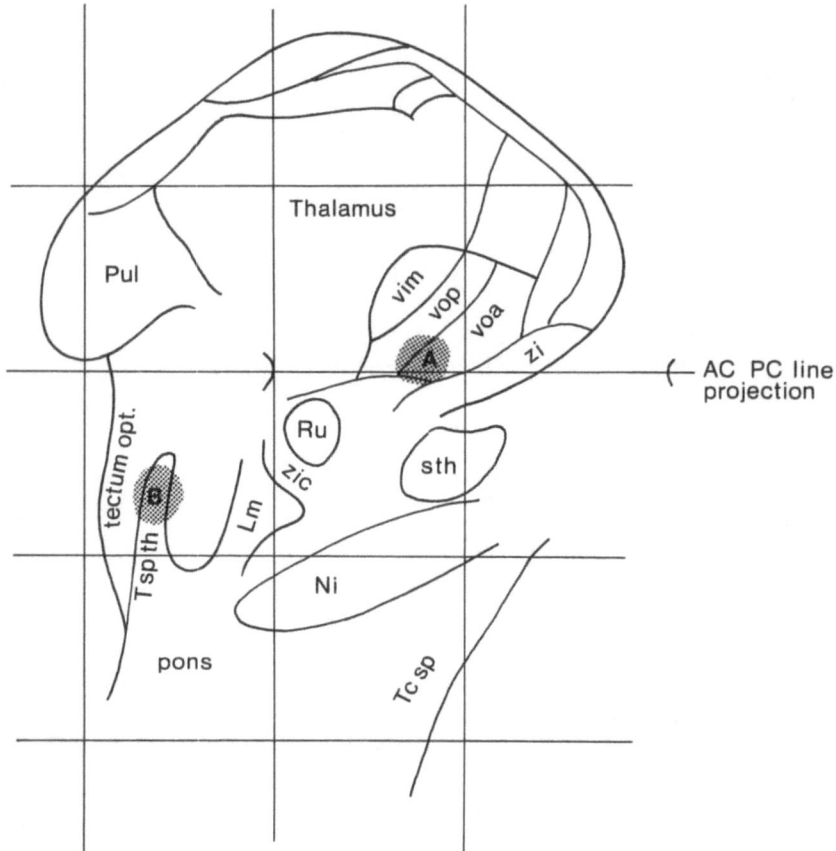

Fig. 126. Line drawing illustrating the topographical anatomy of the ventrolateral thalamus and mesencephalon in sagittal section with a lateral coordinate of 9 mm (after Schaltenbrand and Wahren 1977, Plate 41. With permission). With 1 cm grid. Target area for thalamotomy in tremor treatment is indicated in *A*, and target area in mesencephalotomy for pain in *B*. For abbreviations see Figs. 29 and 30

As is already discussed (chapter 5, sub I), *cerebellar tremor* benefits likewise from thalamic surgery. The target for lesioning is identical, since both the cerebellothalamocortical connections and the pallidothalamocortical fibers run through the target area (Figs. 125 and 126).

## A. Stereotactic Thalamotomy Prior to L-dopa Institution

Although the benefits seem to be greater in Japanese than in Caucasians (Matsumoto *et al.* 1984), nothing points to the possibility that the percentage of benign cases of parkinsonism is higher in Japanese. Some cases, however, run a rather malignant course. These patients are no suitable candidates for surgery or even successful L-dopa administration. In the slowly progressive cases surgical results on tremor and rigidity are very satisfactory, as is evident from many reports. In 90% of the patients the contralateral tremor is abolished after 2 years, and in about 60% after 10 years, whereas in 88% of the patients rigidity in the contralateral side was abolished after 2 years and in about 55% after 10 years (Kelly and Gillingham 1980). Matsumoto (et al. 1984) showed complete alleviation of tremor and rigidity in 61/78 cases (78%) belonging to the grades I–III (according to Hoehn and Yahr 1967), and in only 2/25 cases (8%) in grade IV. The success rate for tremor and rigidity was not significantly less after a second surgical procedure on the other side, as shown in 24 cases with bilateral thalamotomies reported by Kelly and Gillingham (1980). On the other hand, it is well-known, that bilateral surgery is not infrequently associated with speech disturbances, such as reduced voice volume and word blocking (thalamic dysarthria). From the literature it is known, that such speech disorders may follow many other thalamic lesions in the dominant hemisphere (tumors, hemorrhage). Archer (et al. 1981) gives a beautiful description of such a case of thalamic stroke with CT stereotactic localization. Speech complications have become less frequent in recent years with the use of electrical investigation of the target structure and more precise and small lesions. Since the introduction of the micro-electrode technique it has become possible to register the fieldpotential of neurons through a 5–7 micrometer electrode tip at the target site. The firing pattern of any thalamic nucleus can be recorded in that way, and nucleus Vim localized by its synchronous firing with the peripheral tremulous movements (Narabayashi 1983). Small electrocoagulation lesions (with RF heating to 65 °C during 1 minute) in this nucleus will abolish the tremor immediately. Similar rhythmical activity has been recorded in nucleus Vop, however. If lesions are to be made on both sides, Gildenberg (1984) advocates asymmetrical lesions to minimize the risk of side effects to mentation and verbalization.

In order to keep the lesion within the target area, the stereotactic surgeon should be informed about the position of the medial internal capsular border (which is the lateral thalamic border). Hardy (et al. 1979) calculated its position in 130 patients and concluded that this border is lying between 16 and 23 mm lateral from the midplane, depending mainly on the width of the third ventricle. Hitchcock and Cadavid (1984) reviewed 111 normal CT scans and concluded, that pre-operative assessment of the thalamo-capsular distance will much improve the accuracy of the otherwise empiral lateral coordinate.

In his monograph on stereotactic neurosurgery Spiegel (1982) discussed the various targets inside the thalamic complex which have been tried in the last decennia without making a clear choice. From recent studies it has become evident, however, that the target should lie in the Vop or Vim nucleus (Bosch *et al.* 1983, Kelly and Gillingham 1980, Matsumoto *et al.* 1984, Narabayashi 1983, Van Manen *et al.* 1984, Walker 1982 b).

## B. Stereotactic Thalamotomy After L-dopa Institution

Both Spiegel (1982) and Walker (1982 b) recommend conservative treatment *including L-dopa* before a stereotactic operation is considered. We shared their opinion in former years, but due to the serious side-effects which follow protracted medical treatment with L-dopa, have changed our course performing surgery at an earlier stage. After L-dopa treatment during a long period the results of thalamotomy are not as satisfactory according to Matsumoto (*et al.* 1984); our own results in a publication on 18 patients (Bosch *et al.* 1983) confirm this opinion. Especially, the onset or aggravation of tremor on the ipsilateral (non-operated) side is striking (up to 44% according to Van Manen *et al.* 1984) and its mechanism is not clearly understood. Our study is of particular value, because it reports the results of thalamotomy (chiefly at the target Vim) in 18 patients after protracted L-dopa therapy (Figs. 127 and 128). The only comparable study is published by Van Manen (*et al.* 1984) with 32 patients after protracted L-dopa therapy; thalamotomy was carried out chiefly in the nucleus Vop. Impressive is the aggravation of ipsilateral tremor, which was found in 8/18 cases, leading to a percentage of 44%, being the same as found by Van Manen. This aggravation or even appearance of ipsilateral tremor might be considered as L-dopa induced or L-dopa dependent, because in cases which had surgery prior to L-dopa institution this phenomenon is not observed. The decrease in daily intake of L-dopa after surgery (as shown in Table 3) is certainly a positive side-effect.

The results on our patients were assessed between 1 and 3 years postoperatively. There was no postoperative death, which is in conformity with the very low mortality rate in other reports (1 to 0% ; Gildenberg 1984). Postoperative confusion and somnolence was noted in 17% and disappeared within a week. On the treated side the tremor was abolished in 83% and rigidity clearly diminished in 50%. Concerning the other effects, including gait disturbances, dexterity of hand and fingers, speech problems, validity and finally the judgement by the patient himself, the reader is referred to Table 3. Besides the already discussed striking exaggeration of tremor at the untreated side, two other conclusions can be drawn. *Firstly*, 14 out of the 18 patients (78%) were satisfied with the obtained results, which is amazing considering the worsening of the untreated side. *Secondly*, in 12/18 cases (66.6%) the L-dopa (and other drug-) medication could be lowered substantially. In the discussion of the overall results of thalamotomy we also

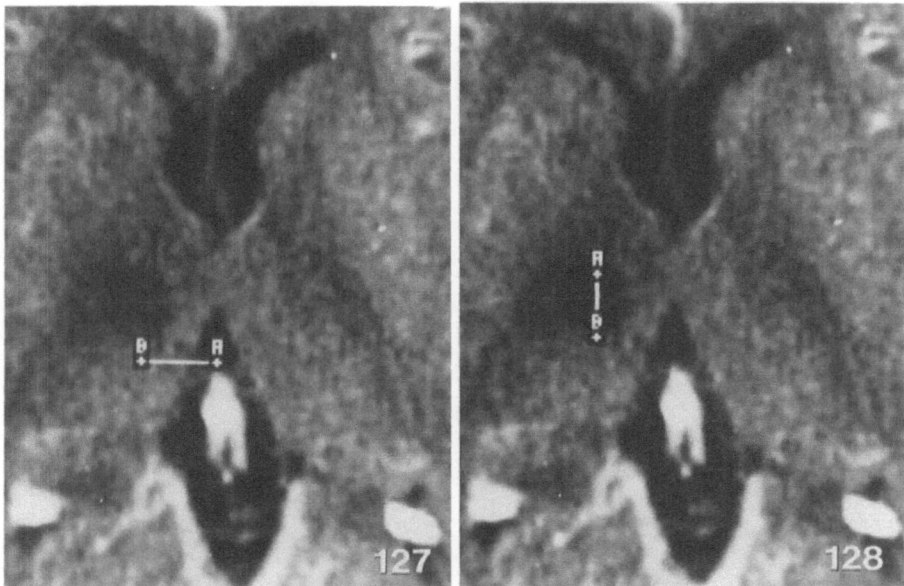

Fig. 127. CT scan picture of lesion after thermocoagulation for treatment of tremor in Parkinson patient. *A–B* is indicating the lateral coordinate (11.3 mm)

Fig. 128. Same case as in Fig. 127. *A–B* is indicating the diameter of the lesion (9.4 mm), as measured 1 week after coagulation

like to stress the great importance of rehabilitation programs, because after surgery some neglect may be seen concerning the treated limbs, a situation which requires training to regain full motor function. Particularly the speed and precision of hand and finger movements ("dexterity") may be decreased after thalamotomy (11/18 of our cases—61%); according to Van Manen (*et al.* 1984) defective hand movements might be seen less frequently with lesions of the nucleus Vop.

To summarize, the ideal candidate for thalamotomy is mentally alert and has unilateral or predominantly unilateral tremor and rigidity. In our opinion the institution of L-dopa therapy should be postponed until it is inevitable because of severe bradykinesia. The patient should take some anticholinergic agents as long as possible. Surgery should always be followed by an intensive rehabilitation program, to achieve maximum validity and dexterity.

## II. Intractable Pain Syndromes

As discussed in chapter 5, sub I B 1 and 2, ablative stereotactic interventions should not be carried out in the "benign" chronic intractable pain syndromes, because life expectancy is normal. Ablative surgery

Table 3. *Our Own Results with Stereotactic Thalamotomy After Protracted L-dopa Treatment (Target Vim)*

| | Sex | Age | Target | Tremor | | Rigid-ity | Dis-turbed gait | Dexte-rity | Dis-turbed speech | Valid-ity | Pa-tient's judge-ment | Medical treatment pre- | post- | Illness pro-gression |
|---|---|---|---|---|---|---|---|---|---|---|---|---|---|---|
| 1 | ♂ | 65 | L* | $r_{00}$ | $l_0$ | —\|— | = | — | + | ↗ | ↗ | eldopa 1,750 disipal 150 | symmetrel 300 parlodel 80 | + |
| 2 | ♀ | 68 | L* | $r_{00}$ | $1_+$ | —\|— | = | — | = | ↗ | ↗ | symmetrel 200 kemadrin 15 | = | + |
| 3 | ♂ | 63 | L* | $r_{00}$ | $1_+$ | —\|— | — | — | = | ↗ | ↗ | madopar 1,125 | madopar 125 cogentin 2 | + |
| 4 | ♀ | 62 | L* | $r_{00}$ | $1_+$ | —\|— | = | = | = | ↗ | ↗ | sinemet 962 symmetrel 200 | sinemet 825 disipal 150 | ++ |
| 5 | ♀ | 61 | R L* | $l_{00}$ $l_{00}$ | $r_+$ $r\_\_$ | —\| | = | — | + | ↗ | ↗ | sinemet 1,237 | sinemet 550 parlodel 50 | + |
| 6 | ♂ | 63 | R | $l\_\_$ | $r_{++}$ | — | = | = | = | ↗ | ↗ | sinemet 825 cogentin 2 | disipal 150 | + |

| No. | Sex | Age | Side | | | | | | | | | | Drug | Drug | |
|---|---|---|---|---|---|---|---|---|---|---|---|---|---|---|---|
| 7 | ♂ | 60 | L* | r00 | 1+ | = | = | = | + | ↗ | ↗ | madopar 1,000 | madopar 750 | + |
| 8 | ♂ | 49 | L* | r++ | 1++ | = | ++ | — | ++ | ↗ | ↗ | sinemet 1,100 | rivotril 2 | ++ |
| 9 | ♂ | 53 | L* | r_ | 1++ | = | ++ | — | + | ↗ | ↗ | sinemet 825 | 0 | + |
| 10 | ♂ | 71 | L* | r00 | 1= | = | = | — | = | ↗ | ↗ | cogentin 3 disipal 150 | disipal 150 | + |
| 11 | ♂ | 65 | L* | r00 | 1++ | ? psychotic reaction | ? | ? | 0 | 0 | ↗ | madopar 625 | = | ++ |
| 12 | ♀ | 50 | L* | r00 | 1+ | = | — | — | 0 | ↗ | ↗↗ | madopar 1,000 | symmetrel 200 | ± |
| 13 | ♂ | 47 | R | l00 | r+ | = | = | + | = | ↗ | ↗↗ | madopar 750 | madopar 250 | ± |
| 14 | ♂ | 56 | R* | l00 | r= | — | = | = | ± | ↗ | ↗ | sinemet 550 | sinemet 825 symmetrel 200 | + |
| 15 | ♂ | 55 | R | l00 | r= | = | + | — | = | ↗ | ↗ | madopar 250 | madopar 250 | + |
| 16 | ♂ | 69 | L* | r00 | 1_ | — | = | — | ± | ↗ | ↗ | norflex 200 | 0 | + |
| 17 | ♀ | 60 | R | l00 | r+ | + | — | — | = | ↗ | ↗ | sinemet 825 | sinemet 412 | ++ |
| 18 | ♂ | 54 | L | r00 | 1++ | — | = | — | 0 | = | ↗ | parlodel 30 | = | + |

Abbreviations: + aggravated; ++ much aggravated; — diminished; —— much diminished; = the same; 0 absent; 00 abolished; ? no assessment possible; * dominant side; ↗ better; ↗↗ much better; ↘ worse; ↘↘ much worse.

Electrode tip diameter 2.1 mm; tip exposure length 2.5 mm.

resulting in a lesion in the pain conducting pathways (as on the spinal level with percutaneous cordotomy) on the other hand is very effective but produces no long lasting pain relief: about 1–2 years at the most. Although many reports (see chapter 3) describe pain relief for sometimes considerably longer periods of time, results on individual patients are no longer reliable after 1–2 years. Even in those cases where the original pains are gone, the success is often eliminated by troubling dysesthesia (or central pain) leading to serious discomfort. Therefore, in cases with normal life expectancy inductive electrical stimulation of deep brain structures (as discussed in chapter 3) may be preferred as well as more peripheral neural stimulation, although the effectiveness is less certain and the underlying mechanisms still unexplained (neuroaugmentative surgery; Kelly 1983). Electrical stimulation with stereotactically placed electrodes is extensively discussed by Adams (et al. 1974), Adams and Hosobuchi (1977), Hosobuchi (1980) and Young (et al. 1985). The target of interest is the nucleus ventralis posterolateralis (VPL) of the thalamus in cases of central deafferentiation pain (such as the thalamic syndrome, anesthesia dolorosa, postherpetic neuralgia and phantom limb pain), and the periaqueductal grey matter (PAG) of the mesencephalon in pains of peripheral origin. For further reading see chapter 14, Sub II, on future applications. Not yet confirmed by others is Levin's conclusion (et al. 1983), that stereotactic chemical hypophysectomy is helpful in the thalamic syndrome.

   Ablative stereotactic surgery for pain syndromes comprises posterior thalamotomy (Cooper 1965 a, Riechert 1960, 1966, Voris and Whisler 1975), mesencephalotomy (Leksell 1966, Nashold 1975, Whisler and Voris 1978), a type of more medially placed (so-called extralemniscal) mesencephalotomy (Amano et al. 1980) and pontine tractotomy (Hitchcock 1973, Barberá et al. 1979). All these reports share the conclusion, that the best results are obtained in cancer pain, mainly because the relief will last during the period of survival. Thalamotomy carries the risk of a higher incidence of postoperative central dysesthesia as compared with mesencephalotomy (Tasker 1982), which is understandable since the first intervention *only partly* destroys a huge complex of somatosensory thalamic nuclei, whereas the latter will cover the whole spinothalamic tract. When studying the respective targets in the Atlasses of Emmers and Tasker (1975) and of Afshar (et al. 1978), the discrepancy between lesioning nuclear matter and tracts will become even more clear. Tasker (1982) also stresses the disappointing results of thalamotomy in dysesthetic (central) pain which will not be relieved by further iatrogenic deafferentiation. Lesions in the mesencephalon or pons will most probably not only include the neospinothalamic but also the paleospinothalamic (= spinoreticular) system, leading to both the destruction of the spinothalamic tract and the extralemniscal short fiber system (Noordenbos 1959, Bowsher and Albe-

Fessard 1963). Therefore the incidence of postoperative dysesthesias might be lower (Barberá *et al.* 1979).

## III. Brainstem Stereotactic Surgery in Cancer Pain

Nashold (1982), reviewing brainstem stereotactic procedures for pain relief, also discusses the importance of partially destroying the spinoreticular pathways plus the spinothalamic tract itself. These pathways may be responsible for the *pain suffering syndrome* and a lesion may reduce anxiety and relieve pain without producing a dense analgesia. However, in clinical practice the surgeon is faced with the problem, that after short-term excellent results unpredictable relapses may occur with (sometimes agonizing) central dysesthesias. Wycis and Spiegel (1962) reported, however, long-term relief in still 31% of 54 patients (over a 14-year-period).

The first indication for stereotactic brainstem procedures is pain of the head, neck, trunk and arm due to carcinoma. Even when pain is not restricted to one side of the body, a mesencephalotomy (eventually bilateral) is successful. Recently, Frank (*et al.* 1982) described 14 treated cases (3 bilaterally) with intractable cancer pain due to lung cancer with as good if not better results as with precutaneous cordotomy. The indication is only relative and in the opinion of the author almost never strong enough in cases of central pain syndromes, because the effect—if present—may fade away after some time, as is the case with peripherally originating benign pains. In fact, a mesencephalotomy has far less side-effects (paresis, bladder dysfunction) than a percutaneous cordotomy, and might therefore also be preferred in cancer pain of the lower limbs. The very precise localization that is possible with stereotactic techniques is responsible for its low morbidity and therefore cordotomies are less frequently performed when one has the choice between both techniques. Moreover, only one puncture track is made in mesencephalotomy, while sometimes many are required in cordotomy. The topographical organization of the different fibre tracts at the various levels (Fig. 67) is such, that there is a safe distance between the spinothalamic and pyramidal tracts in the mesencephalon as compared with the high cervical level. The spinothalamic tract runs throughout the mesencephalon at about 8 mm from the midsagittal plane and the target of choice is situated at about 5 mm posterior and ventral to the posterior commissure (Figs. 129 and 126). When stereotactic mesencephalotomy was first carried out (Spiegel and Wycis 1948) the lesion electrode was introduced using a parieto-occipital approach; this route sometimes produced contralateral weakness of the lower limb, caused by injuring the cortical leg area. Puncture through the quadrigeminal plate may lead to ocular dysfunction (paralysis of vertical gaze; myotic pupils; convergence defects; skew deviation), which almost always disappears within a short

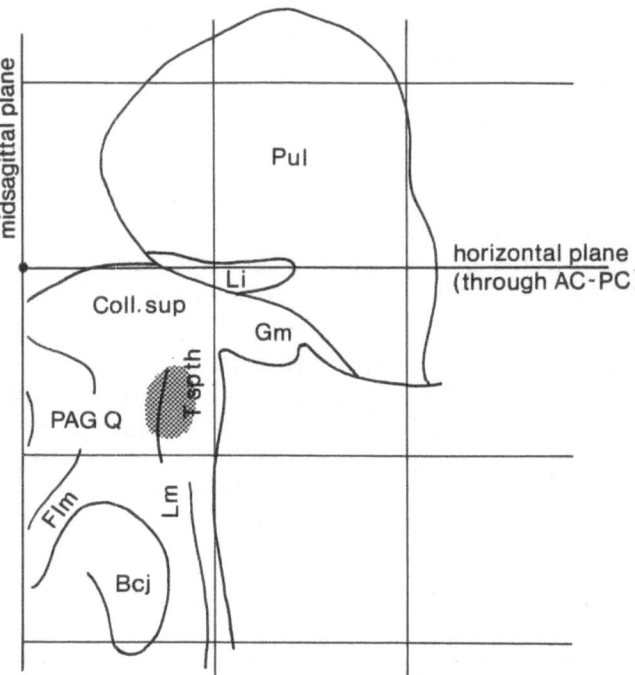

Fig. 129. Line drawing illustrating the topographical anatomy of the rostral mesencephalon (after Schaltenbrand and Wahren 1977, Plate 29. With permission). Frontal section with 1 cm grid. The target area for stereotactic mesencephalotomy is indicated. For abbreviations see Fig. 30

period of time. In recent reports (Nashold 1982, Amano *et al.* 1980, Whisler and Voris 1978) the frontal route is recommended and a burrhole is made more frontal to obtain a puncture track through the third ventricle which intrudes the mesencephalon parallel and at the level of the aqueduct. Ocular symptoms will only seldom be seen and lower limb weakness is never observed with this trajectory (our own results; Fig. 130). Surgery is advocated under local anesthesia to enable careful physiological control of lesion placement, which includes electrical stimulation. According to Nashold (*et al.* 1969), extensive mesencephalic stimulation studies could delineate a more precise organization of somatototrophic regions in the dorsal midbrain. Head, neck and limbs are represented more laterally, while affective and emotional reactions were evoked by stimulation on the border of the periaqueductal grey (PAG), at which site the trunk has its representation. These electrically evoked responses enable the surgeon to place the lesion properly. Micro-electrode recordings were also used. For an overview of localization and lesion data (derived from various authors) the reader is referred to Nashold (1982). Thermistor electrodes (tip diameter

2.1 mm; tip exposure length 2.5 mm) are normally used, with RF heating to 65–75 °C during 30–60 seconds. A properly placed lesion will give instant pain relief without major analgesia. Sometimes the sensation of pinprick and temperature in the treated side will be clearly diminished. The more medially placed lesion will lead to less loss of these sensations and frequently to no clinically detectable analgesia at all. For patients with facial or oral carcinoma, who are anxious and suffer from pain, the more medial lesion is ideal, because it will interrupt both the trigeminothalamic and part of the spinoreticular (extralemniscal) pathways.

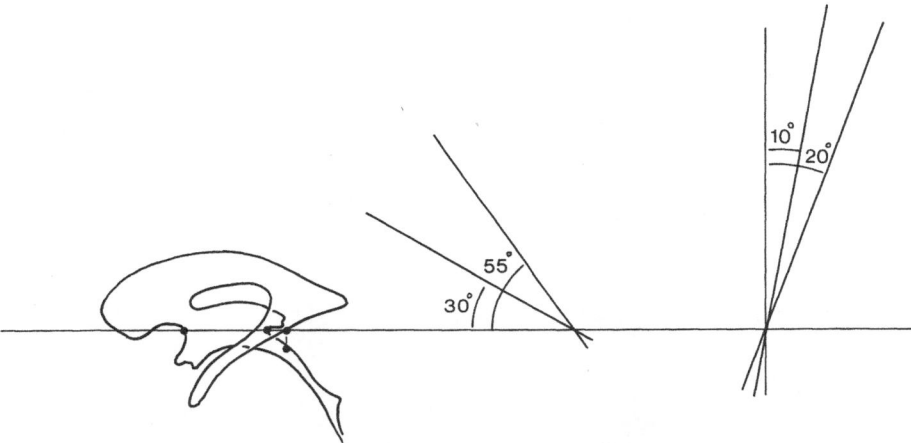

Fig. 130. Schematic drawing showing the target for mesencephalotomy on the lateral ventriculography view, with the variability in angles of electrode introduction (personal results)

Mortality rate following mesencephalotomy averages between 3% and 5%. In the 30 following consecutive cases (our own series), no mortality was met. The morbidity rate was higher (37%), although almost completely due to ocular dysfunction which disappeared within some weeks.

While using the frontal approach (burrhole at the hairbase) we had no cases of leg weakness. In about 50% we could clinically detect some degree of hypalgesia (pinprick and temperature) on the treated side, including the face. This hypalgesia, however, had a patchy distribution and showed no clear relation with the pain relief.

In this series, Table 4, we practiced general anesthesia, because the patients were in a rather bad clinical condition due to the underlying disease or were elderly. We felt that stimulation would threat their well-being as strong emotional reactions and fear may be evoked. For target localization we used intra-operative ventriculography (Figs. 131 and 132), followed by a CT scan of the brainstem after surgery (Fig. 133). This procedure led to

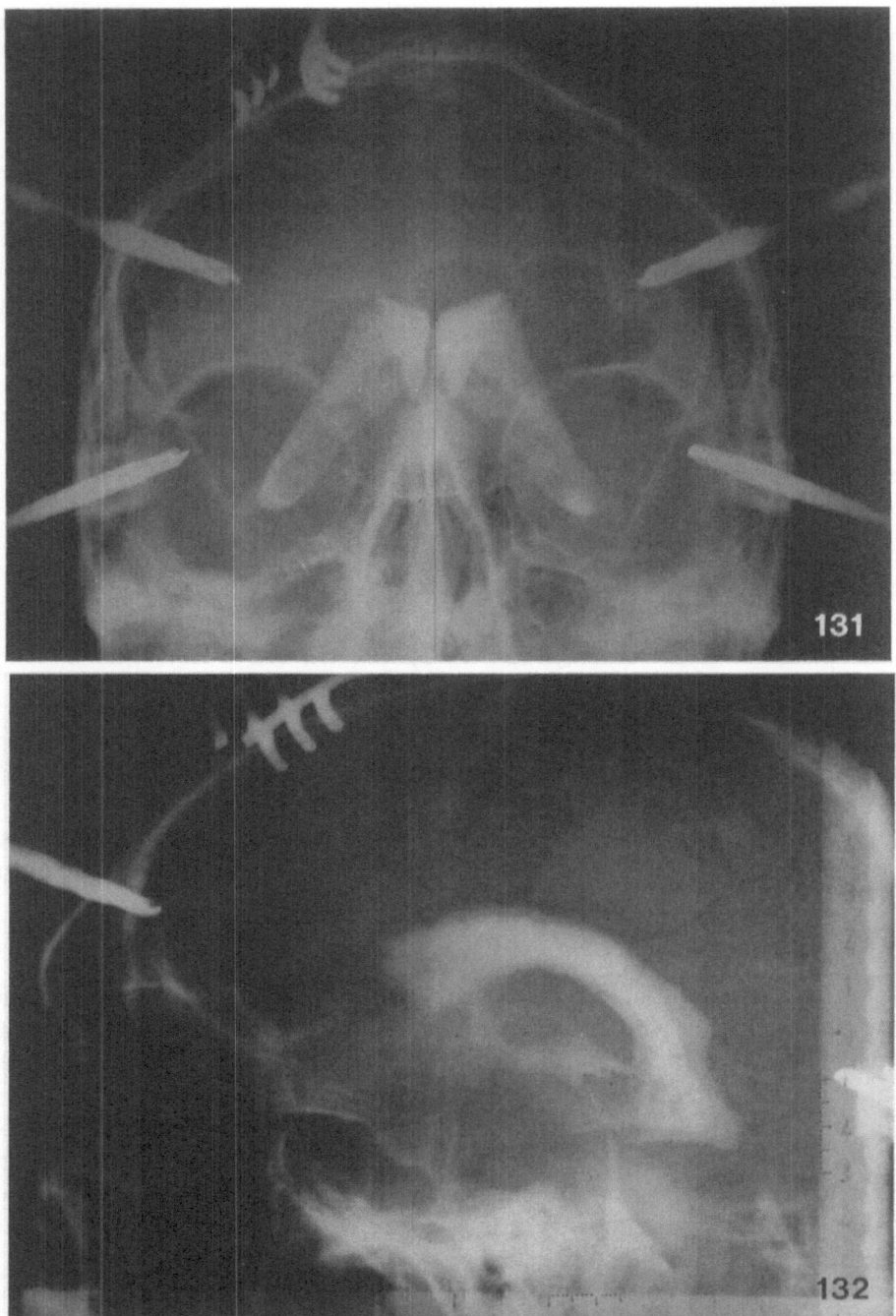

Fig. 131. Stereotactic ventriculography to calculate the target point in stereotactic mesencephalotomy (anteroposterior view)

Fig. 132. Stereotactic ventriculography, lateral view, showing black dots used to calculate target point position for mesencephalotomy

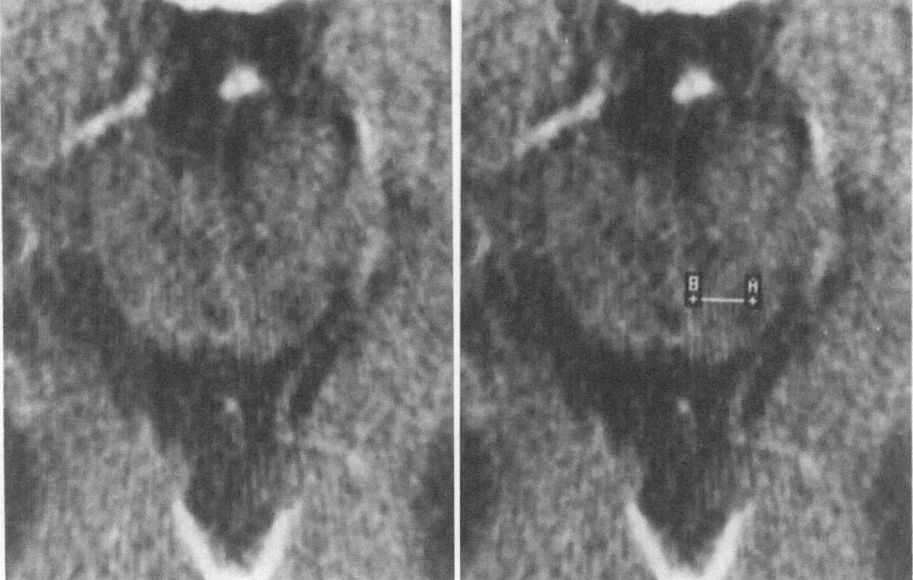

Fig. 133. CT scan picture of mesencephalon, 3 days after performing a stereotactic mesencephalotomy. A hypodense lesion is seen in the left side of the mesencephalon, at the level of the aqueduct. Computer calculation of the lateral coordinate (rightsided picture) gives: *A–B* is 6.4 mm

accurate target calculation and control of the lesion produced. As seen in the Table, our cases (hitherto unpublished) are mostly patients with cancer pains as well as some elderly patients with central pain syndromes. As might be expected, in the central pain cases the results are clearly less reliable (Nashold gives a success rate of only 50%; 1982), and the relief obtained will also wear off with time. Given these results mesencephalotomy in central pain is inadvisable on patients under the age of 70 years. Postoperative dysesthesia was met in 3 cases: 1 thalamic syndrome, 1 postherpetic neuralgia of the trunk and 1 facial postherpetic neuralgia. In the former two patients the dysesthesias were not serious, but the third patient still complains after 3 years of burning and itching sensations in her face. This was the only patient below the age of 70 years, for whom an operation was considered urgent due to serious pains that had otherwise led her to commit suicide. In cancer pains the relief was very satisfactory, except for in 1 case where the electrode did not function correctly. The follow-up period ranges from 3 years to some months and is of minor importance in those patients who do not survive for a longer period of time. In one case we tried to alleviate postoperative dysesthesias by performing a posterior thalamotomy after 1 year. This second intervention had no effect at all on the

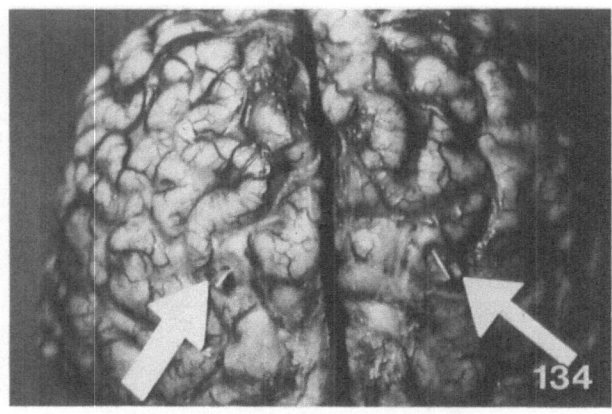

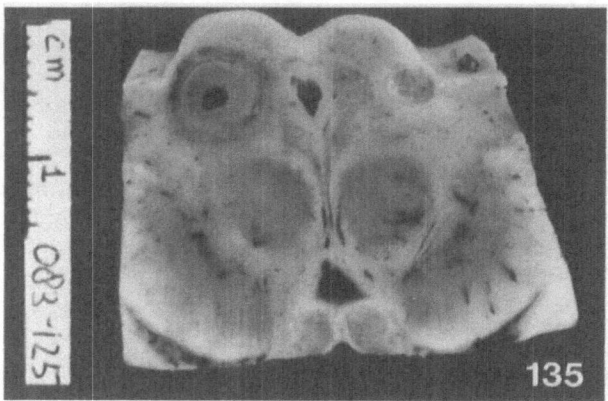

Fig. 134. Frontal brain surface at autopsy after performing a bilateral stereotactic mesencephalotomy. Arrows indicate electrode entrance points

Fig. 135. Specimen of rostral mesencephalon (case presented in Fig. 134), cut through the bilateral lesions. On the right side the first lesion is shown, made 4 months before death, having a diameter of about 4 mm. On the left side the second lesion is visible, made 1 month before death, having a diameter of about 7 mm. Note the relation to the periaqueductal grey. The active process of tissue repair on the left side is evident

suffering. A cervical midline myelotomy (as described by Hitchcock 1970 b, 1974, Schvarcz 1976) did not bring relief either. This case with postherpetic neuralgia of the flank is of particular interest, because the patient also suffered from a prostate carcinoma and a chronic lymphatic leukemia. The pain suffering syndrome has probably been induced by these other invalidating illnesses.

In two instances we performed a second intervention on the same side, since the first only showed a transient effect. This management seems

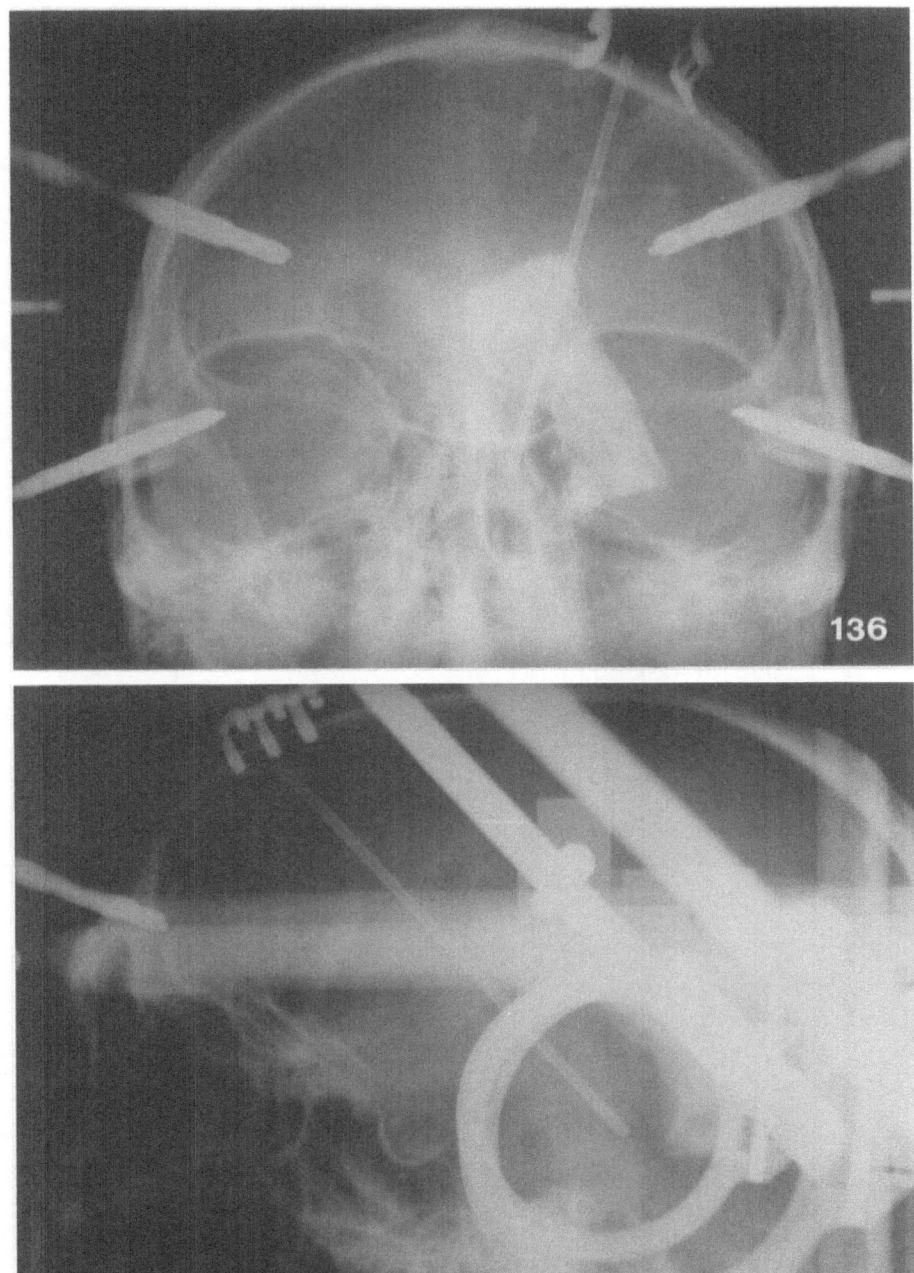

Fig. 136. The position of the lesioning electrode during the stereotactic performance; anteroposterior view

Fig. 137. Lateral view showing the lesioning electrode (tip diameter 2.1 mm) at the target

Table 4. *Our Own Results with Stereotactic Mesencephalotomy in the Treatment of Intractable Pain*

**Cancer pain (21 performances/18 cases)**

Follow-up until death (1–9 months)

| nr. | Sex | Age | Target | Result |
|---|---|---|---|---|
| 1 | ♂ | 50 | R | +++ |
|   |   |   | L | +++ |
| 2 | ♀ | 75 | L | ++ |
|   |   |   | repeated after 6 months | + |
| 3 | ♀ | 45 | R | +++ |
| 4 | ♂ | 76 | R | ++ |
| 5 | ♂ | 65 | L | ++ |
| 6 | ♀ | 75 | R | ++ |
| 7 | ♀ | 49 | L | ++ |
| 8 | ♀ | 68 | L | + |
| 9 | ♀ | 12 | L | +++ |
| 10 | ♀ | 64 | L | ± |
| 11 | ♂ | 70 | L | + |
| 12 | ♂ | 58 | L | + |
| 13 | ♂ | 68 | R (2 ×) | ++ |
| 14 | ♀ | 70 | R | +++ |
| 15 | ♂ | 51 | R | +++ |
| 16 | ♂ | 64 | L | ++ |
| 17 | ♂ | 73 | R | + |
| 18 | ♂ | 50 | L | + |

**Central pain syndromes (7 performances)**

| Sex | Age | Target | Short-term (< 3 months) Result | Long-term follow-up (> 1 year) Result | Postop. dysesthesia | |
|---|---|---|---|---|---|---|
| ♂ | 70 | R | + | 0 | + | thalamic syndrome |
| ♂ | 71 | R | 0 | 0 | 0 | |
| ♂ | 79 | L | ++ | 0 | 0 | trigeminal |
| ♀ | 76 | R | + | 0 | 0 | neuralgia |
| ♂ | 70 | R | ++ | 0 | + | postherpetic |
| ♀ | 64 | R | ++ | + | ++ | neuralgia |
| ♀ | 74 | L | 0 | 0 | 0 | phantom limb pain |

Abbreviations: pain relief; 0 absent; ± dubious; + moderate; ++ good; +++ complete.
Pain located in thoracic wall in cases 1, 8, 12, 13; in pelvis in cases 1, 2, 4, 9, 15, 17; in cervicobrachial plexus in cases 3, 5, 6, 7, 11, 14, 16, 18; in abdomen in case 10.

justified by the effectiveness of the second lesion we obtained. In one case we performed a bilateral mesencephalotomy, with a 2 months interval. This patient with thoracic and pelvic metastasis of carcinoma had no more pains; no narcotic analgesics were necessary any longer and he stayed ambulatory during the last months of his life. Autopsy could be carried out in this case (Fig. 134 and 135). From the figures it is clear, that the fresher lesion is still rather big and in a stage of tissue repair. Untoward sequelae from these lesions were not noted, which is highly interesting when the extent of the lesions is taken into consideration. In order to achieve long lasting relief we recently started performing mesencephalotomy with two lesions at the target site: the first at 2 mm behind and the second at 2 mm before the calculated target point. Both lesions are made with RF monopolar heating up to 75 °C during 60 sec (Figs. 136 and 137). We have the impression, that pain relief lasts longer this way. One of these cases, however, developed a rubral myoclonus, that had to be treated with clonazepam. Regarding the timing of this intervention, we believe mesencephalotomy should be performed prior to the institution of narcotic analgesics. In this way patients will be able to take care of themselves for as long as possible and not become bedridden at too early a stage.

In conclusion, stereotactic ablative surgery for pain should, at least theoretically, be reserved for the treatment of patients with cancer pains. The operation should be carried out prior to the institution of narcotic analgesics and should comprise no nuclear matter but the fiber tracts at the level of the mesencephalon (rostral part). Mesencephalotomy has certain advantages over percutaneous cordotomy regarding technical aspects (equally safe and easily performed under general anesthesia) plus the possibility of making lesions bilaterally. Side-effects are only of minor importance, a persistent diplopia being the worst. The use of general anesthesia seems to decrease the operative mortality rate and, moreover, shows no untoward effects on the pain relief obtained.

# Chapter 10

# Mass Lesions Stereotactics

In chapter 5, sub II we described seven situations in which a mass lesion should be diagnozed by means of a stereotactic biopsy. It is evident, that the availability of CT scan techniques has helped greatly in demonstrating such a situation. CT scan is in fact the only available means (with Magnetic Resonance imaging, which is currently in development) to assess the true position and extent of any mass lesion. Invading of surrounding tissues, such as brain parenchyma, skull base, and falx, is easily detected leading to better clinical diagnosis, although still presumptive without histological proof. In this chapter we will discuss tumor diagnostics, leaving infectious disease (although sometimes presenting as a tumor) for discussion in chapter 11, dealing with localization and aspiration stereotactics. With the assumption, that tumors amenable for stereotactic biopsy are deep seated, a clinical distinction can be made between eight patterns of growth. These patterns are:

| | | | |
|---|---|---|---|
| A | diffuse tumors | B | butterfly tumors |
| C | multiple tumors | D | small tumors |
| E | cystic tumors | F | brainstem tumors |
| G | pineal tumors | H | skull base invading tumors. |

## I. Discussion of Deep Seated Tumors According to Growth Pattern

### A. Diffusely Growing Tumors

Tumors that grow diffusely in the brain (Fig. 138) will have some degree of malignancy and, with bulk resection being impossible because of their deep lying position (Figs. 139 and 141), a quick tissue diagnosis is imperative to discern their origin (glioma, lymphoma, metastatic spreading) and grade of malignancy (Fig. 140). In the group of gliomas this grading is particularly important to be able to decide on further therapy and to give a valuable prognosis. As many deep seated diffuse tumors are shown to be gliomas of low malignancy (astrocytoma grade I, II according to Kernohan) histological confirmation will allow the doctor to propose further treatment with radiotherapy. In most centers this is effectuated by external megavol-

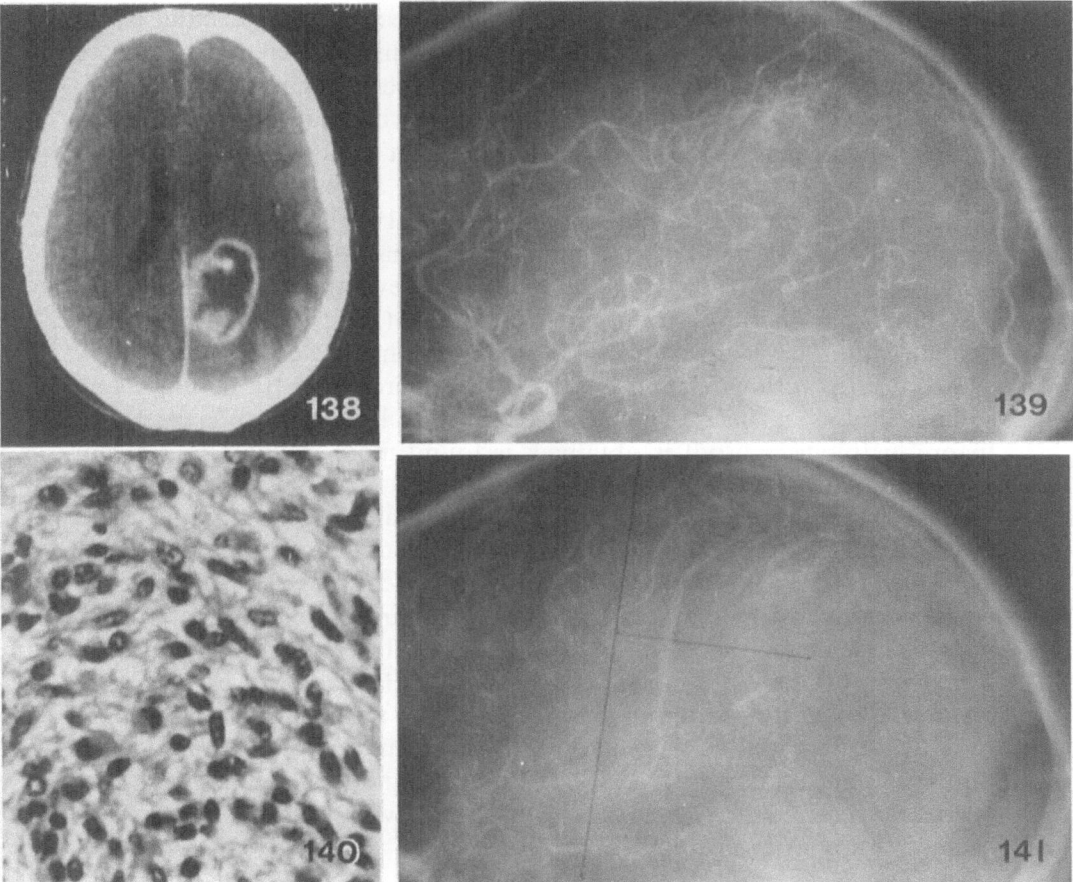

Fig. 138. Postcontrast CT scan showing a deep seated left parietal mass lesion; aspect of malignant tumor with concomitant edema

Fig. 139. Angiography, arterial phase with deep parietal tumor feeding vessels and some early venous drainage

Fig. 140. Biopsy specimen (H & E, 300 ×): astrocytoma grade III (man; 55 years)

Fig. 141. Venous phase with target localization for biopsy

tage irradiation, which will lead to greater 3- and 5-years survival rates (Sheline 1975). Interstitial irradiation (after stereotactic application of various radioactive sources) has been discussed by Mundinger (1982 a, b), Riechert (1980) and may be found in a special monograph edited by Szikla (1979 a). In the case of a malignant glioma (grade III–IV according to Kernohan) the benefit of radiotherapy is doubtful. Sheline (1975) reports a survival rate of 0% after 5 years using surgery alone, whereas only 3–9% is obtained after irradiation following partial resection. As resection is not accomplished in the deep seated tumors we discuss here, the value of irradiation in only biopsied malignant glioma seems negligible. As chemotherapeutic regimens are still in trial phases, we will not discuss its potential future value. If the diffusely growing tumor is not a glioma but a malignant lymphoma, either occurring as a primary or a second malignant tumor (after chemical immunosuppression; Penn 1974, 1976), histological proof is very important. In malignant lymphoma external irradiation will lead to dramatic relief of symptoms and sometimes—eventually combined with systemic chemotherapy—even cure the patient (Henry *et al*. 1974, Mendenhall *et al*. 1983, Neuwelt *et al*. 1983). Lymphoma has a tendency to grow as a butterfly with extension in both hemispheres (sub B). A single and solitary brain metastasis, which is often taken to be a primary brain tumor before histological proof is obtained, is found more frequently in recent years (12/44 neoplasms in the series by Apuzzo and Sabshin 1983). This depends both on earlier detection thanks to CT and MR scanning, and on the increasing number of high risk patients with immunodeficiency syndromes. Although the only option is to resect metastasis completely whenever this is possible, it is sometimes recommendable to handle deep seated single metastasis with further non-surgical treatment, depending on the origin of the tumor (Hildebrand 1980, Gagliardi *et al*. 1983). A metastasis of a Grawitz tumor (hypernephroma) will respond fairly well to radiotherapy as well as secondaries of oatcell tumors of the lung. Other tumor entities as germinoma, Hodgkin disease and leukemia are very rare inside the brain and should also be treated with radiotherapy and/or chemotherapy after histological proof.

## B. Butterfly Tumors

Butterfly tumors of the brain are predominantly involving the corpus callosum and located at the genu or the splenium. Sometimes tumor may involve both hemispheres by spreading through the anterior or posterior commissure. Almost all these tumors are shown to be gliomas or malignant lymphomas. In only 1 case (out of 250 biopsies) we encountered a butterfly metastasis of a squamous cell carcinoma of the lung with unknown primary at the time of the biopsy (Figs. 142 and 143). It is evident, that these tumors cannot be resected and therefore require a biopsy to differentiate between glioma and lymphoma. In the latter case the rest of the body should be thoroughly investigated for the presence of lymphoma outside the CNS, which will influence subsequent therapy. A malignant lymphoma often shows extraordinary distinct enhancement after contrast injection on CT scan, as shown in Figs. 144 and 145.

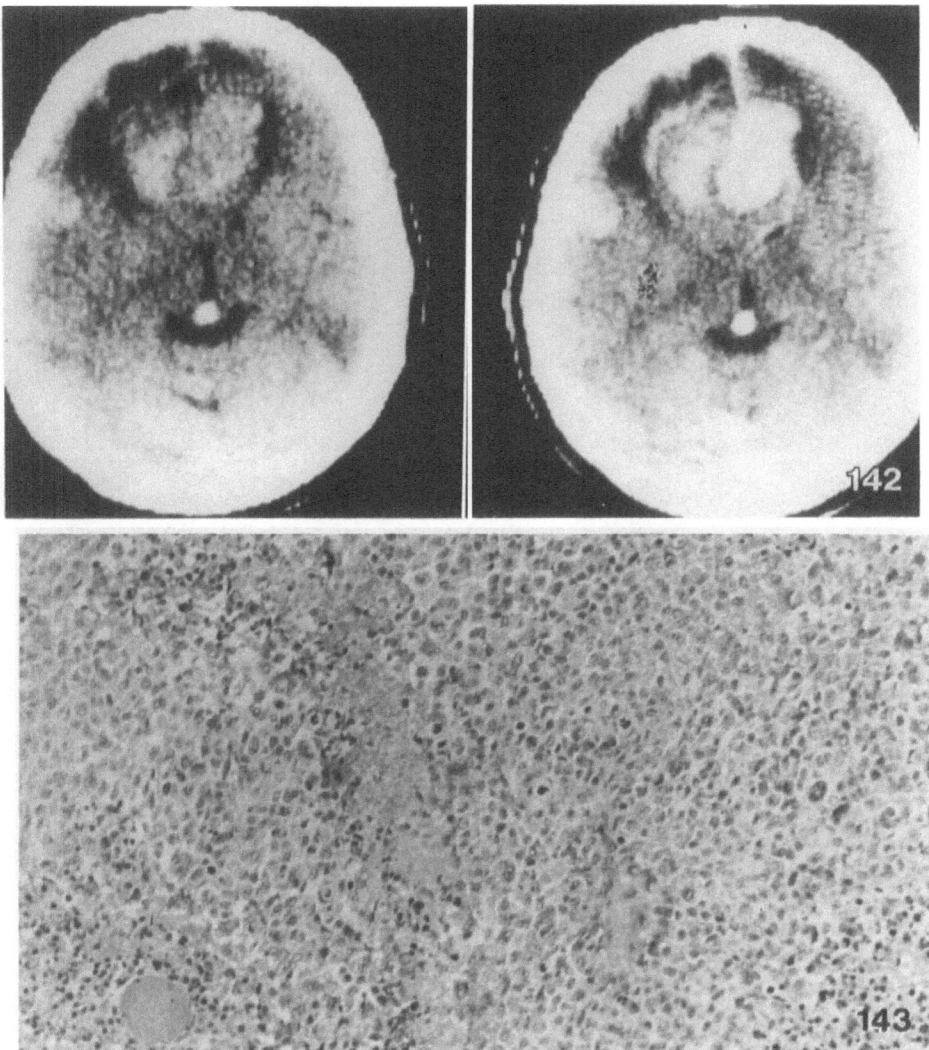

Fig. 142. Pre- and postcontrast CT pictures of butterfly tumor with rightsided frontoparietal second lesion. Man; 32 years

Fig. 143. Biopsy specimen showing metastasis of squamous cell carcinoma (H & E; 200 ×). Later on the primary tumor in the lung was found

## C. Multiple Tumors

Multiple tumors of the brain confront the surgeon with a real problem. First of all it is most important to make sure, that the lesions are tumors and not inflammatory foci [as seen in multiple sclerosis (Fig. 146) and acquired immunodeficiency syndromes—see chapter 3]. Secondly, in our opinion the

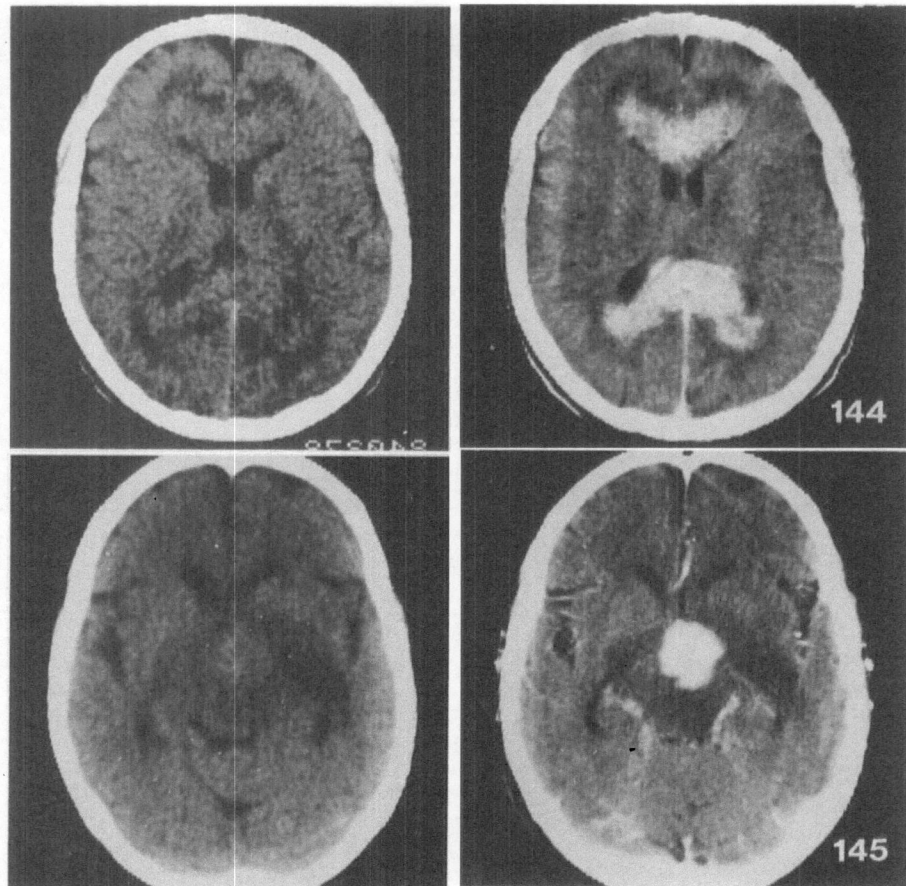

Fig. 144. CT scan pictures (pre- and postcontrast): extraordinary distinct enhancement in a malignant lymphoma case. Woman; 49 years

Fig. 145. CT pictures show a very dense tumor after contrast; malignant lymphoma in a woman, 62 years

absence of a known primary tumor outside the brain is an indication for attaining at least a tissue diagnosis (Fig. 147). Even in cases where at least one tumor could be resected by craniotomy, a biopsy is recommended as a first step, this being much less stressing for the patient and allowing rational planning of further (eventually surgical) treatment. When multiple tumors are diagnosed in a patient with a known primary tumor elsewhere, the validity of a biopsy depends completely on the case history and the prognosis. If the patient was considered to be cured or if proof of intracranial metastasis would alter the therapeutic regimen followed until then, a biopsy might be of great importance.

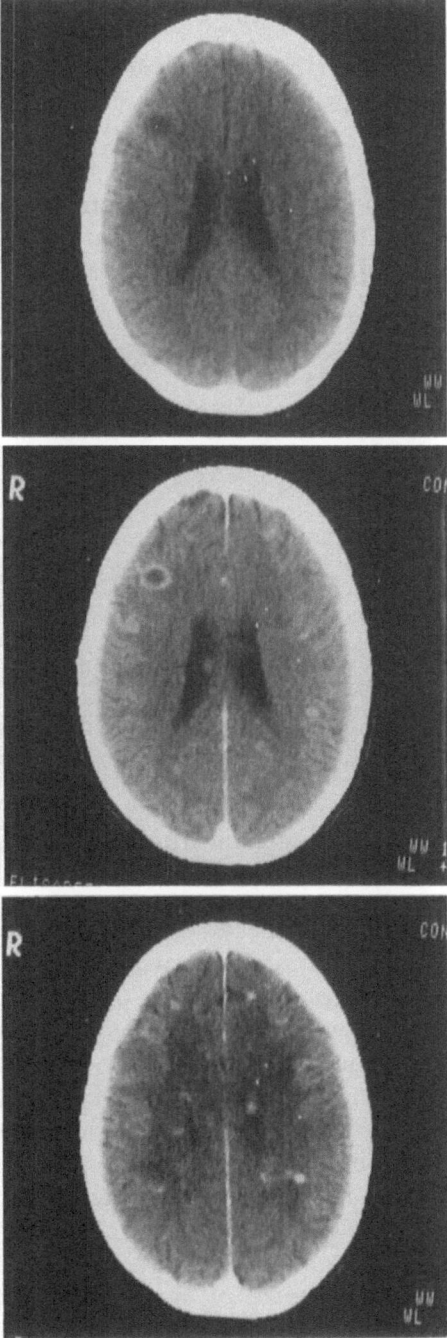

Fig. 146. Case of multiple sclerosis in a female, 32 years. Upper picture without contrast. Multiple enhancing lesions, particularly in the periventricular area (lower picture)

### D. Small Deep Seated Tumors

These tumors form a challenge for advanced stereotactic approach. Although localization is much easier than in the subcortically lying small lesions (chapters 7, sub II C and 8, sub I A), seldom can these be removed by subsequent open craniotomy. These tumors lie in the basal ganglia or thalamus and are therefore not suitable for conventional resection. In the future it will be possible with new instrumentation (chapter 4) to proceed (after biopsy) with stereotactic open resection or endoscopic control and a

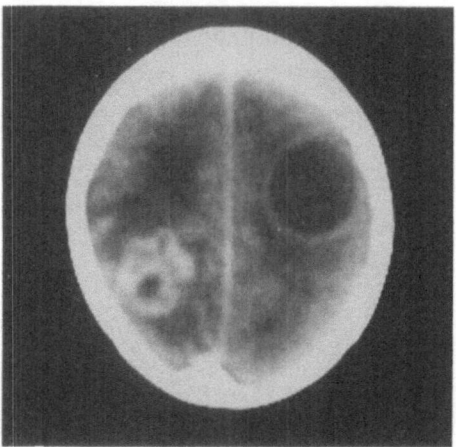

Fig. 147. CT postcontrast. Man, 61 years, with multiple mass lesions. Biopsy revealed metastasis of carcinoma; primary tumor unknown

type of laser beam to vaporize these lesions (Kelly 1983). At the moment the neodymium-YAG laser and argon laser are already adapted to use through the endoscope. Eventually, photoradiation therapy with the use of drugs which form singlet oxygen when exposed to light (such as hematoporphyrin derivatives and tetracycline) may be applied with help of a laser system (Dougherty et al. 1978, Laws et al. 1981). These drugs have been shown to accumulate selectively inside malignant cells and radiation with light at a specific wave length will disrupt the membranes of those cells. It is beyond any doubt, that with help of CT guided stereotactic instruments through the skull opening, needed to perform the biopsy, small deep seated lesions can be destroyed subtotally if not completely in the future. Jacques (et al. 1980) published on stereotactic removal of small lesions such as tumors and arteriovenous malformations with the use of a special "tumorscope" which can be introduced into the brain through a small trephination. They used binocular vision by a specially designed optical system which fitted their tumorscope (a type of speculum).

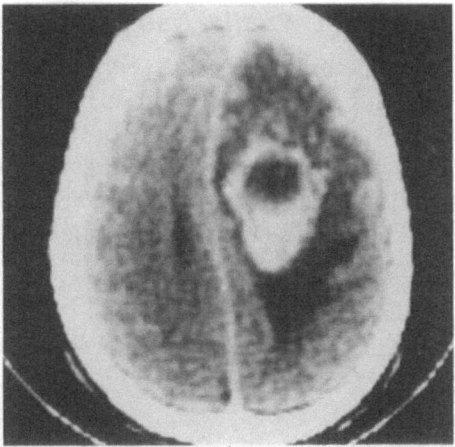

Fig. 148. CT postcontrast. Man, 47 years, known with curatively treated malignant melanoma. Biopsy: metastasis of primary tumor

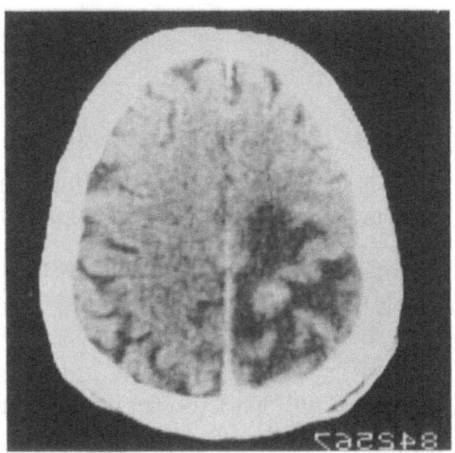

Fig. 149. CT postcontrast. Man, 57 years, with deep seated small tumor and impressive white matter edema. Biopsy: malignant astrocytoma

It is difficult to estimate the histological origin of a small tumor (Figs. 148 and 149) on the basis of neuroradiological investigations. Because of its small size only concomitant brain edema might indicate the presence of a metastasis (or even an abscess). Therefore, histological proof is of utmost importance. We also recommend that some material is investigated for Gram staining and bacteriological culture.

## E. Cystic Tumors

Cystic tumors inside the brain are relatively monomorph in origin. With biopsy almost all these tumors can be classified as astrocytomas grade II or III. Only in the midline and at the base of the brain (hypothalamus) a cystic craniopharyngioma may be found unexpectedly, without suprasellar extension. This ectopic position is very rare, however, and is sometimes suspected because of the presence of small calcifications such as might be seen in the oligodendrogliomas.

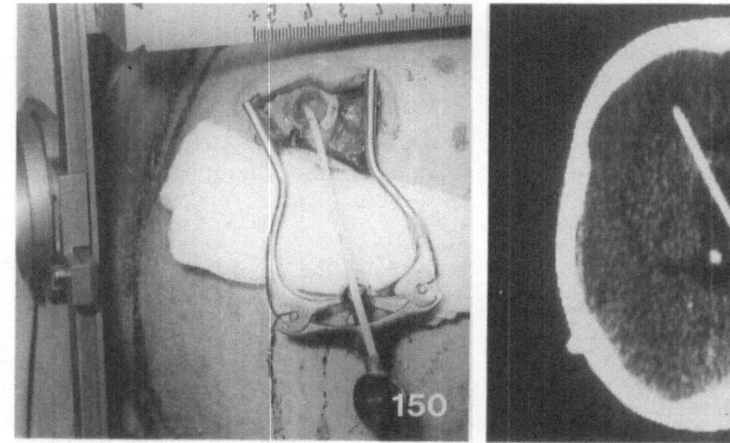

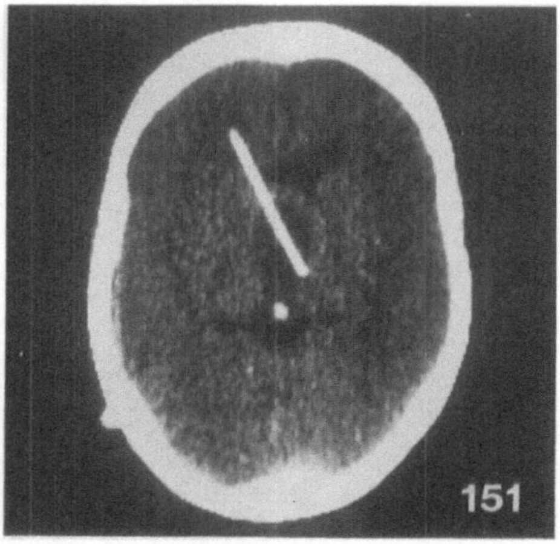

Fig. 150. Stereotactic performance. Introduction of a thin catheter into a recurrent cystic glioma. Note plastic anchor at burrhole site

Fig. 151. CT scan showing the introduced catheter with its tip inside the cyst. Female, 16 years; 2 years after biopsy and radiotherapy for astrocytoma grade II

The stereotactic puncture will lead to escape of fluid before the biopsy forceps or spiral needle can be inserted. All fluid should be aspirated slowly and sent for cytological investigation and bacterial culture. Thereafter the cyst wall can be biopsied easily for performing histological studies. We prefer to replace the stereotactic needle by a section of radiopaque tubing (e.g. ventricular draining tube after Ommaya or Holter), that can be secured in the burrhole to a Rickham reservoir (Fig. 150). This enables the surgeon to repeat evacuation if necessary (Fig. 151), and moreover to introduce radioactive fluid (as $^{90}$Yttrium) when desired. At the same time this marking of the lesion site may be of value for the radiation therapist in planning his booster field. After radiotherapy, which is advisable in the unresectable astrocytoma grade II–III, we sometimes noted—as in the recurrent craniopharyngioma—repeated refilling of the cyst, which can be managed easily in this way in coming years. It sometimes happens that the reaccumulated fluid is so viscous, that disconnection of the reservoir is necessary in order to evacuate the fluid again. A cystic metastasis might also be encountered, although rare, and is frequently a secondary of squamous cell carcinoma of the lung, that has become cystic through necrosis in its center (see Fig. 147).

## F. Brainstem Tumors

It is preferable to approach tumors of the mesencephalon and upper (rostral) pons by stereotactic means (see Figs. 88 and 89). The ponto-medullary region and the medulla oblongata should be explored by open posterior fossa surgery. Because of the distorted anatomy and the vital importance of normal tissue direct vision is essential. Some decennia ago it was believed, that biopsy was too dangerous and therefore radiation therapy without histological proof was carried out under the presumptive diagnosis of brainstem glioma. Further progress in neuro-oncology, however, led to the vital importance of attaining a pathological diagnosis before the institution of proper treatment. Moreover, posterior fossa exploration using microsurgical techniques enabled the surgeon to take tissue samples without serious complications, provided that the manipulation was done within the pathological tissue itself. In recent years general practice has proved stereotactic biopsies to be safe on the condition that the tip of the biopsy instrument, while taking a sample, is lying completely inside the tumor. Before CT scanning was available such a statement could neither be made nor controlled. With CT guided techniques, however, a clearly demarcated tumor in the higher brainstem is easily biopsied (see Figs. 62–64). From clinical experience it is well-known, that many of these tumors are indeed gliomas. However, the grading is important, because it is useless and often positively harmful to the patient to have radiotherapy on a highly malignant tumor. Whyte (et al. 1969), the Mayo Clinic, describes radiotherapy in brainstem tumors in 61 cases; 21 patients had pre-treatment histological verification of an astrocytoma (11 grade I–II; 10 grade III–IV). Their survival rate was 38%. Albright (et al. 1983) discusses the value of biopsying brainstem gliomas in children and concludes that the risk is low and that small biopsies may show representative tissue. Their data indicate that 30% to 45% of children with glioma of the brainstem survive 5 years or longer, after adequate radiotherapy.

## G. Pineal Gland Tumors

Tumors arising in the pineal gland region are notorious for their different growth characteristics (Bosch 1980, Pecker et al. 1978, 1979 b,

Neuwelt *et al.* 1979). This fact is per se a strong indication for attaining histological evidence. As various pineal region tumors are strikingly radiosensitive, open exploration—as advocated by Stein (1979) among others—is not necessary, unless in the case of radioresistant lesions such as dermoid, meningioma, and teratoma. Particularly the germinoma, which is the most frequently encountered in this region, is even curable (Sung *et al.* 1978, Inoue *et al.* 1979), if irradiated with inclusion of the spinal axis (overall survival rate at 5 years of 80%). Germinoma (Figs. 152 and 153), which is

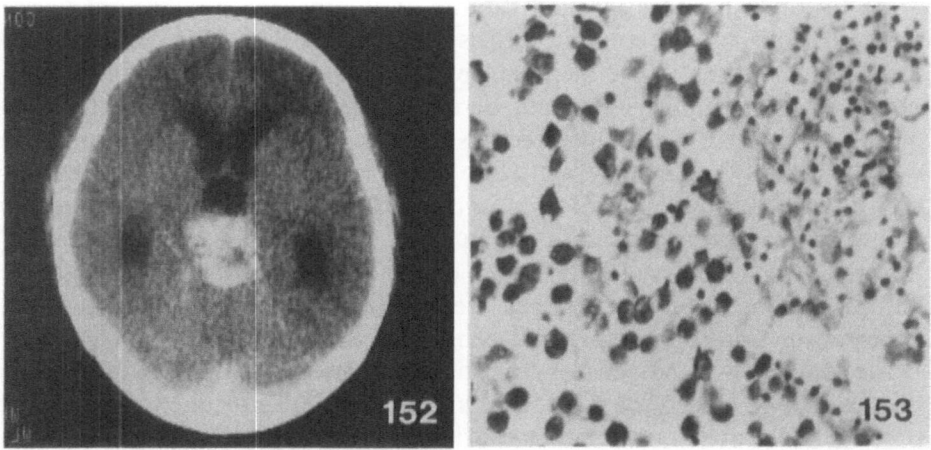

Fig. 152. Postcontrast CT picture of pineal region tumor causing obstructive hydrocephalus. Male, 23 years

Fig. 153. Biopsy specimen of this case. Germinoma (PAS, 250 ×)

also frequently found in the suprasellar region, belongs together with the teratoma to the germ cell tumors and has a remarkably higher incidence in the Japanese (Koide *et al.* 1980). In the old days the germinoma was called pinealoma (with a two-cell pattern), but recent investigations have made clear that there is a strong similarity between this tumor and seminoma, and therefore the name "germinoma" has been introduced. Nowadays the true pinealoma is classified as pinealoblastoma and pinealocytoma, according to the degree of differentiation of the tumor cells. Teratoma is much more radioresistant (Donat *et al.* 1978, Neuwelt *et al.* 1979) as is the endodermal sinus tumor and pinealoblastoma (Chapman and Linggood 1980). These tumors tend to recur after biopsy (or partial removal) and subsequent radiotherapy and may therefore need adjuvant chemotherapy. During the performance of a stereotactic biopsy one should always collect some CSF to send with a blood sample for "tumor marker" detection. Particularly the $\beta$-chain of human chorionic gonadotropin (HCG) and $\alpha$-fetoprotein may be

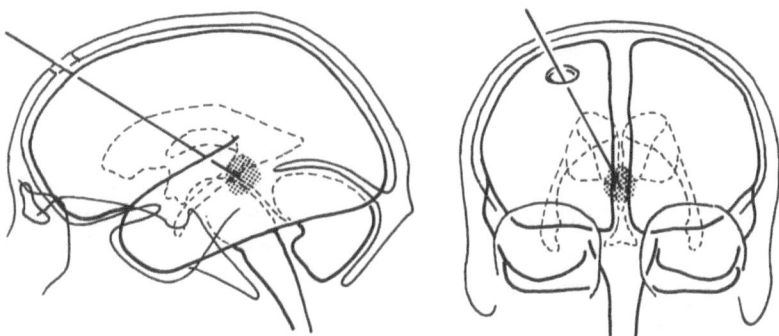

Fig. 154. Schematic drawing illustrating the safest route for stereotactic biopsy of a pineal region tumor

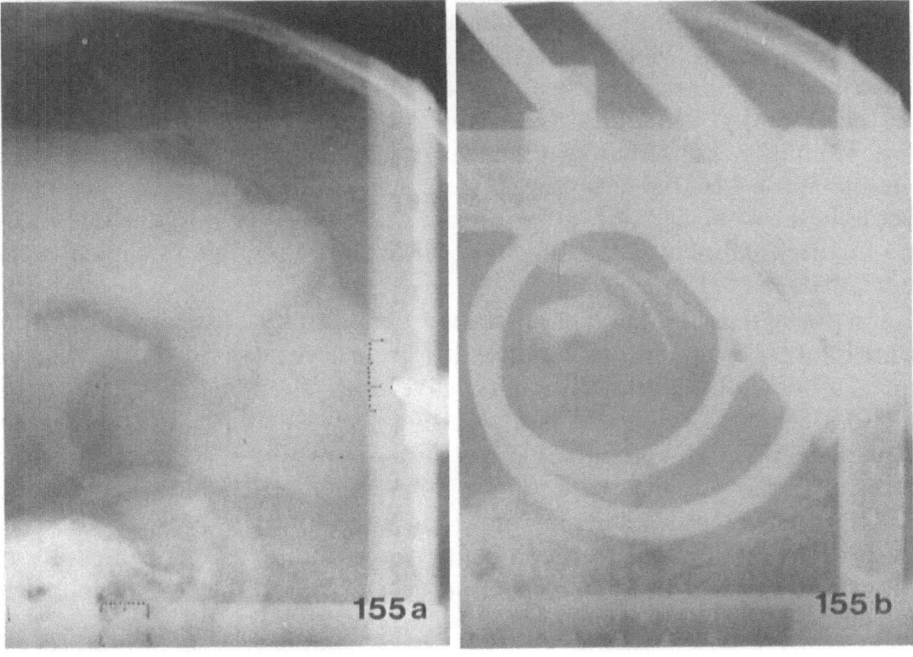

Fig. 155. Stereotactic ventriculography in various cases of pineal tumors. Longstanding obstructive hydrocephalus of lateral and third ventricles (a); already shunted case (b)

of value, because—when present—these markers offer an easy way to test regression of tumor during and after therapy. We would recommend stereotactic ventriculography during the biopsy procedure [as Pecker (*et al.* 1979 b) advocates], because the safest route is through the third ventricle (Fig. 154). In the first place the puncture track should run horizontally enough so as to keep under the third ventricular roof (with the deep cerebral veins), and secondly keep very close to the midsagittal plane to avoid thalamic lesioning and tumor-surrounding vessels that lie predominantly posterolaterally (Rosenthal's veins and precentral cerebellar vein). Ventriculography clearly shows the pathological anatomy in the posterior third ventricle (Fig. 155), which enables the surgeon to recalculate his target if necessary. The frontal burrhole may be used afterwards for insertion of a CSF shunt. As a routine we take CSF samples both for tumor markers and for cytological investigation prior to the ventriculography. Thereafter we perform a tissue biopsy and insert a CSF shunting device (preferably mounted with a cell filter to prevent spreading of malignant cells outside the CNS) under the same anesthesia. About 10% of the germ cell tumors shows metastasis inside the CSF system. Further treatment is determined after histological verification of the tumor's origin. In those cases, which are not radiosensitive (about 20% of all pineal gland tumors) open excision is to be considered, unless in the case of harmartomatous lesions. Bosch (1980) described 2 hamartomas on 6 pineal gland tumors, both requiring no further therapy. Sequential CT scans are recommended with a 1–2 year interval in the case of hamartoma, the actual diagnosis sometimes being a glioma grade I that grows very slowly. One of the above mentioned cases actually shows a very slow growth; today, 6 years after stereotactic biopsy no further treatment is yet indicated, since after shunting all clinical signs have disappeared.

In pineal region tumors preoperative angiography is even more essential than in other brain tumors, because this site is notorious for the presence of an arteriovenous malformation or cavernous angioma (Vaquero *et al.* 1980). In chapter 8, sub II A, such a pitfall is presented (see Figs. 112–116). Angioghraphy will sometimes show the arteries that feed the tentorium, indicating the presence of a tumor demanding a rich blood supply (as usually seen in tentorial meningioma; Fig. 156 shows these arteries in a case of pinealoblastoma). After complete neuroradiological documentation, biopsy of a pineal tumor presents no greater a risk than other biopsies, which means an operative mortality of about 2%.

## H. Skull Base Invading Tumors

Skull base invading tumors are typically lesions that should be biopsied first, so as to understand their origin and enable the planning of a valid strategy of treatment. We only observed cases of metastasis, which had either invaded the skull base from below (carcinoma of sphenoidal sinus) or invaded the skull base from the basal meninges. Often a biopsy is better performed by the ENT-surgeon, when the lesion is situated in his field. Occasionally invasion originating in the basal cisterns and meninges is

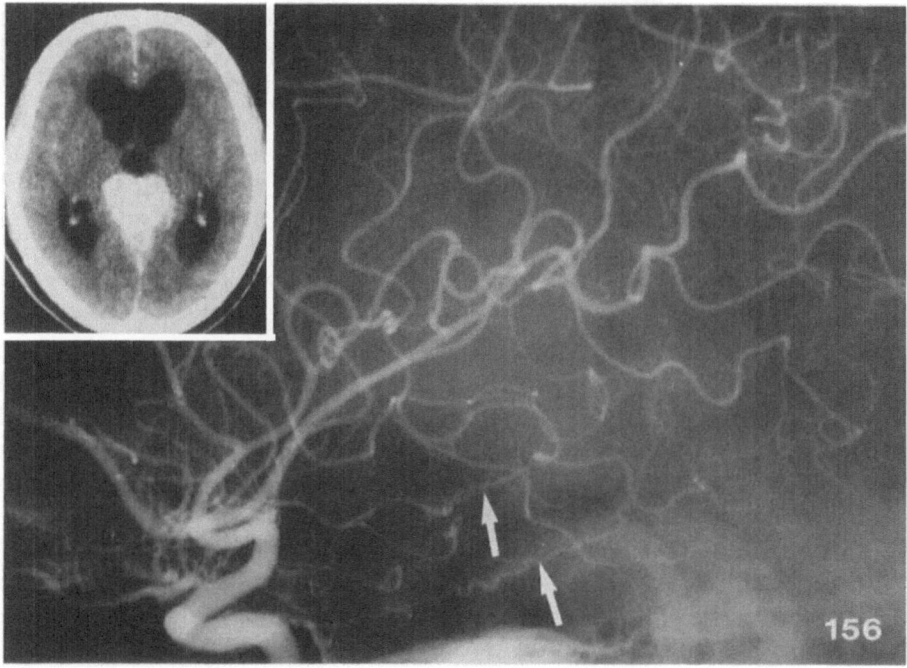

Fig. 156. Pinealoblastoma case; man, 39 years. Angiography, arterial phase, shows feeding arteries to the tentorium (arrows), which supply the tumor with blood. Insert: postcontrast CT picture

found, which should not be biopsied by the ENT-surgeon, because it carries the risk of CSF leakage and subsequent infection. Since many of these processes are clearly malignant and almost always secondary to a (unknown) primary tumor elsewhere in the body, a stereotactic biopsy is the safest way to histological verification. Further treatment will often consist of palliative radiotherapy and/or chemotherapy. In Figs. 157–159 we show a skull base invading meningeal metastasis of mammary adenocarcinoma in a 60 year old woman.

## II. Presentation of Our Own Material and Discussion of Other Reports

During the period 1978–1984 we performed about 250 stereotactic biopsies on tumors, which according to the already discussed growth patterns had been diagnozed as deep seated. From our data on all cases with intracerebral mass lesions we concluded, that in about 20–25% of all intracerebral tumors a stereotactic biopsy performance was indicated. This percentage of course depends largely on the type of surgery the surgeon prefers, but open surgery was always carried out in cases where at least substantial removal was thought to be feasible. Another important factor is the influence of CT scanning on clinical practice; particularly small and deep seated (thus silent) tumors are more often discovered, leading to stereotactic diagnostic interventions. For the purpose of statistical analysis of the material the first consecutive 100 cases were studied (Bosch *et al.* 1982) and will be presented here. All interventions were carried out with Leksell's instrument and under dexamethasone protection. Local as well as general anesthesia were used, depending on age and clinical state. Complications were rare: 2% of the patients died due to the intervention itself. The first due to fatal bleeding from a feeding vessel at the biopsy site in an angiographically silent, but nevertheless present sclerotic hemangioma (see Figs. 84–86) in the mesencephalon, and the other due to tearing of the sylvian arachnoid with the spiral needle, resulting in bleeding from a medial artery branch and lethal brain swelling. In 4% we met complications that were not life-threatening: twice hemiparesis developed (presumably due to some bleeding at the target site), 1 case presented an oculomotor palsy due to lesioning the nucleus (a case of hamartoma of the posterior third ventricle), and 1 case developed an acute obliteration of CSF pathways with obstructive hydrocephalus after biopsy of a thalamic malignant glioma. False positive results were obtained in about 1.5% and false negative results in 6.4% (see chapter 8, sub II B for detailed discussion).

Greenblatt (*et al.* 1982) reported 4 false negative and 1 false positive diagnosis on a total of 24 procedures; their percentages are significantly higher, but they used CT guided *non-stereotactic* needle biopsy. Moreover, their complication rate is higher, with 1 death due to hemorrhage and 2 intratumoral hematomas. This report is of utmost importance, since it stresses that stereotactic biopsy is much more reliable and safer than any kind of non-rigid probe insertion, whether CT guided or not.

Table 5 representing the various histological diagnoses illustrates, that in 13% no tumor, but other mass lesions were present. The 13 cases could be diagnozed as: hematoma (3), infarction (2), infection (2), cysts (2), and non-representative material (4). One of the infections was a herpes simplex encephalitis and could be verified within some hours virologically with immunofluorescence techniques (see also Lunsford *et al.* 1984 b). The 4 failures include one technical and two sampling errors (i.e. 3 false negative results) and one biopsy, that showed compact stroma with Rosenthal's

---

Fig. 157. Postcontrast CT pictures of skull base invading tumor; female, 60 years, known with mammary adenocarcinoma

Fig. 158. Angiography, arterial and venous phase, with tumor surrounding frontopolar artery and venous shift

Fig. 159. Histological specimen (PAS, 400 × ), revealing metastasis

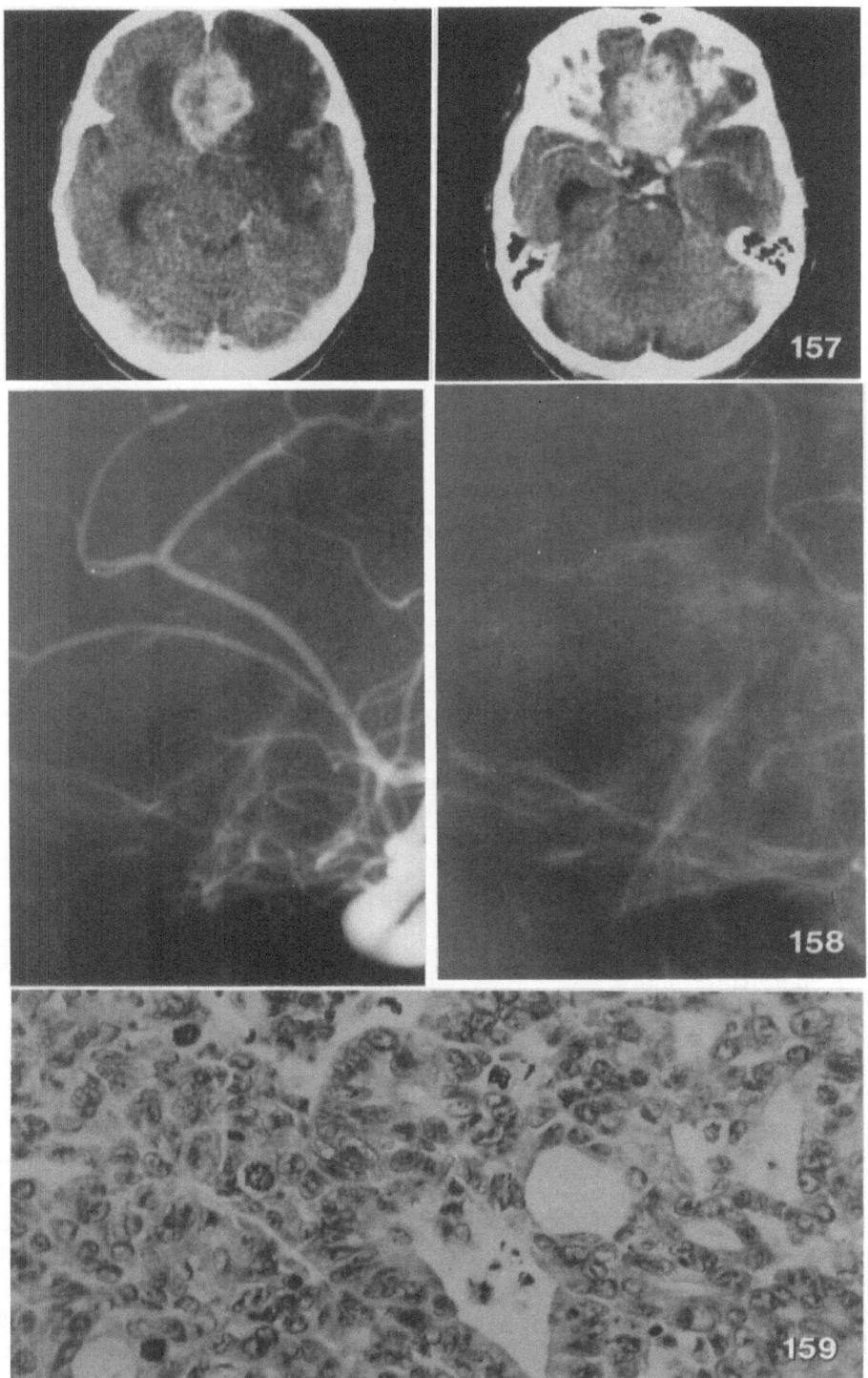

Figs. 157–159

Table 5. *Analysis of the First Consecutive 100 Cases of Stereotactic Biopsy in Clinically Suspected Tumors*

Our own results in deep seated mass lesions; Bosch 1980, *et al.* 1982.

| | | | |
|---|---|---|---|
| 62 | glioma | 27 | malignant, grade III–IV |
| | | 24 | low grade malignant, grade II–III |
| | | 9 | benign, grade I–II |
| | | 2 | monstrocellular, in Bourneville's disease |
| 11 | pineal region | 4 | germinomas |
| | | 2 | ependymomas |
| | | 3 | hamartomas |
| | | 1 | teratoma |
| | | 1 | cystic lesion |
| 7 | metastasis | 5 | with unknown primary tumor |
| | | 3 | multiple |

3   malignant lymphomas

2   craniopharyngiomas

1   germinoma in thalamus

1   sclerotized hemangioma in mesencephalon

1   hamartoma in hypothalamus
    (with Von Recklinghausen disease)

1   cystic lesion in lateral ventricle

3   hematomas

2   infarctions

2   encephalitis

| | | | | |
|---|---|---|---|---|
| 4 | non-representative | 1 | technical error | false |
| | | 2 | sampling errors | negative |
| | | 1 | nondiagnostic | negative |

100 biopsies          87 tumors          10 non-neoplastic mass lesions

3 unproved tumors = false negative

fibers from a lesion that presumedly is a tumor, although after 6 years no sign of growth was noted. In 4 cases only necrotic tissue was obtained, but nevertheless these tumors were listed as malignant gliomas because of the pathological shunting vessels at angiography. Theoretically these cases should, however, have been listed as non-representative. Taking into account the cases with a false negative result, the final percentage of non-neoplastic biopsies will be 10%.

This percentage of 10 non-neoplastic biopsies is of great importance, as it indirectly shows that the clinical diagnosis of tumor requires a histological verification. Without the availability of stereotactics in most of these 10 cases radiotherapy would undoubtedly have been suggested as the sole treatment modality left. This so-called blind irradiation is of course positively harmful to a patient who does not harbor a tumor. Ostertag (et al. 1980) published on 26 non-neoplastic biopsies, 3 abscesses and 3 colloid cysts, eliminating tumors in 32/302 cases. This percentage of 10.6% closely resembles our figure of 10%. Kleihues (et al. 1984) also presents 11% of non-neoplastic biopsies (66/600 cases). Apuzzo and Sabshin (1983) published a consecutive series of 71 patients, 44 cases harboring a neoplasm, the other cases being infectious (20) or vascular (7). From their report, however, it is not clear in how many cases the diagnosis "tumor" was handled preoperatively. It is obvious, that with the recently developed new generation CT scanners preoperative differentiation between tumors and non-neoplastic mass lesions has become easier to make. This will also lead to a decrease of the 10–11% figure.

Nevertheless, in the future a presumedly low percentage of non-neoplastic cases will be observed after a clinical diagnosis of tumor, having consequences for further therapy planning. Moreover, metastasis with an unknown primary tumor will be found incidentally: in 5 of 7 metastasis patients (out of our first 100 cases) this was completely unexpected. Broggi and Franzini (1981) reported 4 metastasis on 35 tumor biopsies, 3 of these being unsuspected preoperatively. This makes the incidence of unsuspected metastasis 5% in our own series and 8.6% in the other. In the extensive studies published by Ostertag (et al. 1980) and Edner (1981) no incidence of unsuspected metastasis at biopsy is given. Particularly in small mass lesions a radiological differentiation between glioma and metastasis is almost impossible, as shown in Figs. 147–149. In both situations marked white matter edema may be present. The histological diagnosis of malignant lymphoma is also of great importance, because of the possibility of a much longer survival or complete cure, which is achieved with irradiation and—if indicated for treatment of further spreading—chemotherapy. Fig. 34 shows a butterfly tumor, which proved to be a malignant lymphoma. After adequate treatment the follow-up scan (4 years later) showed complete regression (case1; chapter 12) and the patient was able to return to active life. In the inaccessible craniopharyngioma verification plus cyst drainage offers a good (though essentially palliative) treatment with long-term survival (Mann et al. 1983).

In our series of the first 100 consecutive cases we observed a 5% incidence of vascular lesions, by that time unsuspected before biopsy. Small intracerebral hematomas will always present a real pitfall, as these may occur as a manifestation of cryptic arteriovenous malformations or venous angiomas [venous malformations according to Huang (*et al*. 1984)]. A review has been written by Becker (*et al*. 1979), in which 18 angiographically occult cases are reported, based on histologically proven vascular malformations of the brain. Follow-up of our cases for more than 3 years confirmed the non-neoplastic origin (Fig. 160). There was no operative morbidity after biopsy in these cases.

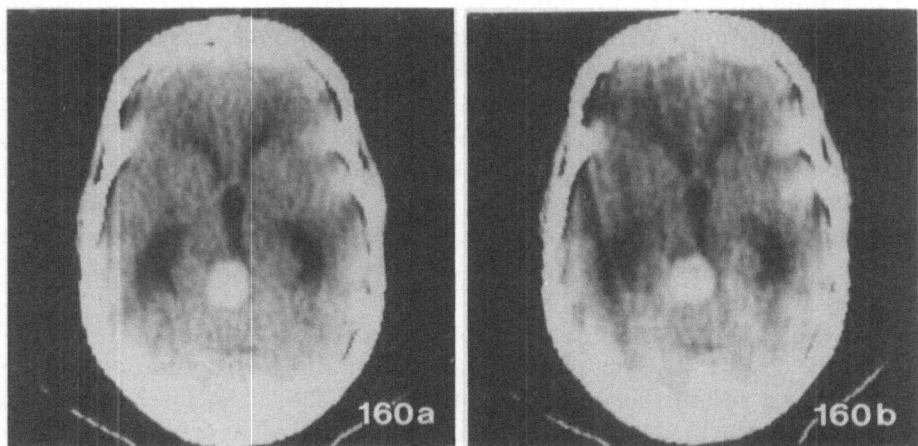

Fig. 160. Pre- and postcontrast CT pictures (a, b) of hematoma in a female, 30 years, presumably caused by a cryptic vascular malformation. Clinical signs of headache and raised intracranial pressure subsided within a week and follow-up CT showed no abnormalities

As is obvious from clinical experience, the great majority of cases represented gliomas: 62%. Grading (according to Kernohan's criteria) was not always possible, but a clinically useful differentiation between clearly malignant (27), dubious or low grade malignant (24) and benign (9) could be made. In 2 of the 62 gliomas a typical Bourneville tumor at the foramen of Monro was found; in one of these cases signs of this disease were also found elsewhere in the body.

The grading was useful for further therapy planning: in the group of clearly malignant gliomas radiotherapy was deliberately withheld, because bulk resection was not feasible. The Bourneville—gliomas responded fairly well to radiotherapy, although the histological characteristics are rather polymorphous with giant glial cells. Because colloid cysts of the third ventricle (see chapter 11, sub II) also show contrast enhancement on CT, sometimes a Bourneville glioma may be mistaken for a colloid cyst, as in one of our own cases, without any other sign of tuberous sclerosis (Fig. 161 and 162). Ostertag (*et al*. 1980) found a 70% incidence of gliomas in his large group of patients, which leads to a percentage of at least 30% of

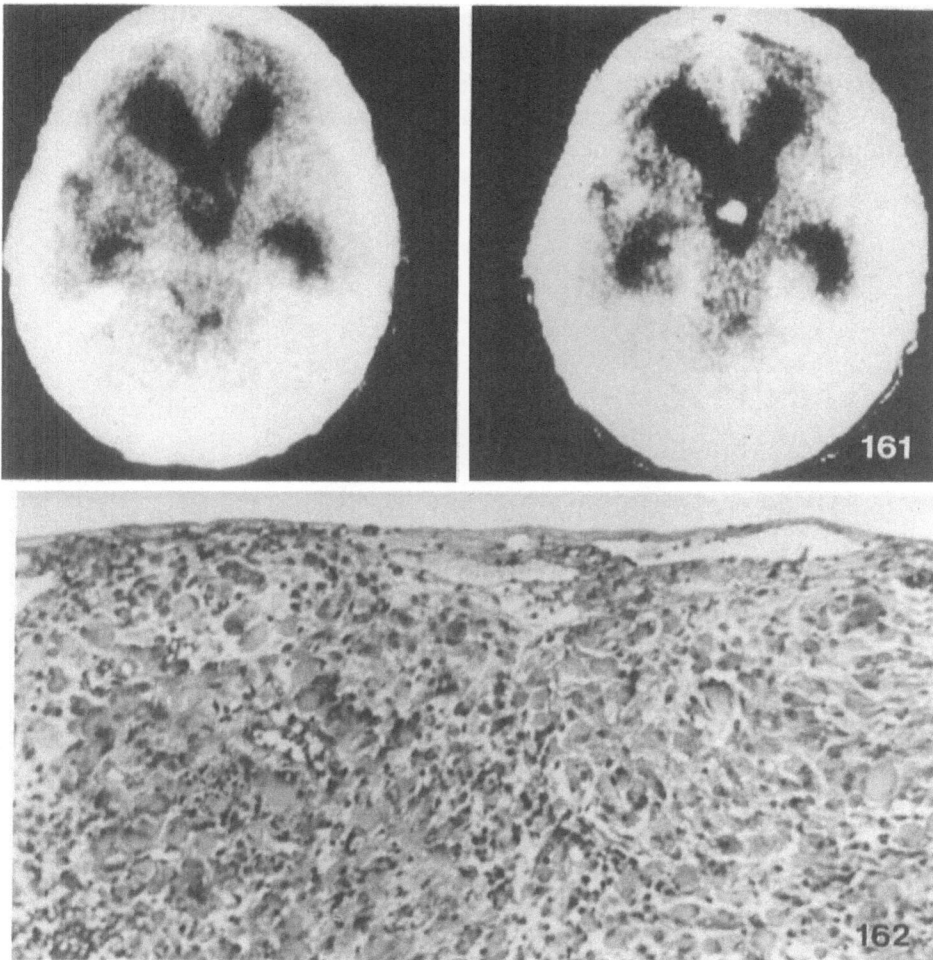

Fig. 161. Pitfall: man, 48 years, with anterior third ventricle tumor, enhancing after contrast injection (right). Presumptive diagnosis: colloid cyst. Stereotactic aspiration was carried out

Fig. 162. Histological specimen of extracted tumor sample: monstrocellular glioma, typical for Bourneville's disease (H & E; 250 ×)

histologically verified non-glial mass lesions. From the neuro-oncological point of view these data obviously offer a more sophisticated treatment planning than was ever possible in the past where stereotactic biopsy techniques were non-existent. The great advantage using these techniques is best illustrated with the pineal region tumors. Germinomas of this region are found in 4% of all deep seated mass lesions in the brain, which is in about 50% of all pineal tumors (Bosch 1980, *et al.* 1982, Ostertag *et al.* 1980). Knowledge of the histological diagnosis may then lead to cure of the patient. Our second series of 150 patients treated by biopsy for deep seated mass lesions (not published) supports the hitherto made conclusions. All reports share the view of the extreme importance of this field of clinical neurosurgery. Real progress in neuro-oncology will never be achieved without histological evidence.

# Chapter 11

# Stereotactic Localization with Subsequent Lesion Treatment

## I. Introduction

Stereotactic localization is often the only possibility open to the surgeon for reaching the lesion of interest. Although in fact all stereotactic interventions use localization techniques, for the purpose of clarity we would like to discuss separately *those* lesions, which after localization can be treated by aspiration or microsurgical resection. One reason for this subdivision is, that these lesions are not necessarily tumors, and that the pertinent literature on this subject shares only the localization technique with stereotactic diagnostics. The main reason, however, for setting the lesions apart, which nowadays can be treated with combined stereotactic and microsurgical techniques, is the evident progress made possible by this methodology in clinical neurosurgery. A new era will be ushered in in cerebral lesion management with the methodological advances in this field.

The progress has been made very recently and began after the development of high resolution CT scan and computer equipment, making both the identification and the stereotactic treatment feasible. As already reported in general in chapters 3 (sub III), 4, 5 (sub IV), and 6 (sub IV), the lesions we have in view include small subcortical lesions which can be aimed at stereotactically for subsequent microsurgical resection (tumors, arteriovenous malformations) as well as small deep seated lesions which can be treated by aspiration (colloid cysts, primary hematomas, abscesses). For stereotactic removal of foreign bodies the reader is referred to Hitchcock and Cowie (1983) and Riechert (1980: pp. 84–89).

In this chapter we will discuss the stereotactic treatment of colloid cysts of the third ventricle, primary deep seated hematomas, and small subcortical AVM's and illustrate these sections with our own material.

## II. Colloid Cysts of the Third Ventricle

In 1978, Bosch, Rähn and Backlund described the first group of (four) patients, successfully treated by stereotactic aspiration. Thereafter more experience has been collected by these authors, which confirms their initial conclusion that longlasting (follow-up now 7 years) decompression can be

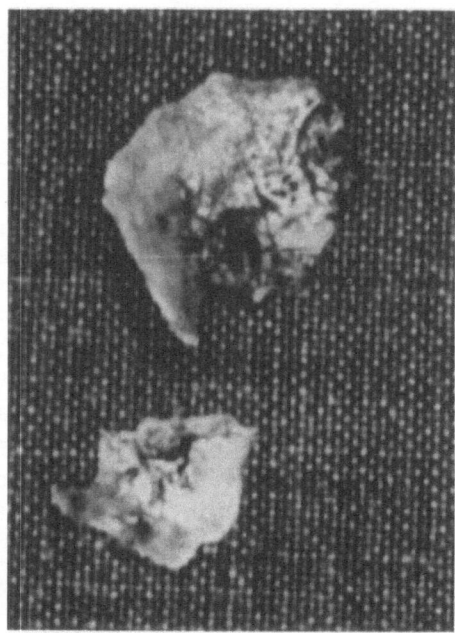

Fig. 163. Extracted tumor specimens in case shown in Figs. 161 and 162

achieved by this simple and safe technique. Essential for obtaining a good result is the pre-operative neuroradiological work-up, including angiography.

Although colloid cysts are rare and represent less than 1% of all intracranial tumors (Ferry and Kempe 1968), the correct diagnosis should be made, because the symptoms may be dangerous and cure from these benign lesions is attainable. Although the CT scan picture is often suggestive, arteriography is obligatory because the lesion should be avascular to be treated successfully with strong vacuum aspiration. On angiography localized elevation of the anterior portion of the internal cerebral vein, closure of the venous angle, and depression of the internal cerebral vein may be found (Sackett et al. 1975). The neuroepithelium, which is considered the embryonic origin of a colloid cyst, is located in the tela choroidea of the roof of the third ventricle and receives its arterial supply primarily from the posterior medial choroidal arteries. The lesion itself is, however, not vascular. This is in contrast with a rare case of AVM presented by Britt (et al. 1980), in which situation a transventricular microsurgical resection was obligatory. We actually met one case simulating a colloid cyst, that with stereotactic aspiration proved to be a tumor (Bourneville's glioma; see Figs. 161 and 162). This patient should not have been treated in that way, as the tearing of a vessel is possible with life

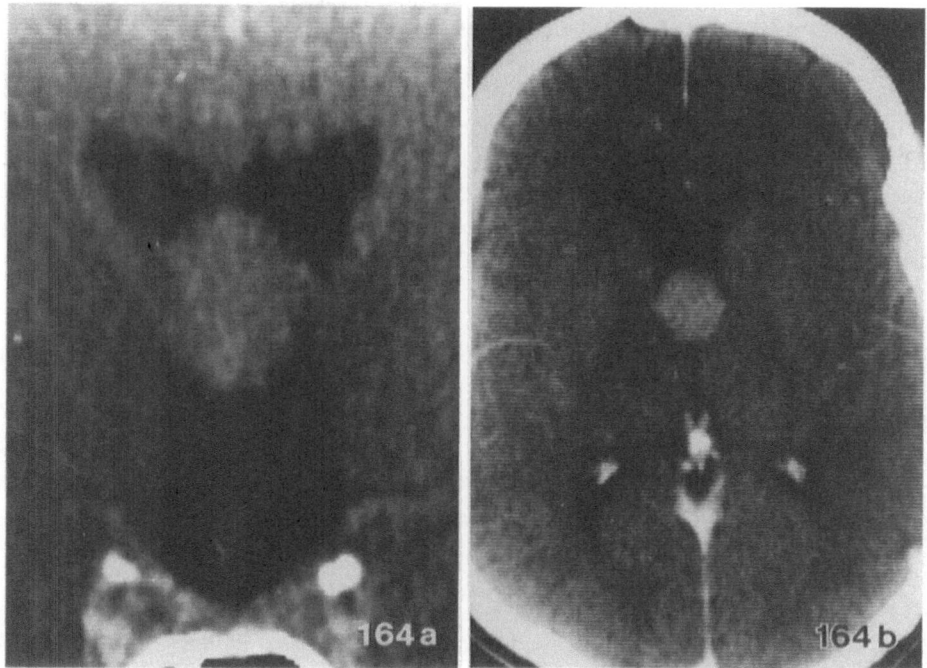

Fig. 164. Typical case of colloid cyst of third ventricle; male, 24 years. Coronal picture without contrast (a), axial picture with contrast (b)

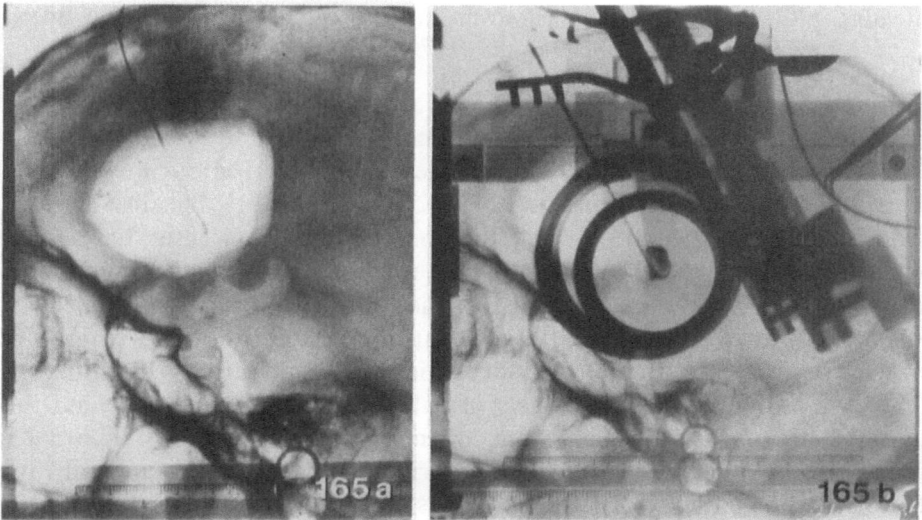

Fig. 165. Stereotactic evacuation of cyst contents in third ventricle colloid cyst. Stereotactic air ventriculography (a); Cystography after evacuation (b). Case published in Surg. Neurology 9, 15–18 (1978) by Bosch et al.

threatening complications (Fig. 163). On CT scan colloid cysts show diffuse enhancement after contrast injection and signs of obstructive hydrocephalus of the lateral ventricles (Fig. 164). After evacuation of the cyst's contents hydrocephalus will usually subside and therefore a CSF shunt is almost never required. Gildenberg (1982 b) discusses colloid cysts among the lesions, which may be managed completely by stereotactic aspiration. Treatment of benign cystic tumors of the third ventricle by free-hand introduction of a catheter has been described by Gutierrez-Lara (*et al.*

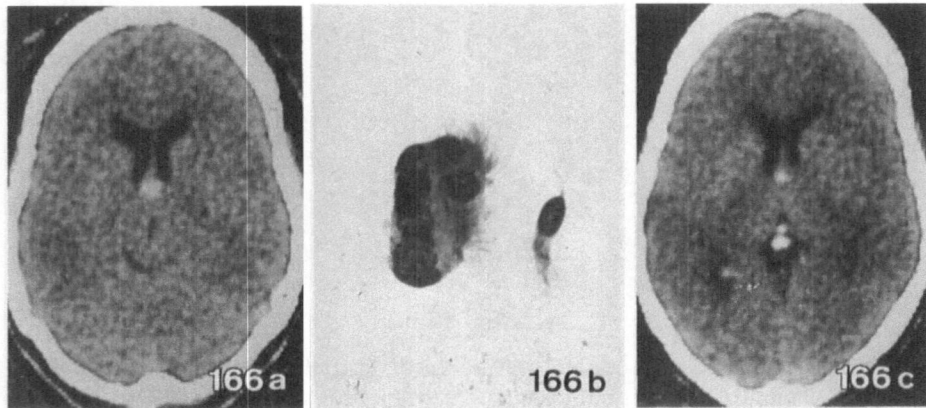

Fig. 166. CT scans immediately before (left) and one week after the evacuation (right) show the decrease of the size of the cyst. Picture in between shows specimen of cubic epithelium with cilia, which forms the cyst wall. Case published by Bosch *et al.* (1978)

1975). Among the five cases presented colloid cysts and ependymal cysts were found. In contrast with their experience we preferred the introduction of a guided, and large cannula (1.5 mm inner diameter), because the cyst wall is not easily penetrated and the contents are so viscous that strong aspiration is needed for evacuation. We recommend stereotactic guidance instead of free-hand puncture, because the cyst is a centrally lying and small lesion. As shown in Fig. 165 after evacuation of the contents a cystography may be performed with metrizamide, which clearly delineates the situation. The cyst wall (Fig. 166 b) consists of cubic epithelium with cilia, and the contents are a protein rich substance with some phagocytes. Follow-up CT scan (Fig. 166 c) shows decrease of ventricular dilation and almost always restoration of patency of CSF pathways.

Lunsford (*et al.* 1982) presented one successfully treated case of colloid cyst with CT imaging during the stereotactic performance. Apuzzo (*et al.* 1984 a) also treated a colloid cyst uneventfully with CT guided stereotactics.

Open surgery, as was advocated by McKissock (1951) before stereotactic management became known, presents the danger of damaging the internal cerebral and thalamostriate veins with subsequent infarction of the basal ganglia, or of uncontrollable bleeding. Stereotactic treatment proved to be less dangerous and in our cases no complications at all have been met. Also seizures, which after transcortical operations may sometimes complicate recovery, are never seen.

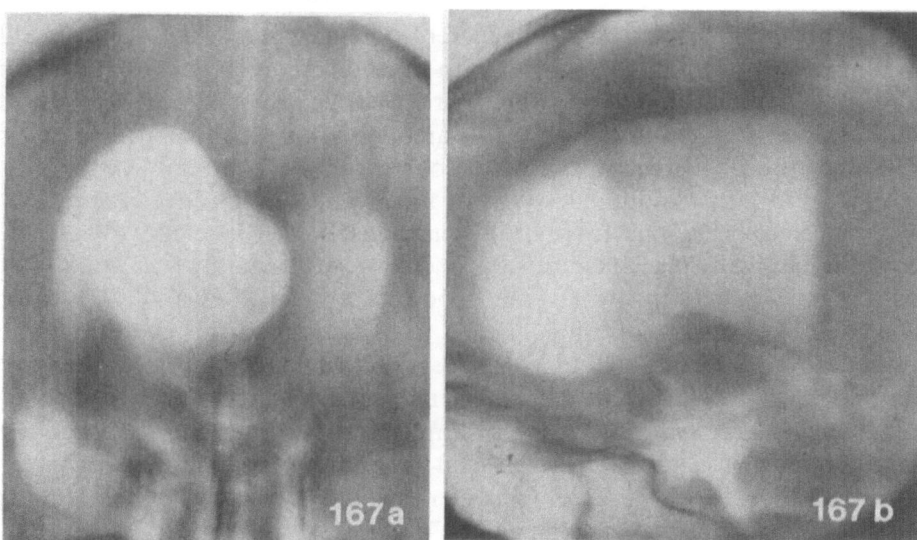

Fig. 167. Air ventriculography, anteroposterior and lateral view (a, b), revealing anterior third ventricle tumor (colloid cyst). Case published by Bosch *et al.* (1978)

Although computed tomography is the diagnostic procedure of choice to establish the presence of a lesion in the anterior third ventricle, and the diagnosis of a colloid cyst can nowadays be made without (Fig. 167) ventriculography (Apuzzo *et al.* 1984 a), stereotactic exploration may sometimes lead to an unsuspected tumor. Histological diagnosis will then disclose the tumor's nature and form a firm basis for transcortical transventricular open surgery in those cases, which benefit from resection (papilloma, meningioma, hemangioma).

Because all mass lesions at the foramen of Monro are clinically malignant and colloid cysts are completely benign lesions (Hirano and Ghatak 1974), stereotactic exploration is the optimal treatment, at least to start with. Angiography is recommended as a safety precaution. Even with possible refilling of the cyst we would advocate a second stereotactic aspiration. Underestimating the incidence of refilling and thus clinical recurrence is no longer a danger with repeated CT scanning during follow-up.

Recently, Rivas and Lobato (1985) presented another study of colloid cysts treated successfully in this way, using an even larger cannula (1.8 mm in inner diameter). On the basis of collected evidence it seems justified to treat these lesions only stereotactically.

### III. Primary Deep Seated Hematomas

Stereotactic evacuation of intracerebral hematomas was first practized by Backlund and Von Holst (1978) with subtotal clot removal (70/100 ml) in a primary hematoma patient, who after 1 week of critical illness showed an impressive and rapid improvement thanks to this approach. They deserve merit for their construction of a stereotactic probe, that can even handle clotted blood: an Archimedes-type of screw and suction instrument, that has proved to be very useful in the evacuation of clots. Attempts to aspirate by stereotactically placed cannulas are only successful in the first minutes of hematoma formation, when the blood is still liquid, and also after considerable periods of time due to liquefaction of the contents. The presentation of Backlund and Von Holst (1978) deserves appraisal, because of the new instrumentation, which enables the stereotactic surgeon to remove clotted hematomas using a simple method. This also reopened the discussion on the desirability of surgical intervention. In the following pages a differentiation will be made between primary hypertensive hematomas and non-hypertensive hematomas.

### A. Hypertensive Intracerebral Hematomas

Although the question whether spontaneous hypertensive hemorrhage should be operated upon remains a matter of discussion, during the last years several reports have shown favourable results of surgery. Particularly the Japanese neurosurgeons have made clear, that early operation for hypertensive hemorrhage (mainly in the putamen; Fig. 168) may lead to good functional recovery (Kaneko et al. 1983). Their operative technique makes use of both transsylvian and transtemporal approaches with craniotomy and a 10–15 mm cortical incision to evacuate the hematoma and coagulate the bleeding points (mostly the lenticulostriate branch in hypertensive cases) with microsurgical instruments. They stress the importance of early surgery (up till 3 hours after the onset of symptoms!), so that in a way their patients can be compared with those presenting postoperative intracerebral hemorrhage after some type of craniotomy. According to Kaneko (et al. 1983) the indication for surgical intervention is stupor and semicoma (scores 6–12 as judged by the Glasgow Coma Scale).

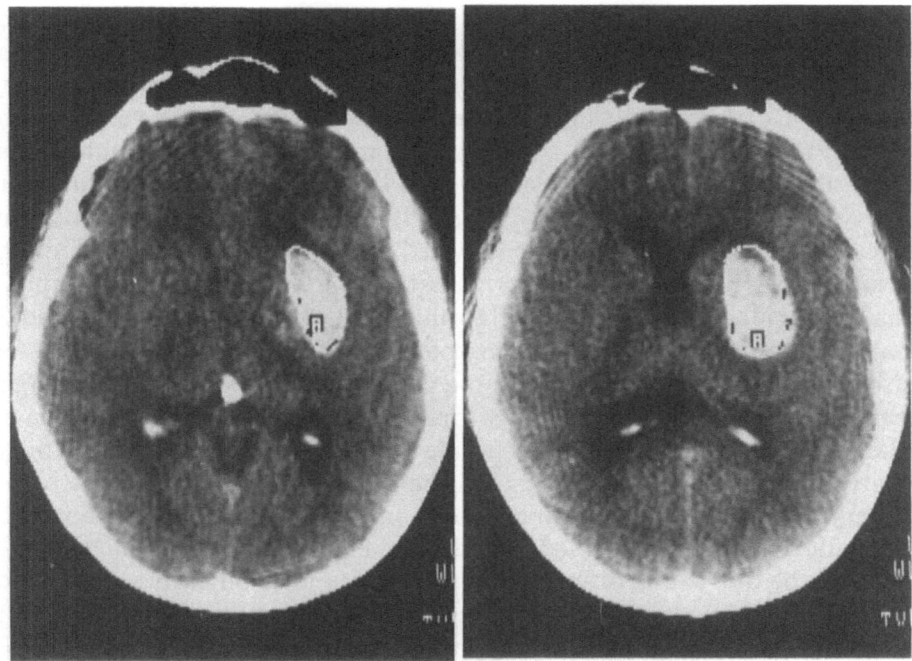

Fig. 168. CT scan pictures without contrast showing a spontaneous hypertensive putaminal hematoma. Measured surface volume $A$: 4.36 cm$^3$ (left), and 6.10 cm$^3$ (right)

Their impressive results (mortality rate 7%, and useful recovery at 6 months 83%) depended in the first place on the early timing of surgery, because with delayed surgical treatment (Kanaya *et al.* 1978) a mortality rate of 28.6% and a useful recovery of 62.8% were reported.

As in these putaminal hemorrhages (Kaneko *et al.* 1983) in the strictly lobar hematomas arterial hypertension is the main cause. Intracerebral hemorrhage caused by arteriovenous malformations or aneurysms should be demonstrated by CT scan and angiography and be treated by the appropriate means. Lobar hypertensive hemorrhage is discussed by Kase (*et al.* 1982) and according to these authors indications for surgery are in fact the same: candidates for surgery are patients with medium or large size lobar hematoma, who are in an obtunded or lethargic state of consciousness, worsening after admission. Early surgery is then the best option, because otherwise the development of brain edema will interfere with the intended recovery.

From these reports it follows, that several authors agree as to the indications needed for performing surgery in primary hypertensive hematoma. However, no agreement has yet been made regarding the surgical technique that should be followed. Open surgery is safe and offers the possibility to coagulate the bleeding points under visual control, which seems to be essential in early surgery. In delayed surgery, however, stereotactic clot removal is preferable, because rebleeding will very seldom occur (Broseta *et al.* 1982, Kandel and Amano: personal communications 1983). Recently, Kandel and Peresedov (1985) published a report on their own cases in which they discussed the safety and effectiveness of stereotactic evacuation. Out of 32 patients 25 survived, 23 with useful recovery. Timing of surgery was: 21 patients within the first 3 days, 9 within 4 to 9 days, and 2 finally after 3 weeks. There were 16 putaminal, 14 internal capsule, and 2 thalamic bleedings, with penetration of blood in the lateral ventricle in 19 cases. In all but 4 cases the hematoma could be removed totally, although rebleeding occurred in 5 cases. To prevent rebleeding, the authors have taken preliminary steps to try and inflate a Silastic balloon in the hematoma cavity with hitherto good results. On the other hand results of early open surgery have proved slightly more promising than with delayed stereotactic evacuation (Kaneko *et al.* 1983, Kandel and Peresedov 1985), which might, however, be due to the difference in timing. Reports on early stereotactic evacuation of hypertensive intracerebral hemorrhage have not yet been published, except for the report by Matsumoto and Hondo (1984), describing 16 out of 51 cases, which were operated within 12 hours after onset of symptoms. These authors also assessed the outcome for different preoperative grades of consciousness, and not only evacuated the clots but also delivered urokinase inside the cavity at repeated intervals. As compared with the results after open surgery no significant difference in mortality rates between the two procedures is seen. Similar results were observed on patients graded in group 1, 2, or 3, but the comatose (grade 4) cases showed better results after craniotomy, presumably due to the fact that these had very large hematomas, which could not be evacuated completely by aspiration. On the other hand, the deep seated (thalamic) hematomas seem to benefit more from stereotactic surgery, because of the invasiveness of open surgery.

The stereotactic instruments for evacuation [the Backlund aspiration screw and the Higgins (*et al.* 1982) modification] will aspirate both liquid and solid hematoma by application of a fluid irrigant under pressure, in combination with screw rotation and suction. One of our own cases of spontaneous intracerebral hematoma is shown in Figs. 169 and 170.

To reduce the risk of rebleeding this instrumentation may be completed with endoscopic instruments that enable the surgeon to inspect the cavity for bleeding points (Apuzzo and Sabshin 1983). Possible bleeding with fiberoptically transmitted laser instrumentation could be controlled (Kelly 1983). Also Jacques (*et al.* 1980) published on the successful removal of hypertensive intracerebral hematoma with stereotactic instruments.

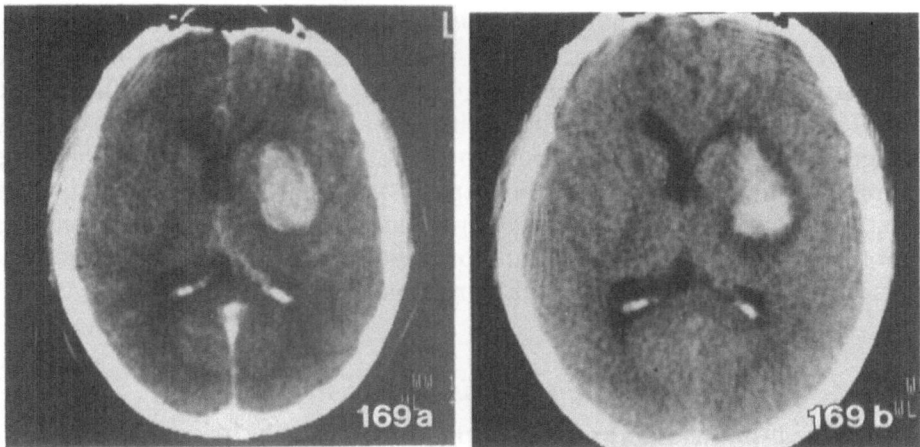

Fig. 169. CT [postcontrast in (a) and precontrast in (b)] pictures of hematoma before and after subtotal evacuation. Evacuation was stopped after removal of the calculated volume. However, more blood is present (b)

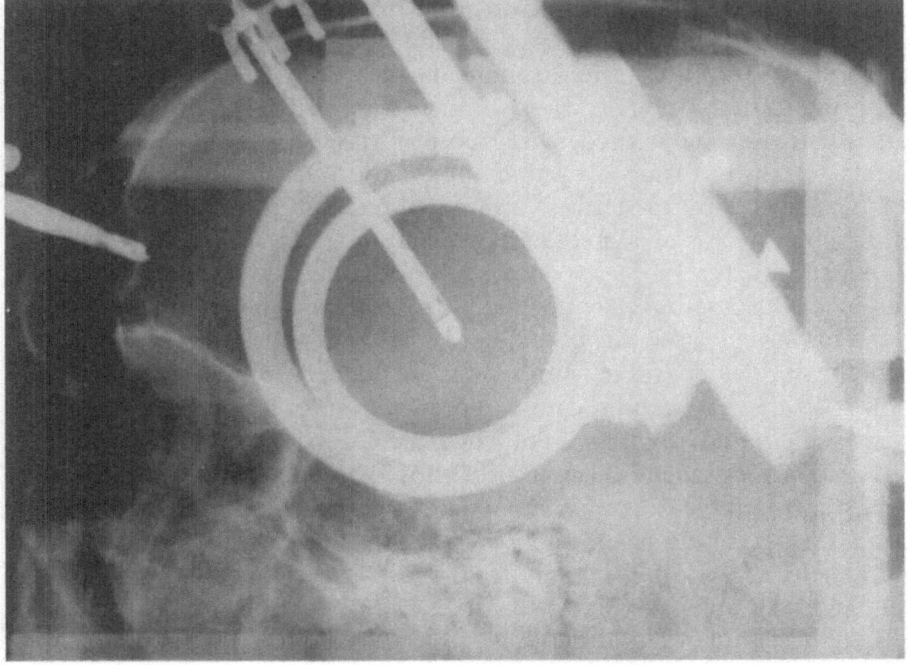

Fig. 170. Stereotactic evacuation of spontaneous putaminal hematoma with the aid of an Archimedes screw (type Backlund)

To summarize, the only relative contra-indication for stereotactic early hematoma evacuation in hypertensive hemorrhage is the risk of rebleeding. However, with completion of the Archimedes screw with a fiber optic endoscope and a (argon or neodymium-YAG) laser beam bleeding can be controlled. With the availability of these instruments even in cases of early surgery stereotactic intervention is to be preferred to open evacuation. This applies particularly for the more deep seated hematomas, which cannot be reached without damage to overlying structures. It is expected, that results yet to be published will contribute to a better understanding of the natural history of primary intracerebral hemorrhage.

## B. Primary Brainstem Hematoma

It is well-known, that primary hematoma of the brainstem has no clear relation to hypertension (O'Laoire et al. 1982, Durward et al. 1982). Causative factors include small arteriovenous (cryptic) malformations and venous angiomas (Huang et al. 1984). In fact, seldom the cause can be detected, as the hematoma obscures the vascular anomaly. Acute pontine hematoma forms only 10% of all primary intracerebral hemorrhage. With conservative treatment mortality is high: 76% in a series of 25 cases (Sano and Ochiai 1980) and 80% in another report describing 15 cases (Bryan and Weisberg 1982). With surgical treatment a 80% recovery has been achieved, according to the review of Mattos Pimenta (et al. 1981), who discussed 24 patients who were operated. Until recently surgery has been performed in the classical way (using the subtemporal approach to the lateral mesencephalon or the fourth ventricle approach to the pons), except for two case reports on successful stereotactic evacuation (Beatty and Zervas 1983, Bosch and Beute 1985). Open surgery has the disadvantages of being complicated, sometimes giving incomplete recovery with permanent injury to the brainstem (as in the case described by Durward et al. 1982). Injury might be observed particularly after having taken biopsies of the hematoma wall. Also the time required to explore the lesion with open surgery is a drawback compared with stereotactic evacuation. On the other hand, the stereotactic approach to this vital area should be carried out preferably with a small size cannula (less than 2 mm in diameter), which might be useless in the acute stage, clotting being active. A thin sized screw with the facilities the Archimedes screw offers, might be of great help in such cases. Although technically feasible, such an instrument has not yet been constructed.

The successful evacuation in the two cases reported (Beatty and Zervas 1983; Bosch and Beute 1985: Figs. 171 and 172) could have depended on the timing of surgery, which was 2 days or more after the bleeding. As most reported cases of brainstem hematoma present a (rapidly) deteriorating neurological state, conservative treatment is not justified and the deteriora-

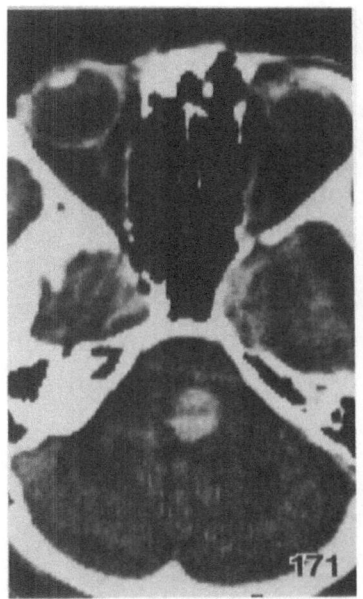 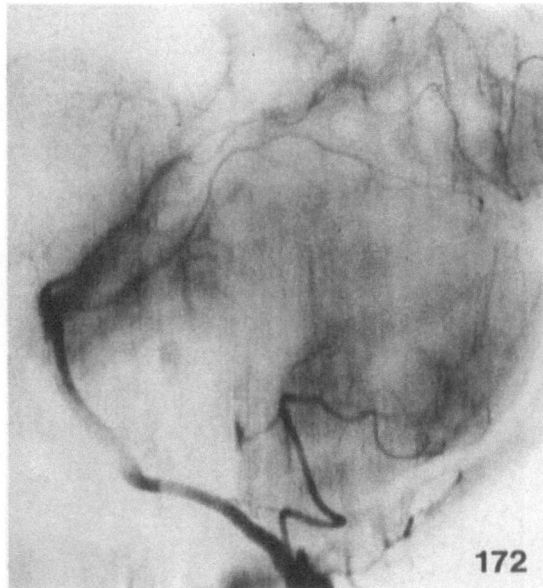

Fig. 171. CT scan demonstrating a hyperdense lesion (without contrast) in the left pontomedullary junction, suggestive of a primary hematoma; Female, 25 years (Bosch and Beute 1985)

Fig. 172. Vertebral arteriogram revealing bleeding from a perforating branch of the left posterior inferior cerebellar artery

tion itself is in fact the main indication for surgical intervention (O'Laoire *et al.* 1982). As compared with the less deep seated putaminal and lobar hematomas, the brainstem hematoma is much more difficult to approach by open surgery. This forms a relative indication for stereotactic evacuation, because the method is simple and complications tend to be less. Moreover the procedure can be carried out under local anesthesia (Beatty and Zervas 1983). It is obvious, that difficult cerebral transit can be avoided by choosing stereotactic surgery, making this type of operation even suitable for the elderly and critically ill patients. As reported by Matsumoto and Hondo (1984), particularly in the early hours after onset of bleeding clotting is present, preventing complete removal by aspiration alone. In those cases, where acute surgery is necessary due to rapid deterioration, the surgeon might try to place a small catheter stereotactically inside the hematoma cavity after apparent incomplete hematoma removal, to start postoperative local infusion of urokinase (as studied by Matsumoto and Hondo 1984). Urokinase in a solution of 6,000 IU/5 ml is recommended by these authors to liquefy the blood and repeated aspiration of residual hematoma may be attempted at a 6–12 hour interval with CT scan control.

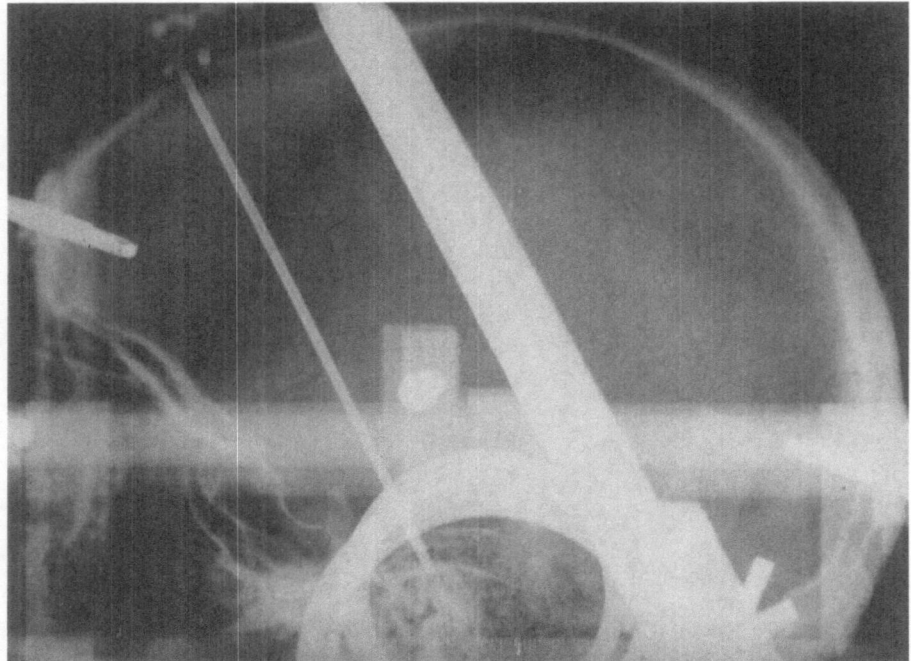

Fig. 173. X-ray film showing the tip of the stereotactic puncture needle inside the hematoma

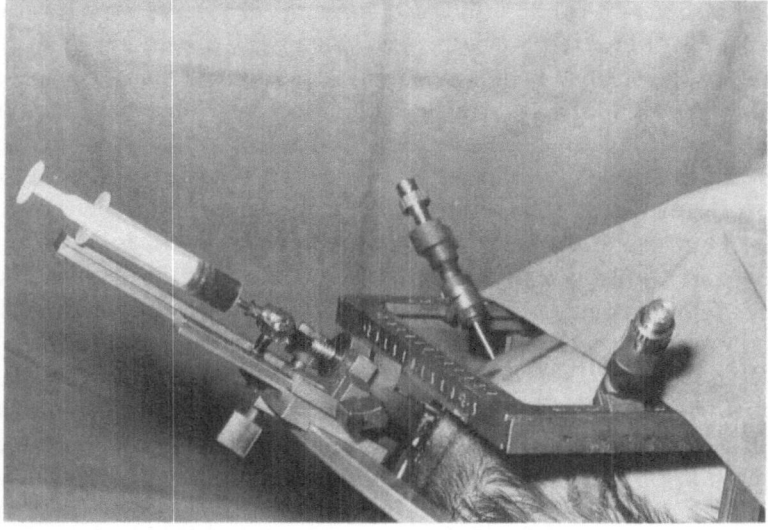

Fig. 174. Evacuation of blood by aspiration via the needle mounted on the Leksell stereotactic apparatus

The stereotactic approach to the mesencephalon should be from anterior, as described by Beatty and Zervas (1983). To the lower brainstem (the pontomedullary region) the stereotactic approach should preferably be from posterior, to minimize injury due to penetration of the brainstem over a longer trajectory. The positioning of the patient for the posterior

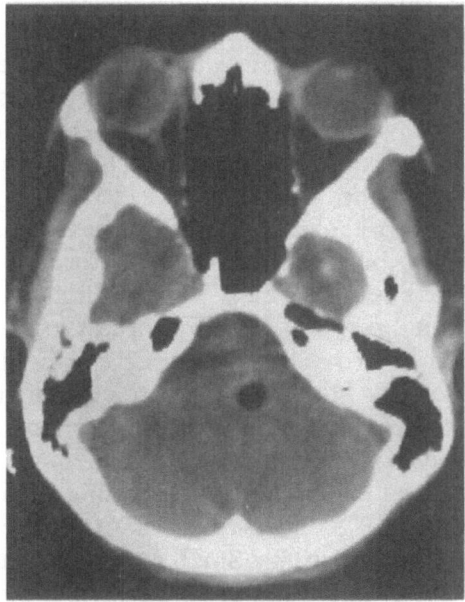

Fig. 175. CT scan picture 1 hour after surgery demonstrating air at the target area. There is no blood visible (Figs. 171–175 were published in the J. Neurosurg. *62*, 153–156; 1985)

approach may be relatively cumbersome, however, depending mainly on the stereotactic instrument used. Moreover, the suboccipital trepanation takes more time compared to a frontal burrhole, justifying the frontal route (Figs. 173 and 174) in an emergency case (as reported by Bosch and Beute 1985). From functional stereotactic studies, including mesencephalotomy and pontine tractotomy (Hitchcock 1973), it is well known that little harm is done to these structures by penetrating electrodes. In our case a postoperative anisocoria is explained by the use of the frontal route (Fig. 175).

We conclude, that in deep seated and life-threatening primary hematoma stereotactic surgery is strongly indicated and may safe life with good functional recovery.

## IV. Deep Seated Small Arteriovenous Malformations

### A. Introduction

Many years ago Riechert (1962) and Riechert and Mundinger (1964) disclosed the effectiveness of combining open surgery with stereotactic aiming techniques. Their early description of so-called combined interventions regards the management of deep seated angiomas and arteriovenous malformations. A review is given by Riechert (1980) in his monograph on stereotactic brain operations, in which he stresses the value of completing open surgery with stereotactic methods. The way of treatment often advocated some decennia ago, i.e. occlusion of feeders, has proved to be inappropriate, however, and Riechert's presentations are therefore obsolete as far as indications are concerned. Large AVM's seldom need stereotactic localization and should be resected totally if possible. The methods proposed and practiced by Riechert have remained untouched, however, and have only been refined for the treatment of small and deep seated AVM's. Reasons being the easy finding of the lesion and its afferent vessels, and the minimal cerebral resection necessary to reach and handle the lesion. Moreover, the route of preference can be discussed and even computer simulated in the stereotactic approach that uses CT guidance. Eloquent brain can be spared by choosing an alternative transit, whenever the malformation is lying in a critical brain area.

In discussing his great experience in the management of arteriovenous malformations, Drake (1979) stresses the importance of AVM size in relationship to the initial symptoms. Small malformations have a tendency to bleed, being 3 times higher than the large ones (more than 3 cm in diameter), according to Waltimo (1973). This observation is confirmed by others (Graf et al. 1983) and has led to the overall opinion, that patients with small malformations are candidates for surgery and should be operated after the first bleeding (Drake 1979, Luessenhop and Rosa 1984, Wilson et al. 1979). However, whether surgery is indicated in malformations that have not bled is a point yet to be settled. The risk of hemorrhage is only known in symptomatic AVM's, as the prevalence of asymptomatic AVM's is not known. The risk of bleeding in symptomatic AVM's is discussed by Graf (et al. 1983); he concluded, that the tendency for spontaneous bleeding inversely varies with size. The risk of hemorrhage in small malformations is estimated to be 10% at 1 year and 52% at 5 years, while large malformations might have a risk of 0% at 1 year and 10% at 5 years (this study dealt with 71 cases of unruptured but symptomatic AVM's). Ruptured malformations may lead to intracerebral hematoma or subarachnoid hemorrhage. As already discussed sub III, some spontaneous hematomas (particularly in the brainstem) may be induced by cryptic AVM's, that can no longer be detected with angiography after rupture. As Wilson (et al. 1979) describes,

CT scanning with and without contrast infusion may sometimes visualize a ruptured AVM, which is not detected with angiography; 3 cases of intracerebral hematoma (2 thalamic and 1 in the caudate nucleus) proved to be cryptic AVM's during exploration. The occult cerebrovascular malformations, not demonstrable with angiography, are reviewed by Becker (*et al.* 1979). CT scanning is more effective than angiography in detecting these small malformations, as shown in 18 histologically proven cases. It is

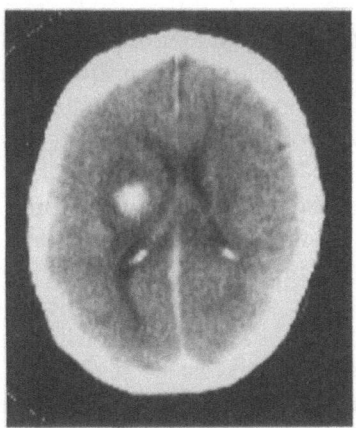

Fig. 176. Case of spontaneous hematoma formation in a man, 32 years. At puncture 2 cc of blood were collected. Angiography showed no abnormalities. Clinical diagnosis: cryptic vascular malformation

interesting to note, that on exploration partial thrombosis was always found as well as evidence of old hemorrhage. From these data it is apparent, that exploration should be considered in intracerebral hematoma well localized by CT (Fig. 176), even when the arteriogram is normal and a malformation cannot be demonstrated. For this reason one might consider stereotactic hematoma evacuation (as discussed sub III) only acceptable when having fiberoptical and laser instrumentation at hand.

Particularly in the young, normotensive, patient who presents acute neurological symptoms of intracerebral hemorrhage, arteriovenous malformations are successfully resected preventing further bleeding with substantial morbidity. Although no exact data are available on the percentage of occult malformations that are the cause of spontaneous intracerebral hematoma, Becker (*et al.* 1979) suggests this percentage will be significant.

In conclusion, small arteriovenous malformations are particularly dangerous. Whenever they bleed and cause rapid deterioration due to hematoma formation, surgical intervention is mandatory. The small and deep seated ones should be localized stereotactically so as to continue with resection in stereotactic space. As will be discussed sub B this kind of surgery is done with microsurgical and laser instrumentation. On the other hand, the group of AVM's to be treated this way is relatively small, and up till now only case histories have been published.

## B. Stereotactic Aiming and Open Surgery in Stereotactic Space in Small and Deep Seated AVM's

It is only in recent years that experience has been published on the stereotactic approach to these small malformations. Cahan and Rand (1973) published the first case report on stereotactic coagulation of a paraventricular arteriovenous malformation. Their attempt, however, was only partly successful.

It is generally accepted, that total excision of the malformation is preferable to ligation or coagulation of its feeders. The following reports (Garcia de Sola *et al.* 1980, Yamada *et al.* 1983) describe localization of small AVM's with stereotactic means as the first stage of open surgery to resect the lesions. The advantages are clear: total excision of the AVM core is made possible without the necessity of finding and following feeding arteries that may lie in critical brain areas; the cerebral transit route of choice may also be calculated. In fact, stereotactic localization may be the safest starting procedure in total resection of subcortically lying AVM's.

Although stereotactic radiosurgery of small AVM's (Backlund 1979, Kjellberg *et al.* 1983) forms a good alternative, it has the disadvantage that the shunting vessels are only occluded after about 1 year (a period of substantial morbidity due to rebleeding). Therefore, whenever the small AVM can be reached safely with stereotactic open techniques, it is advisable to resect it with microsurgical techniques—even in thalamic lesions—(Fig. 177).

The open stereotactic method for the total excision of deep seated malformations has become popular since the reports of Jacques (*et al.* 1980) and Kelly (*et al.* 1982 b, 1983) were published. Jacques used a small trephination and various dilators to reach the depth of the lesion, followed by the introduction of a new type of speculum into the brain, which is opened at the target. Small lesions, including 1 very small arteriovenous malformation (only detected by CT scan), were completely removed with the help of a series of specially designed instruments for use in this speculum ("tulip"). Kelly described a specially designed self-retaining retractor for use with the microscope, and laser instrumentation for precision resection of deep seated malformations by stereotactic and computer monitored open surgery. This technique includes CT scanning and angiography with the stereotactic instrument fixed onto the skull. During craniotomy the lesion is placed in the center of the stereotactic apparatus for precise aiming of the instruments (Todd-Wells system) using the computer collected data.

To achieve this sophisticated way of treatment one should be equipped with a stereotactic system, that allows for CT guidance, and with computer software connected to the CT scan, which produces information during surgery regarding the area of interest and the progress being made in resecting. On the other hand, with only using stereotactic localization and

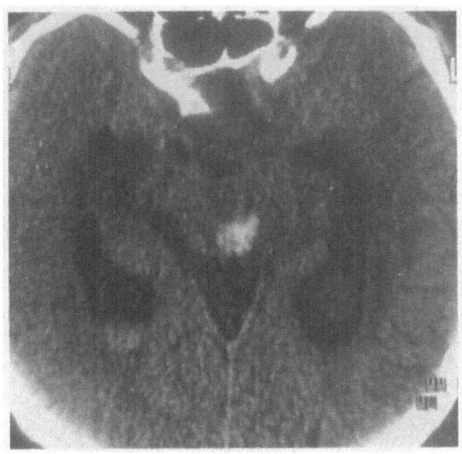

Fig. 177. Small mesencephalic hematoma (man, 62 years), caused by tiny arteriovenous malformation (visualized with angiotomography). Indication for stereotactic radiosurgery

subsequent conventional craniotomy, resection with microsurgical instruments with the help of the operating microscope will give similar results (Garcia de Sola *et al.* 1980, Yamada *et al.* 1983, our own unpublished results). Figs. 178–181 show one of our own cases.

## V. Stereotactic Aiming and Open Surgery in Stereotactic Space for Small and Deep Seated Tumors

Open craniotomy in the stereotactic apparatus after careful localization and three-dimensional reconstruction from CT pictures of the lesion's shape, size, and position in relation to the stereotactic environment has also been reported by Jacques (*et al.* 1980), Shelden (*et al.* 1980, 1982) and Kelly (*et al.* 1982 a, 1983, 1984 a, b).

This sophisticated way of tumor treatment has to be regarded as a major future development in stereotactics and is discussed in more detail in chapters 13 and 14. However, as biopsy in these procedures is only the first

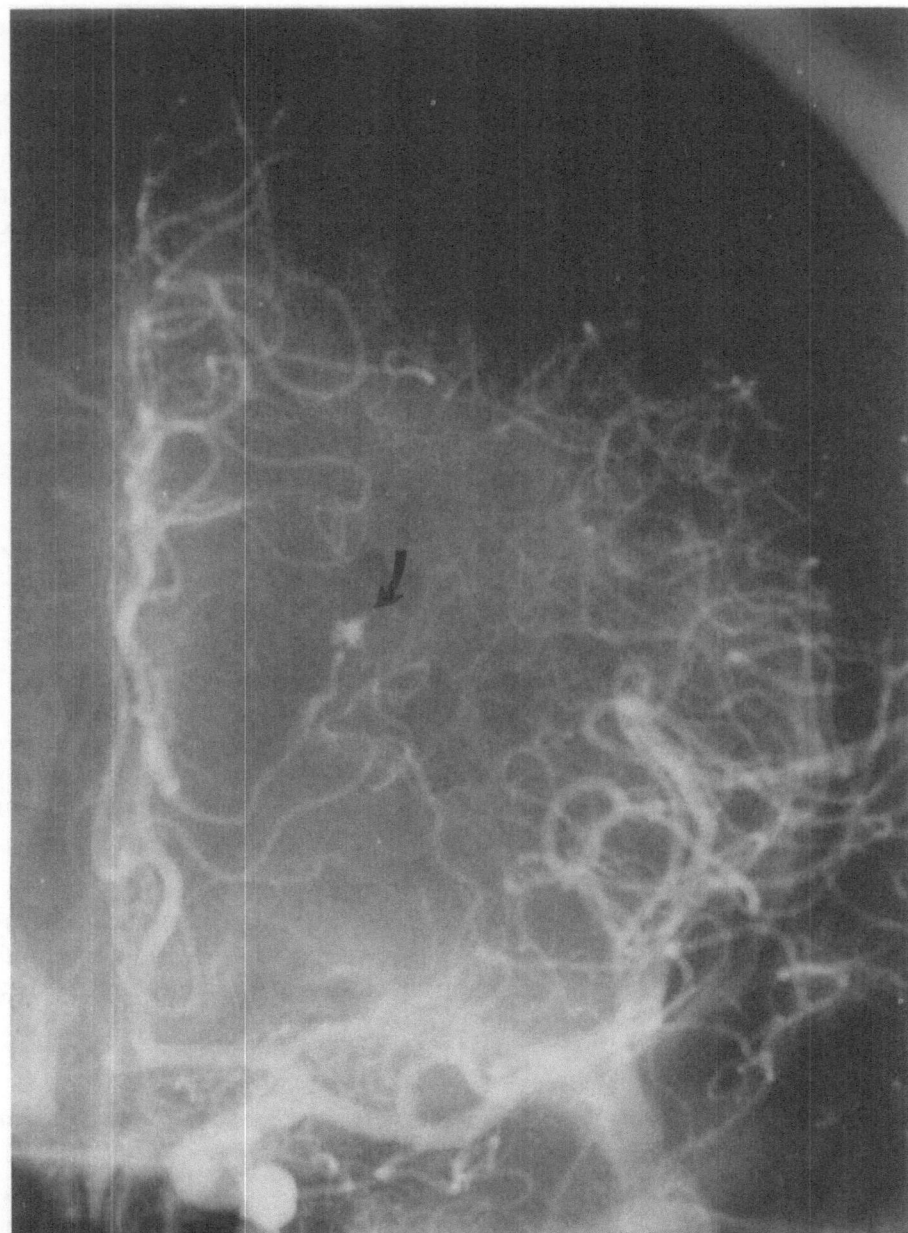

Fig. 178. Deep seated small arteriovenous malformation. Anteroposterior view. Lying in the wall of the lateral ventricle and draining through the thalamostriate vein. Man, 51 years, submitted with the clinical state of subarachnoid hemorrhage

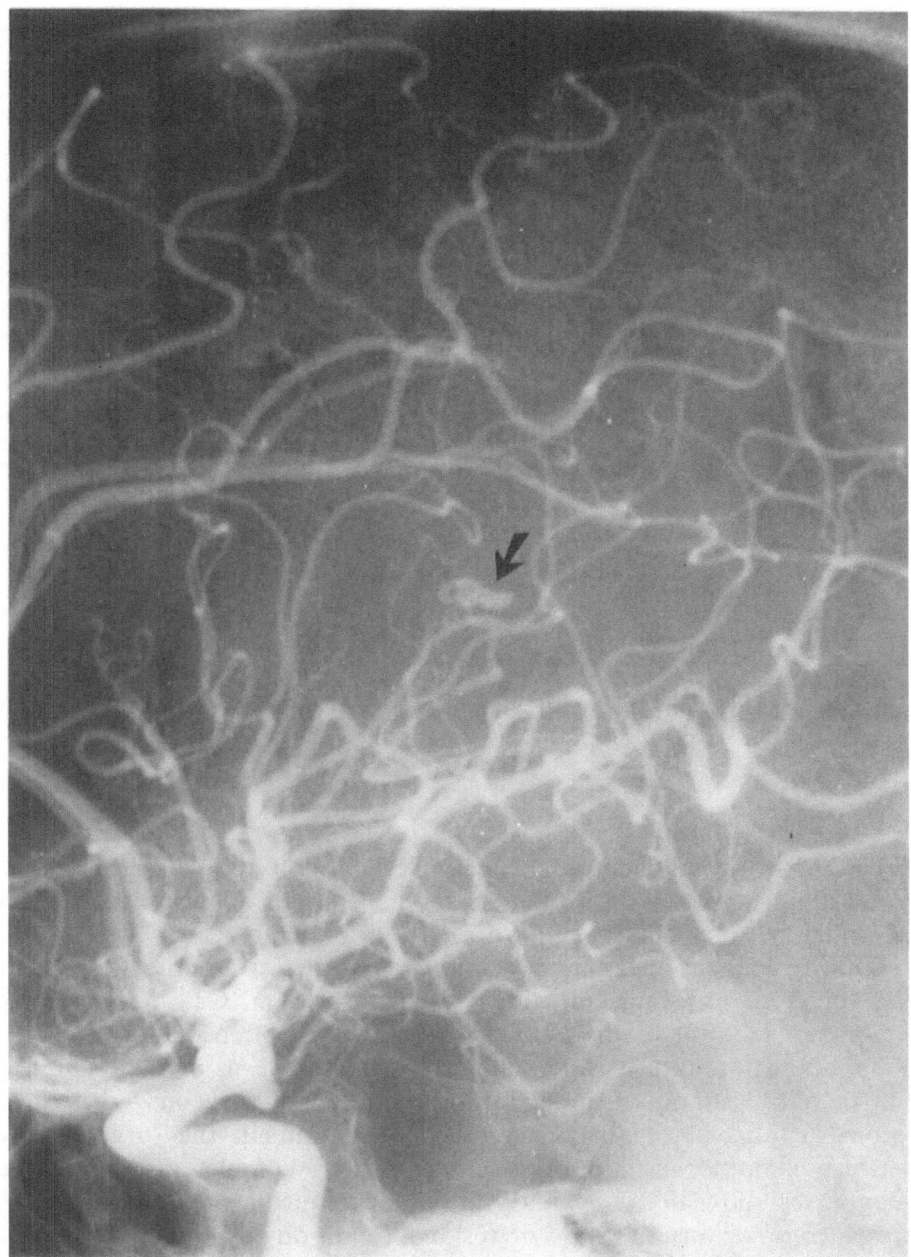

Fig. 179. Case presented in Fig. 178, lateral arteriogram. Further draining is seen through the internal cerebral vein. Indication for stereotactic localizing and subsequent resection

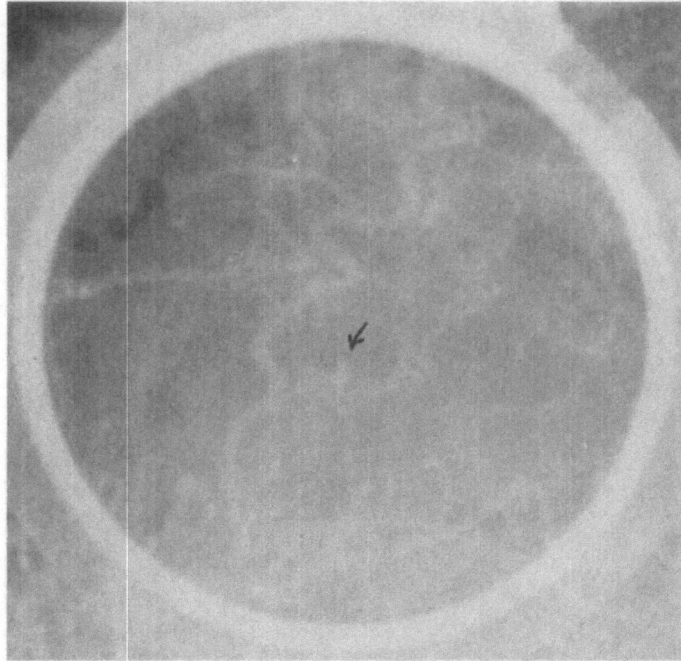

Fig. 180. Arteriography during the stereotactic localizing procedure (left common carotid injection), visualizing the AVM (arrow)

step, diagnostic information being directly followed by treatment, i.e. craniotomy to resect the tumor as far as CT can delineate it, a short introduction at this place is appropriate.

During conventional surgery tumor boundaries are frequently unclear and therefore unreliable on direct visual inspection. CT and Magnetic Resonance pictures of the lesion in question will often demonstrate the boundaries more clearly, and computer reconstructions of these pictures will therefore supply essential information to the surgeon. With these reconstructions placed in a stereotactic environment the surgeon may perform computer monitored resections that are complete as long as the imaging technique does not fail. With this technique the mentioned authors presented resections that show no residual tumor on postoperative CT, this being a great advance in surgical technique regarding deep seated cerebral tumors.

On the other hand, one should realize the limited value of so-called complete removal in malignant disease, as spreading of tumor cells outside these boundaries, as assessed with scanning, cannot be detected. MR imaging may become more important in the delineation of tumor as

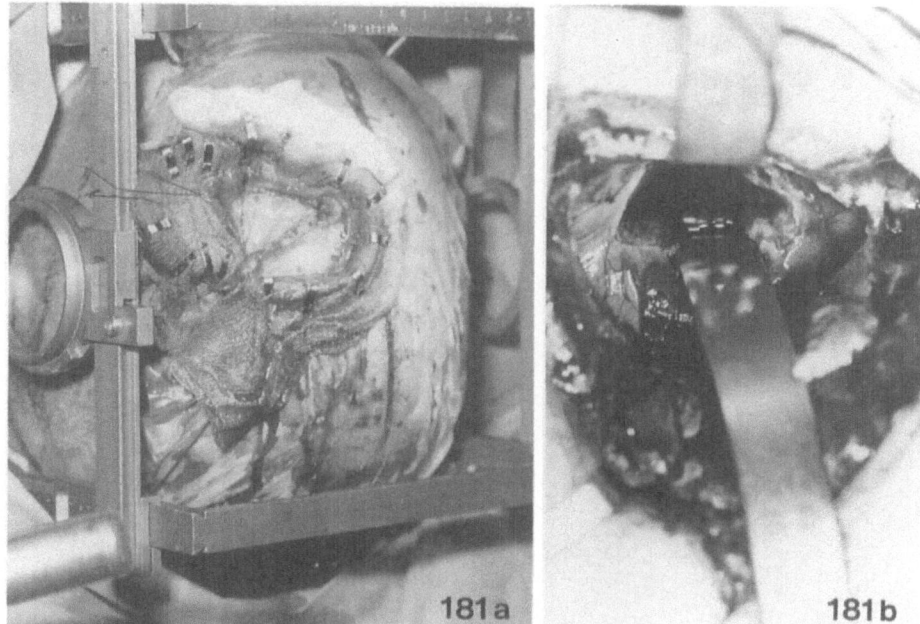

Fig. 181. Combined surgery for resecting deep seated AVM. A small craniotomy is performed in the stereotactic instrument (a), and through a small corticotomy (b) the lesion is approached with microsurgical techniques

compared with CT. However, this will give no technical problems as the CT guided stereotactic systems can also be used with MR guidance (chapter 4).

It is evident, that with this methodological advance in neurosurgery a completely new surgical strategy may be developed regarding the management of cerebral tumors. Cure of small and deep seated intracerebral malignancies could be within reach in the future, as local adjuvant therapies (see chapter 14) might complete this type of resection. Particularly, postoperative interstitial irradiation after computer simulation of the best available source positions (Kelly *et al.* 1984c) as well as local photo-radiation therapy (Laws *et al.* 1981, Shelden *et al.* 1982) are promising developments.

All these new technical advances may well usher in a new era in neuro-oncology.

Chapter 12

# Illustrative Cases

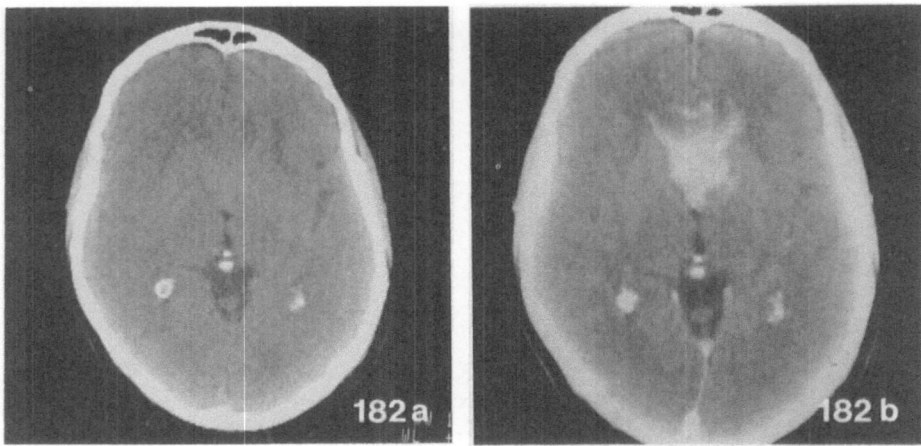

Fig. 182. **Case 1.** Male, 62 years. Presenting headache and mental changes with absent-mindedness. CT scan pictures (pre- and postcontrast; a, b) reveal a strongly enhancing tumor, growing as a butterfly, through the anterior commissure. Biopsy proved the tumor to be a malignant lymphoma. Histology is shown in Fig. 191. External radiotherapy was given and courses with intrathecal methotrexate

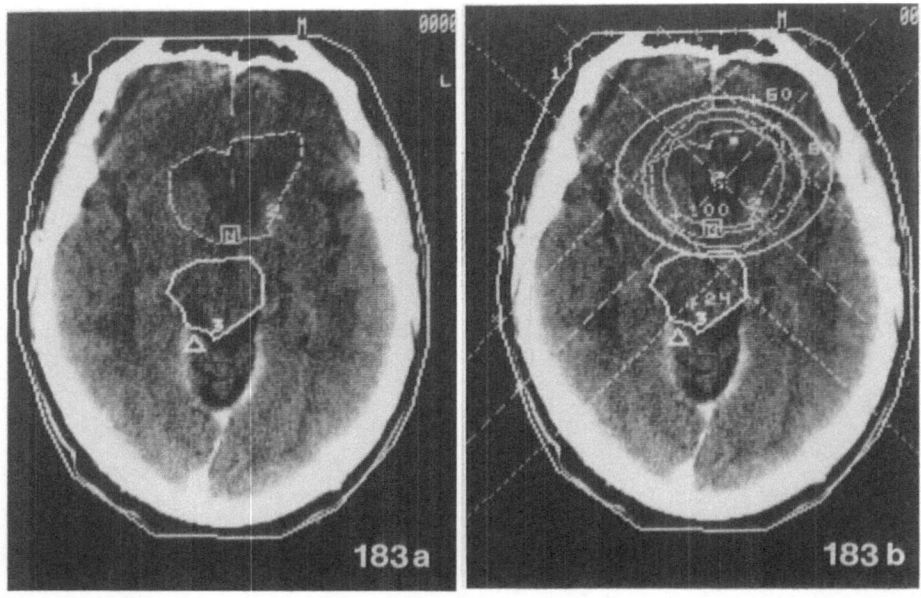

Fig. 183. Computer reconstructions superimposed on CT pictures, revealing the situation 4 years later. The patient is cured; postcontrast pictures demonstrating no residual tumor (a). Computer reconstructions show the tumor area with isodose curves (b) and the brainstem area that is radiosensitive (by courtesy of D. Bakker, K. Kersten, L. van Buul and M. Crommelin; Philips, Eindhoven)

---

Fig. 185. CT (pre- and postcontrast) demonstrates large left thalamic tumor, with some enhancement of the outer edge. Stereotactic biopsy was carried out and revealed a germinoma. Histology is shown in Fig. 192. Treatment was started with radiotherapy: a total dosis of 40 gray at the tumor area, and of 30 gray along the cerebrospinal axis. CSF cytology was positive

Fig. 186. Follow-up, 6 years later, reveals that the patient is cured. CT pictures (pre- and postcontrast) demonstrate no residual or recurrent tumor. At the site of the tumor a cystic area is found

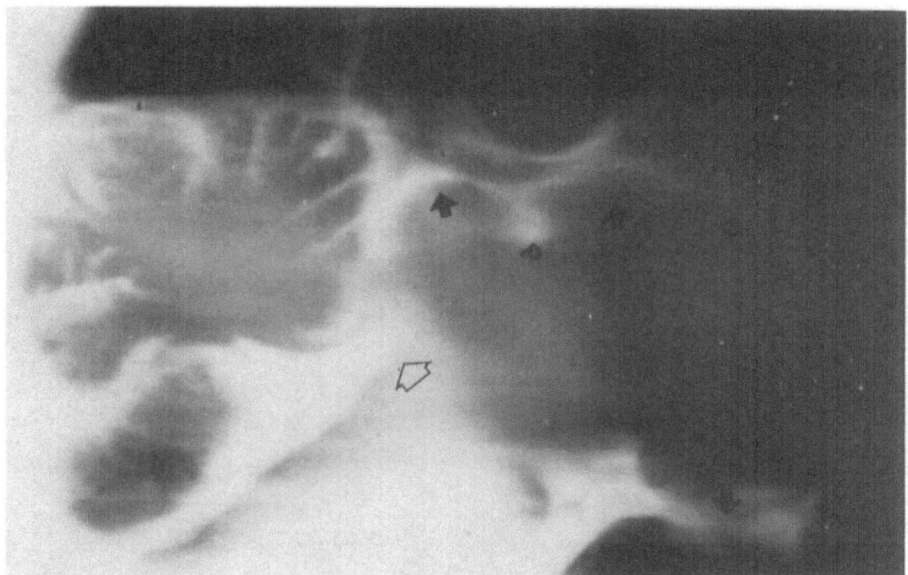

Fig. 184. **Case 2.** Male, 23 years. Presenting headache due to obstructive hydrocephalus. Papiledema. Ventriculocardial CSF shunt was inserted after ventriculography that demonstrated obstruction at the aqueduct (open arrow) and a thalamic tumor occupying most of the third ventricle (arrows)

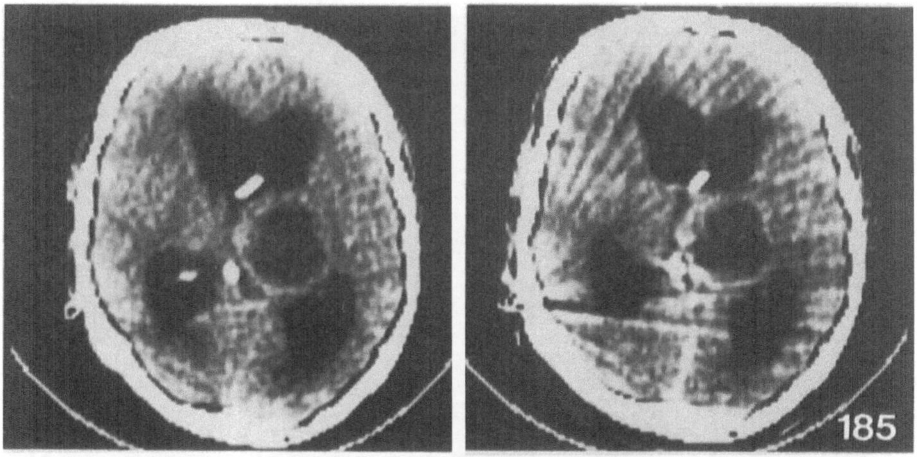

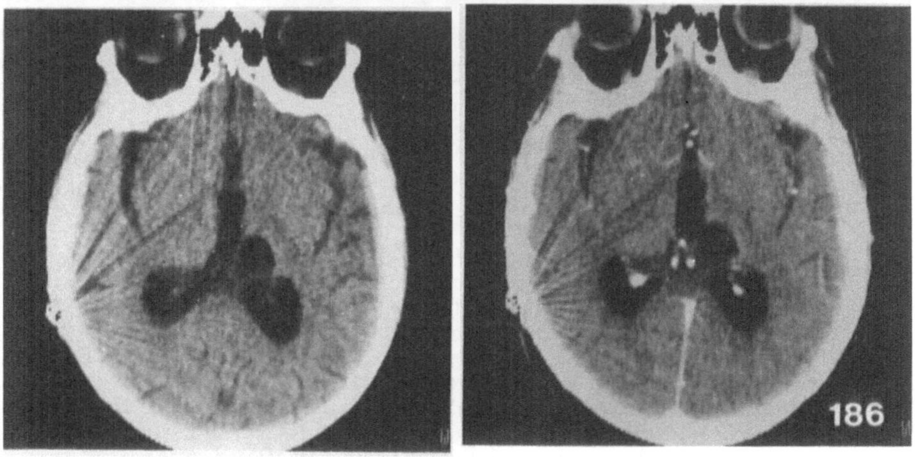

Figs. 185–186

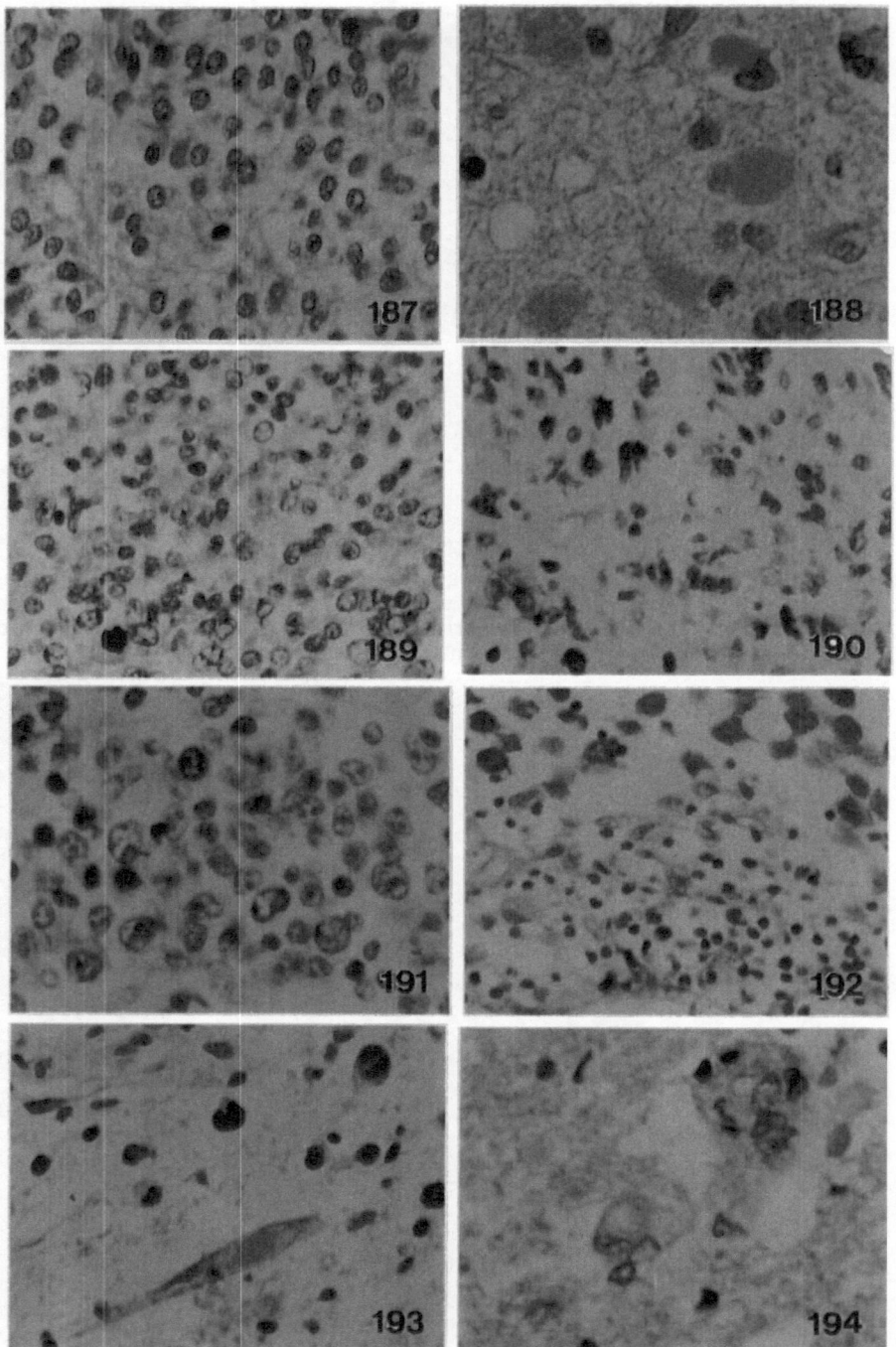

Fig. 187. Oligodendroglioma II, female 33 years. H & E 400 ×
Fig. 188. Gemistocytic astrocytoma II, male 47 years. H & E 600 ×
Fig. 189. Astrocytoma II, male 4 years (see Fig. 205). H & E 400 ×
Fig. 190. Astrocytoma IV, female 35 years (see Fig. 46, 78 and 79). PAS 400 ×
Fig. 191. Malignant lymphoma, male 62 years (see Fig. 182 and 183). H & E 600 ×
Fig. 192. Germinoma, male 23 years (see Fig. 184–186). PAS 250 ×
Fig. 193. Brainstem astrocytoma II, female 33 years (see Figs. 62–64). H & E 400 ×
Note pigmented nerve cell (substantia nigra)
Fig. 194. Anemic infarction, female 59 years. H & E 600 ×

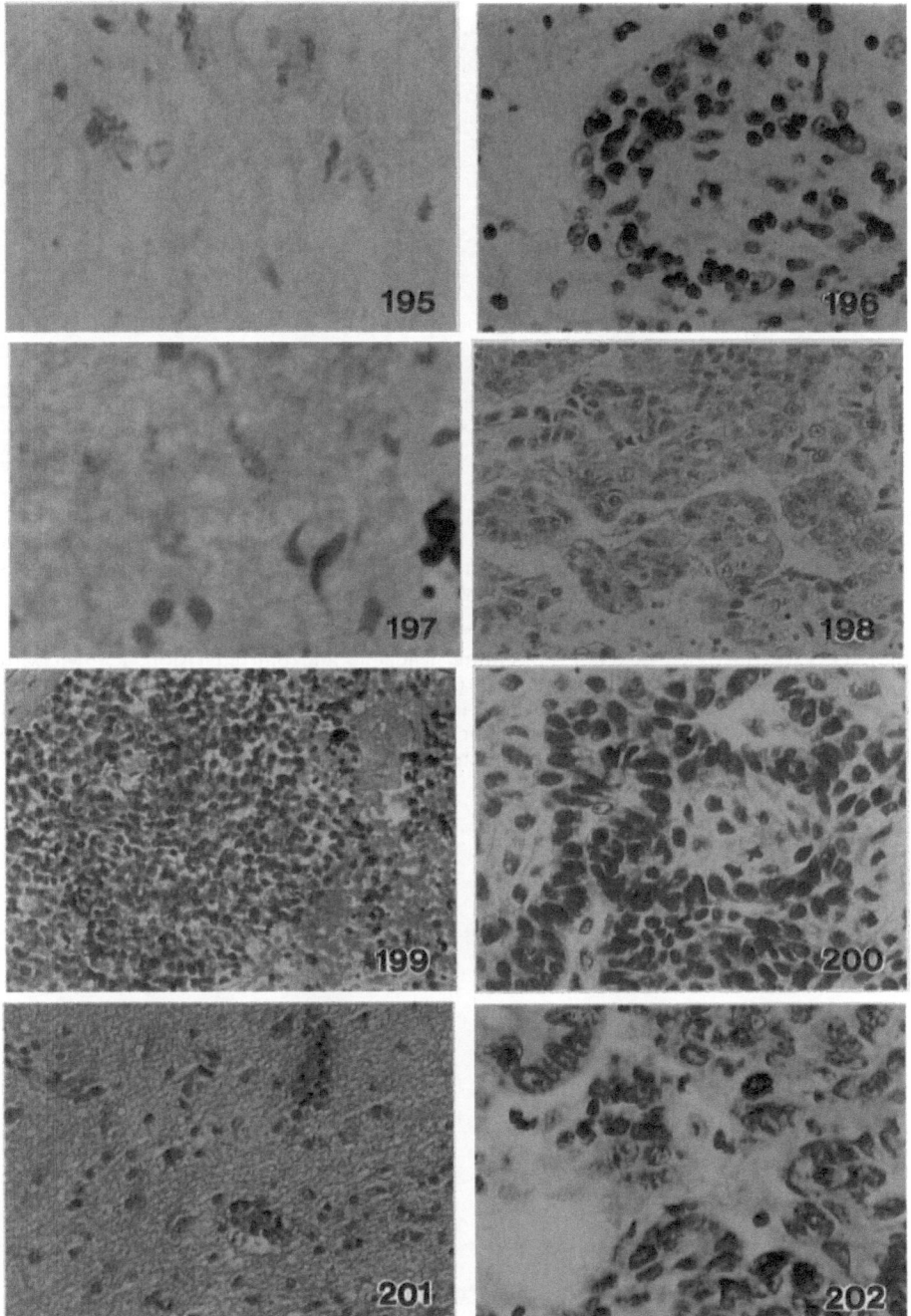

Fig. 195. Temporal gliosis (birth trauma), male 16 years (see Figs. 69 and 207). PTAH 600 ×
Fig. 196. Reactive lymphocytes, male 35 years (see Fig. 73). Klüver-PAS 400 ×
Fig. 197. Prenatally contracted matrix bleeding, female 18 years (see Figs. 77 and 203). Perls
600 ×
Fig. 198. Metastasis of papillary adenocarcinoma, male 61 years. H & E 300 ×
Fig. 199. Metastasis of anaplastic carcinoma, male 56 years known with larynx carcinoma.
H & E 200 ×
Fig. 200. Craniopharyngioma, male 43 years (see Fig. 204). H & E 400 ×
Fig. 201. Herpes encephalitis, female 15 years (virologically proved). H & E 200 ×
Fig. 202. Metastasis of adenocarcinoma of the breast, female 51 years. PAS 400 ×

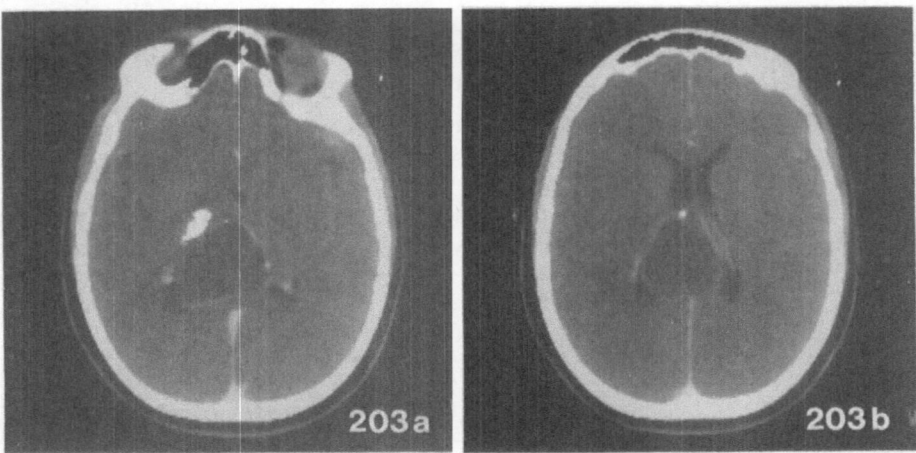

Fig. 203. **Case 3.** Female, 18 years. Presenting large subependymal cyst with some calcifications (different scanning levels: a, b). Biopsy of the cyst wall showed (see Fig. 197) abnormalities compatible with a prenatally contracted bleeding in the subependymal cellular matrix. After biopsy a catheter was left in situ (see Fig. 77), but repeated fluid evacuation has not been necessary (follow-up 2 years)

Fig. 204. **Case 4.** Male, 43 years. Presenting headache and blurred vision. Known with genuine epilepsy for years. CT scan pictures (postcontrast) demonstrated the presence of a suprasellar mass lesion (pictures a, c), being unresectable. Biopsy proved the tumor to be a craniopharyngioma (see Fig. 200) and radiotherapy was given. Inactive tumor rests are shown on the pictures b, d; 2 years later

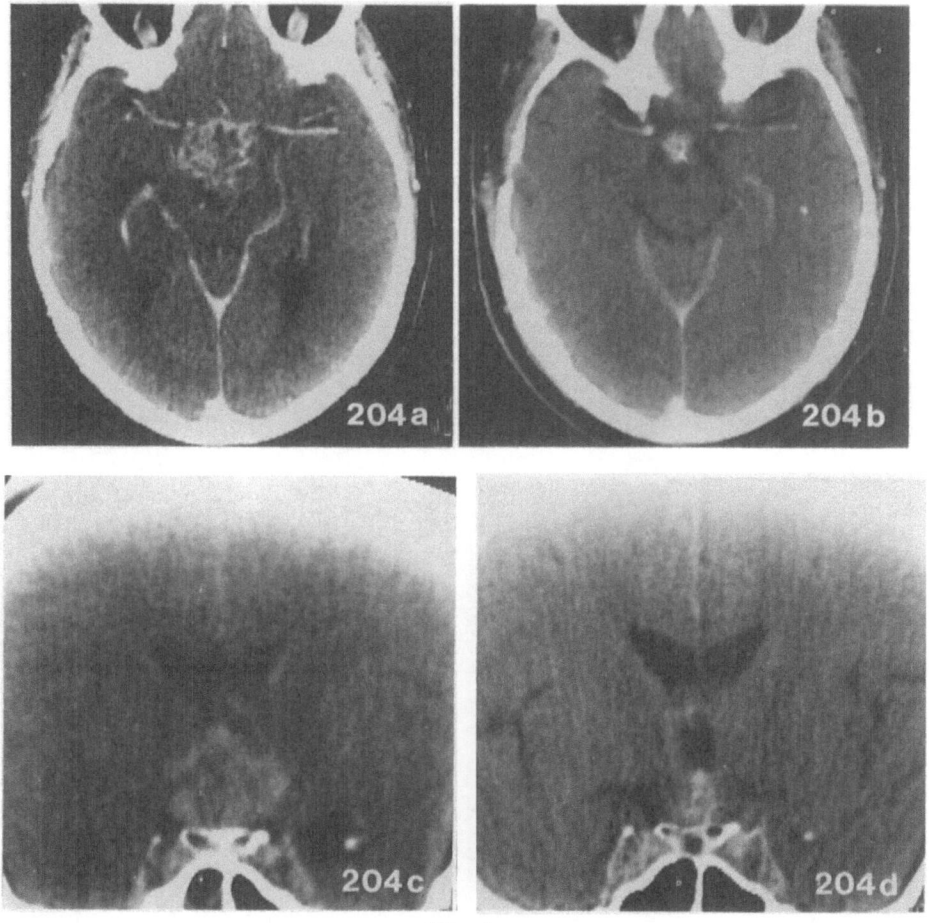

Fig. 4

Fig. 205. **Case 5.** Boy, 4 years old. Had an epileptic fit and was brought to the hospital. CT scan (a and b) pictures, pre- and postcontrast, revealed the presence of a tumor in the right parietotemporal area. A biopsy was performed (see Fig. 189), which showed an astrocytoma grade II. 1 year after radiotherapy local recurrent growth was noted (c) and the patient died

Fig. 206. **Case 6.** Boy, 4 years old. Presenting endocrine disturbance with obesitas and polyphagia. CT scan (a and b) pictures, pre- and postcontrast, showed a strongly enhancing tumor mass in the right hypothalamus. Biopsy demonstrated a pilocytic astrocytoma to be the cause. Radiotherapy was started and after 4 years (c) tumor remnants are inactive

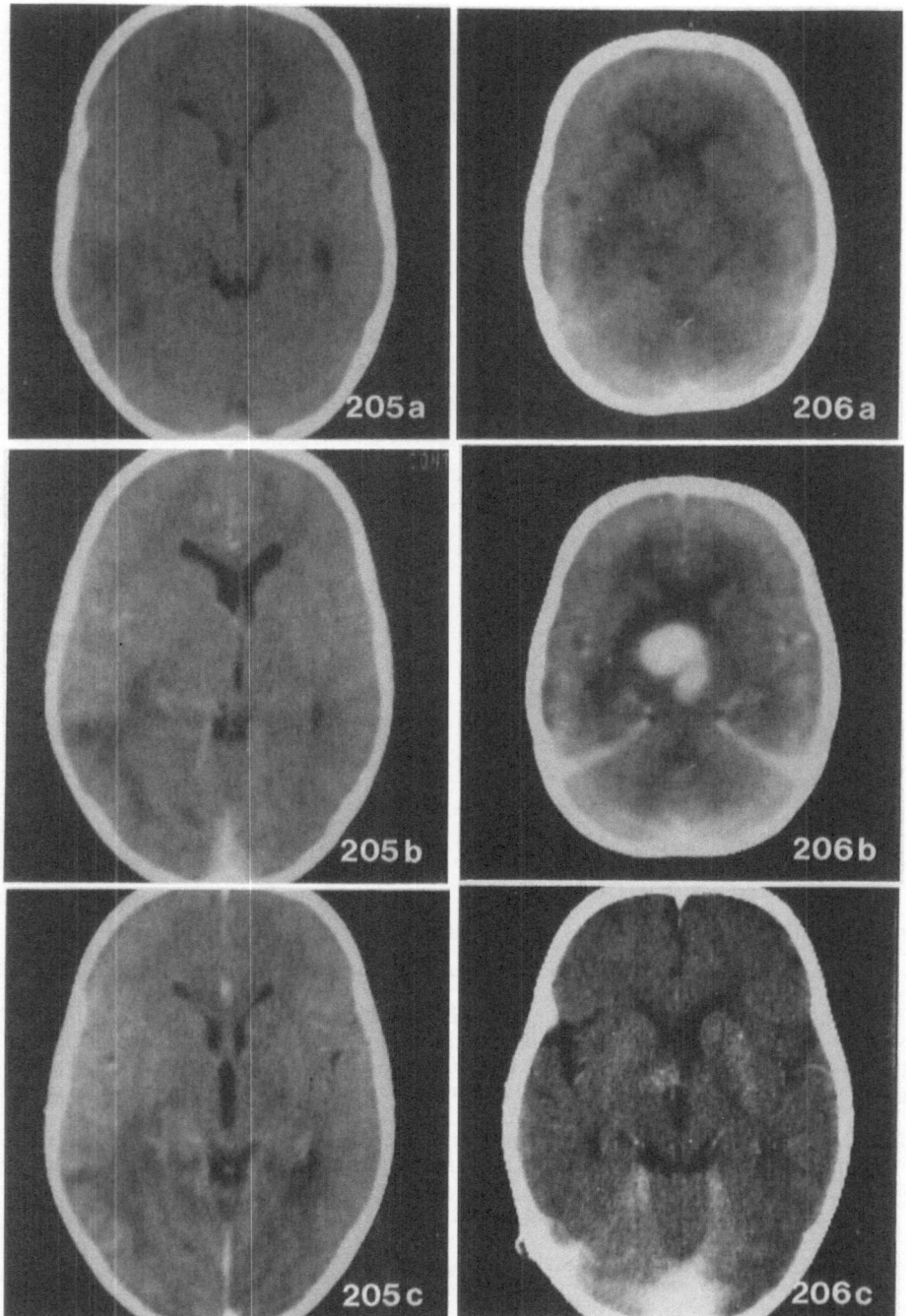

Figs. 205–206. Legends see p. 225

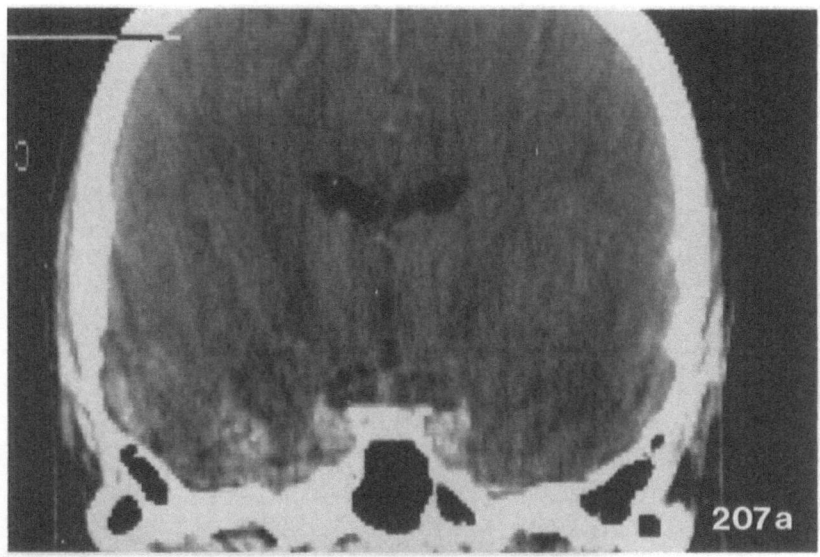

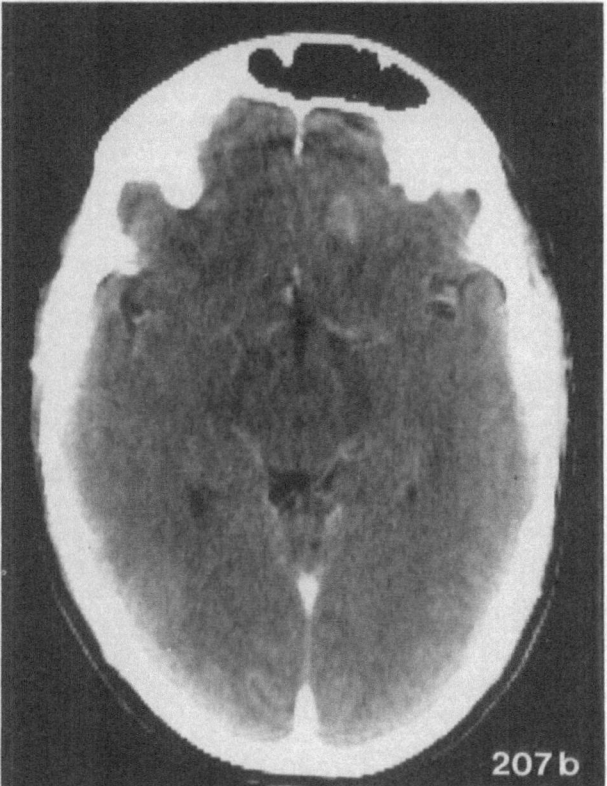

Fig. 207. **Case 7.** Male, 16 years. Known for years with genuine temporal epilepsy. EEG showed rightsided epileptic activity and CT (coronal picture: a) confirmed the presence of an enhancing lesion. CT (axial picture: b) also demonstrated a small leftsided frontobasal lesion. To rule out the possibility of tumor biopsies were carried out (see Fig. 195), which proved the lesions to be gliotic scarr tissue due to anoxia

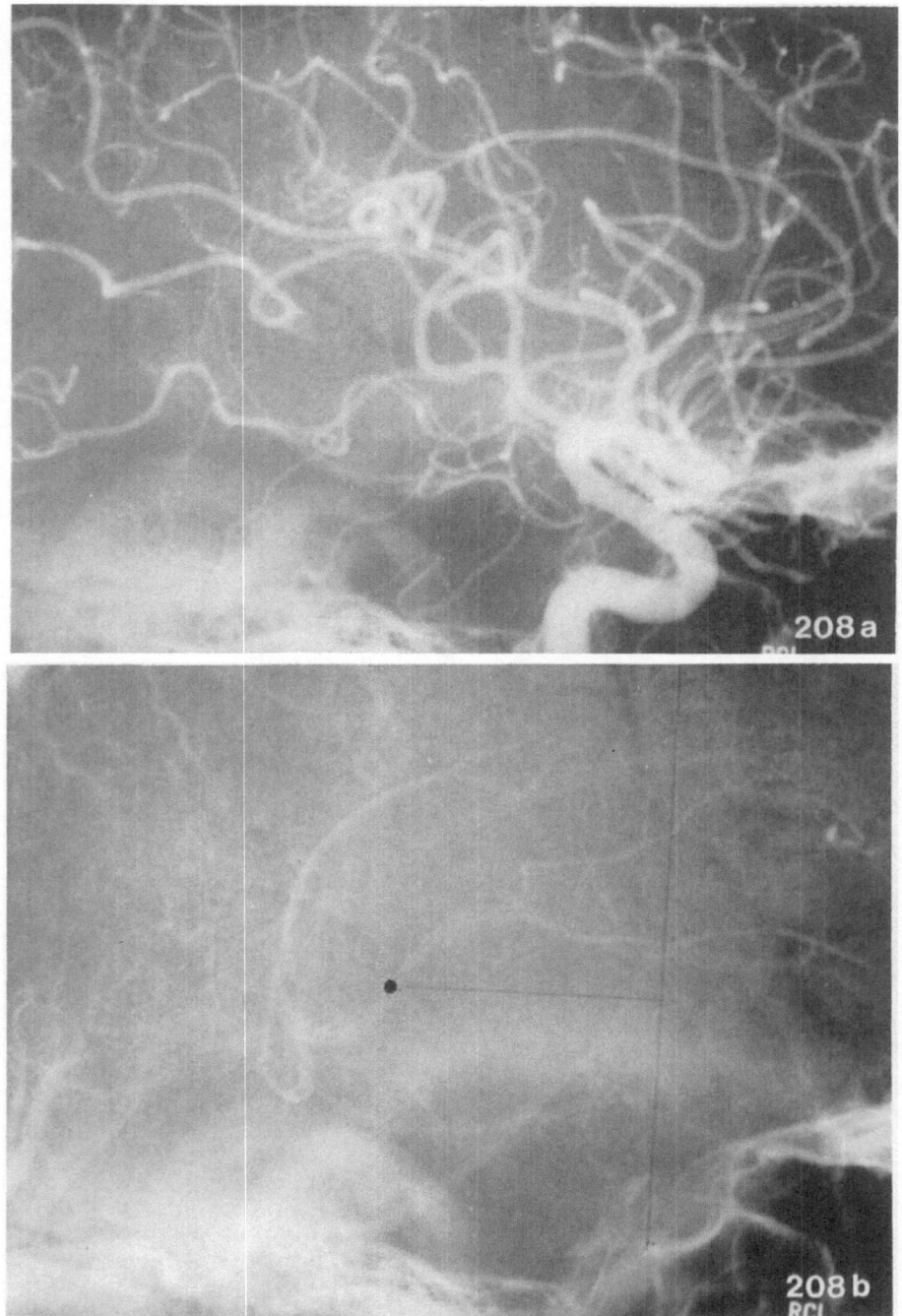

Fig. 208

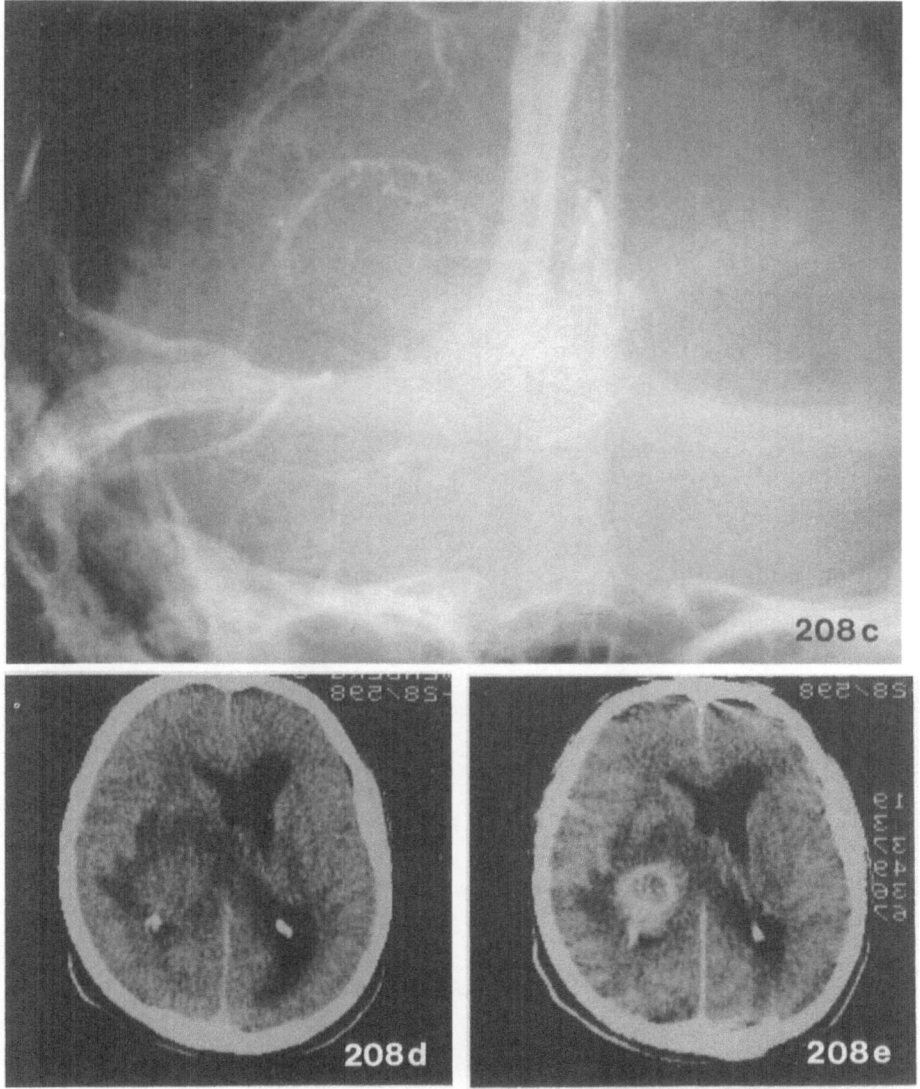

Fig. 208. **Case 8.** Male, 55 years. Headache and increased intracranial pressure with leftsided hemiparesis. Cerebral angiography demonstrated in arterial and venous phases (a–c) tumor surrounding vessels without distinct pathological shunting vessels. CT (pre- and postcontrast; d) and e) showed clearly enhancing lesion with marked midline shift to the left. Biopsy (black dot) was performed and revealed an astrocytoma grade III

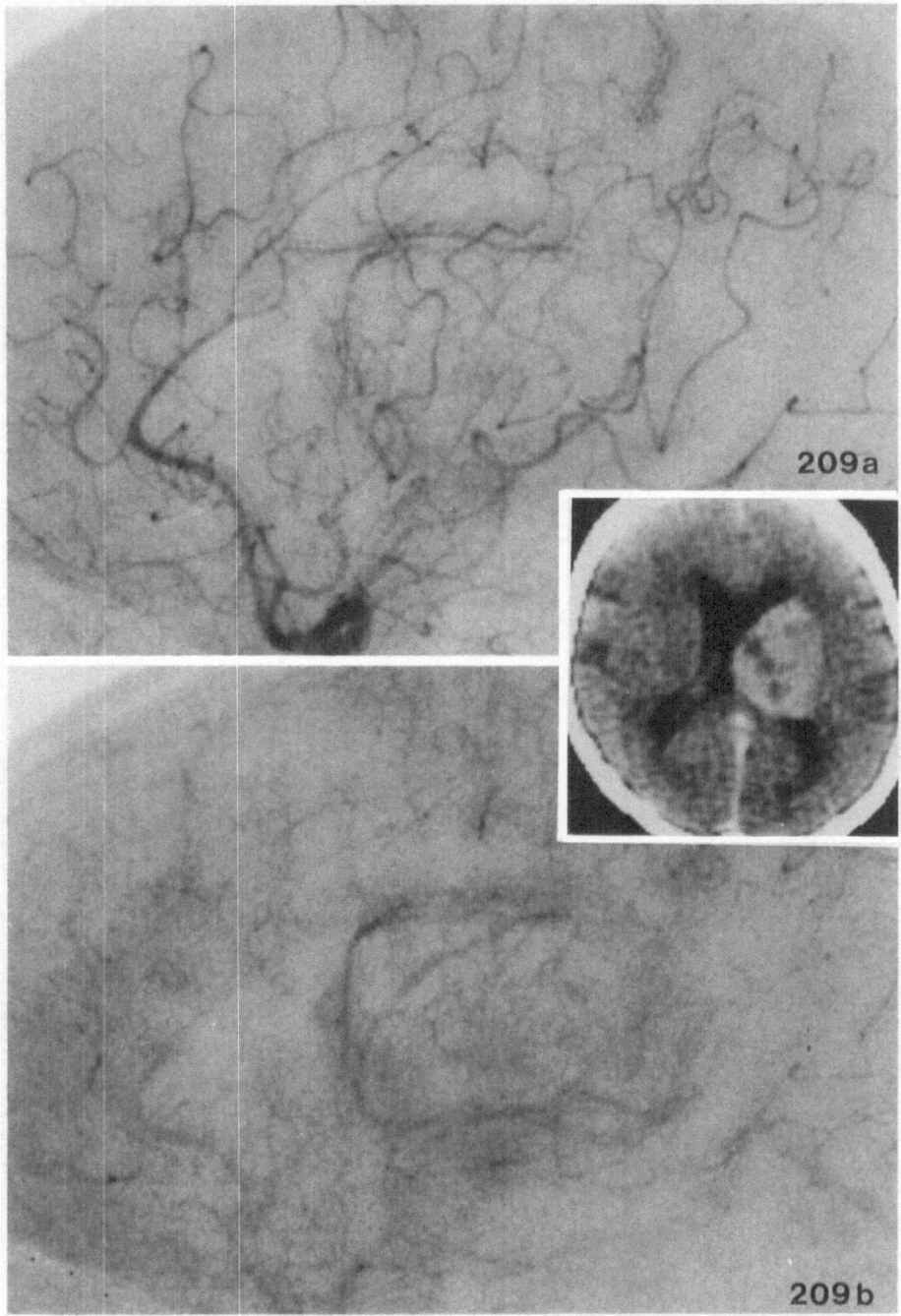

Fig. 209. **Case 9.** Female, 68 years. Leftsided deep seated tumor with necrotic parts (see insert) is seen on postcontrast CT picture. Angiography demonstrated a highly vascular tumor with pathological vessels and early venous drainage. Biopsy showed the presence of a malignant astrocytoma (grade IV)

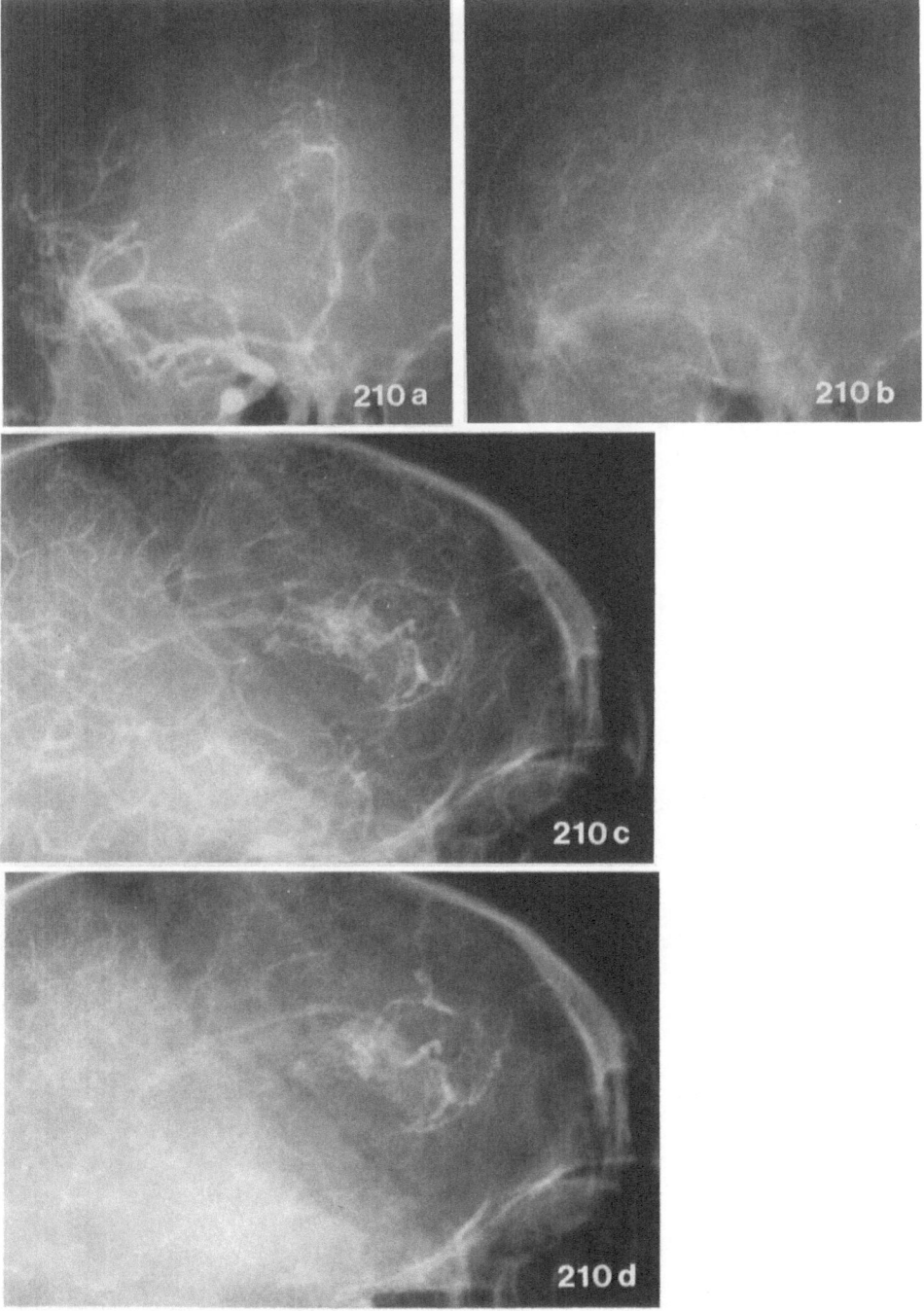

Fig. 210. **Case 10.** Male, 58 years. Presenting mental changes and headache. No paresis. Angiography, arterial (a, c) and venous (b, d) phases, reveals arteriovenous shunts inside the tumor, which at biopsy proved to be an astrocytoma grade III. Tumor is growing as a butterfly in the corpus callosum

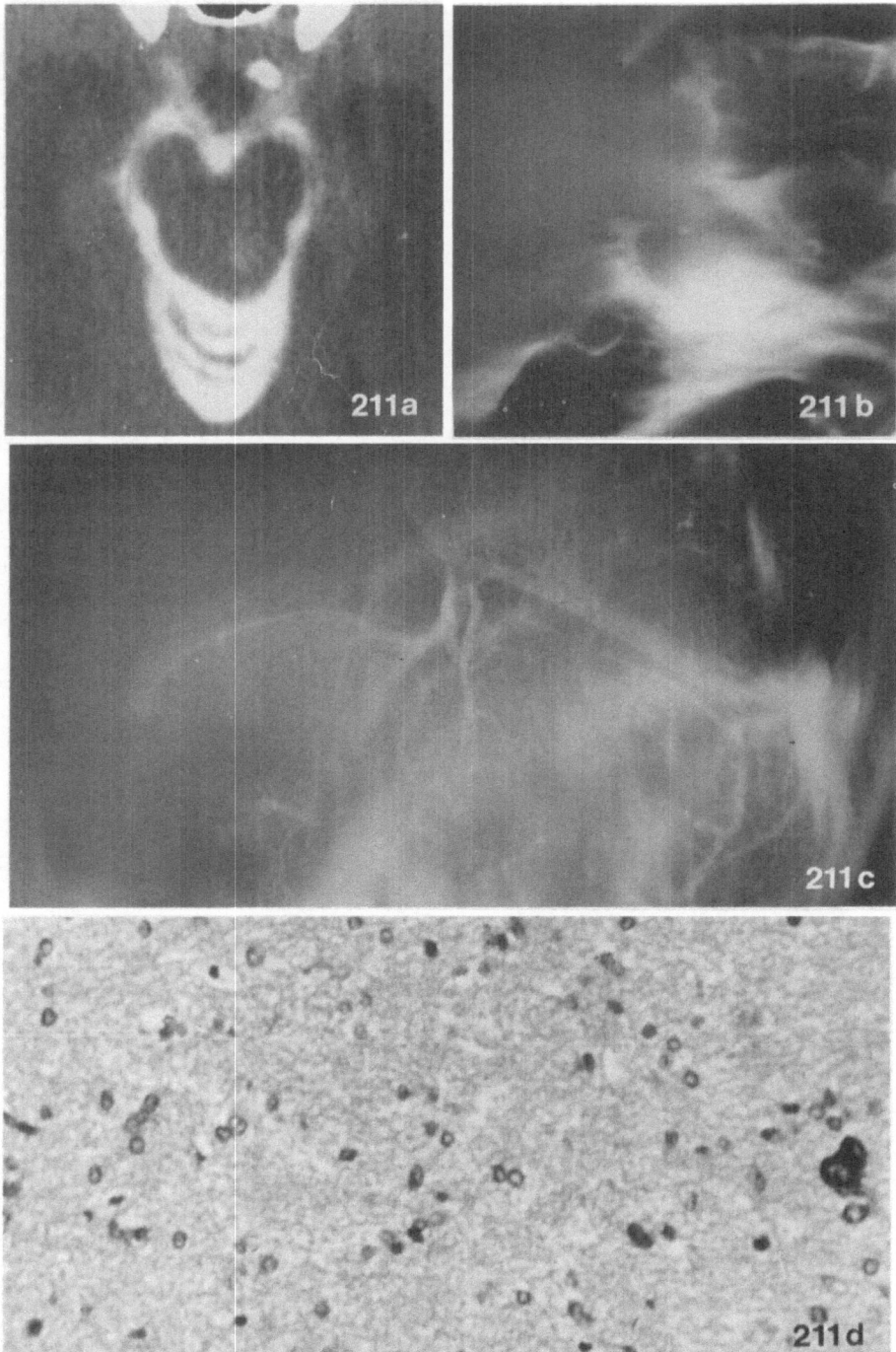

Fig. 211. **Case 11.** Boy, 7 years. Known for years with hydrocephalus and treated by then with a ventriculoperitoneal shunt. Presented "so-called" shunt dysfunction, but with reexploration and testing the shunting device showed to be patent. CT cisternography (a) was carried out and demonstrated a leftsided enlargement of the rostral brainstem. X-ray tomography with positive contrast (b) showed obstructed aqueduct due to mesencephalic mass. Angiotomography (c) showed abnormal course of draining veins and it was decided to perform a stereotactic biopsy. Histological examination (d) showed the presence of an astrocytoma grade I (H & E, 200 ×)

Chapter 13

# Integration of Stereotactics in Clinical Neurosurgery

## I. Introduction

Seen from a historical point of view stereotactic surgery has initially been developed as a tool to a better understanding of normal brain function, i.e. neurophysiology. Stereotactic instruments were built for brain research in animals and the use of the stereotactic method has in fact much contributed to a better understanding of deep brain structures (nuclear substance and conducting pathways). The logical consequence of these neurophysiological experiments was the application of the stereotactic method to functional treatment of various syndromes in man. This step has been taken by Spiegel and Wycis in 1947 with the first stereotactic intervention to alleviate otherwise intractable pain. Subsequently stereotactic surgery became an accepted method of treating patients with so-called functional syndromes. Some neurosurgeons learned the technique and became known as stereotactic neurosurgeons. Not infrequently this meant, that these neurosurgeons lost their interest in general neurosurgical problems and procedures.

Consequently, until recently stereotactics has been held to be a rather isolated form of surgery, without any connection to general neurosurgery.

After about two decennia, interest in brain tumor treatment with non-surgical means (i.e. radiotherapy) increased considerably and one felt the necessity of acquiring information as to the true nature of tumors. Histological examination of tumor samples and grading protocols became popular. Moreover, deep seated tumors could be biopsied safely with stereotactic means. This breakthrough rose the interest of general neurosurgeons in the stereotactic method, and slowly the process of integration started. All over the world this opening was accepted eagerly and one began applying stereotactics to mass lesion diagnostics. Thus a disconnection took place between functional and stereotactic surgery. Although functional surgery remained stereotactic, stereotactic surgery became a methodology in general neurosurgical practice.

## II. The Computer in Neurosurgery

Within the following years computerized axial tomography became available and gave a firm basis for localization and visualization of mass lesions inside the brain. Targets made visible (chapter 2, sub V A 2) with X-ray studies, such as angiography, were clearly depicted with these new techniques and exact positioning of the target in stereotactic space with calculation of the extent of the lesion became feasible. A true integration of stereotactic in general neurosurgery was within reach.

The subsequent development of high resolution scanners and magnetic resonance imaging of the brain have provided neurosurgeons with essential information during the last years. Technically speaking, imaging of pathological processes inside the brain has no limits, and three-dimensional reconstruction from data collected with the scanning procedure is possible (Bertrand 1982). Indeed, as Gildenberg states (1983), "the marriage of computerized tomographic (CT) scanning and stereotactic surgery opens up new technical possibilities". Stereotactics has matured from a more particular method into a fullgrown methodology presenting the interested neurosurgeon with the tools to manage pathological conditions which would otherwise have been (too) difficult to localize.

Even conditions, which should be managed with microsurgical and open techniques may benefit from stereotactic localization and three-dimensional reconstruction techniques with the aid of the computer. Open surgery will then follow computer guided study of the position of the lesion and the best approach to reach it. Thanks to the computer which provides a precise three-dimensional data base, many neurosurgeons are now revising their operative techniques so as to take advantage of this precision. This precise surgical control within three-dimensional space will lead to more and more general applications of stereotactic methodology to neurosurgery (Kelly 1983). Besides the great value of CT scanning for stereotactic surgery (chapter 4), the computer itself and laser and ultrasound techniques will become incorporated into stereotactic procedures, because of their high precision that is particularly suited to combination with the exact spatial control offered by stereotactic techniques. These technical advances do not only apply to target localization control, but also to functional stereotactics in which the target must be deduced from the patients cerebral anatomy.


## A. The Computer and Functional Stereotactics

As Hardy (*et al.* 1983) has described, computer assisted stereotactic surgery in the field of functional disorders is rapidly developing. A computer generated stereotactic atlas of the brain may be superimposed on CT scan slices of the patient's brain. The computed tomography scan may even become "a labeled atlas of the individual patient's brain" (Kelly 1983). Afshar and Dykes (1982) reported three-dimensional computer recon-struction of the human brainstem and discuss its applicability to functional stereotactic surgery. The technique enables the surgeon to visualize and calculate any target wanted as well as the electrode trajectory.

Hardy (*et al*. 1983) developed computer software that stores stereotactic brain maps from the Schaltenbrand and Wahren Atlas (1977) in the system's memory, and allows the operator (i.e. the surgeon) to call any specific section from the atlas and display it on the graphics terminal. Afterwards the displays can be manipulated according to references taken from the patient's ventriculogram (intercommissural point and brainstem coordinate system of axes, etc.), to match the patient's anatomical dimensions.

The hardware support for their computer graphics terminal in the operating room has become portable, which implies easier handling of the computer for clinical use. It is thought, that in the near future it will be possible to have a system which can store, manipulate, and selectively display CT images in the theatre, even if the stereotactic CT studies (with the base frame fixed onto the skull) are performed in the CT-suite before transporting the patient to the operating room.

### B. *The Computer and Diagnostic and Therapeutic Stereotactics*

Whilst a stereoscopic series of angiograms gives the surgeon a depth impression as to the position of the tumor if pathological course of certain blood vessels is present, a CT image offers only a two-dimensional image of the lesion. Using imaging derived from different neuroradiological investigations in combination with computer techniques an integrated stereoscopic image of blood vessels, tumor, and simulated instrument trajectory may be observed. This method has been developed successfully by Suetens (*et al*. 1984) using a fixed position of the stereotactic instrument to the skull during both the investigations and the surgical performance. Similar results may be obtained with the computer based method of Kelly (*et al*. 1984a), in which an operating room computer allows the precise determination of tumor volume and can display its three-dimensional configuration.

An additional stereotactic stereo-angiography may then be carried out to feed the computer with the course of important vascular structures.

These methods undoubtedly make the introduction of a biopsy probe or forceps safer and allow biopsy trajectories to be simulated beforehand. Kelly makes use of this biopsy method to take serial samples up to, through, and beyond the CT defined tumor boundaries and is able in this way to obtain the true histological boundaries, which will not always be alike.

A method for translation of any tumor volume defined by CT into stereotactic space is described extensively by Kelly and co-workers (Kelly *et al*. 1984b). This reconstruction of tumor volume with the computer is particularly important for patients undergoing computer assisted stereotactic resection (e.g. laser vaporization) of their neoplasm (Kelly *et al.* 1982 a, 1983). Moreover, computer simulation of isodose configurations produced by isotope sources to be placed inside the tumor may lead to the best source position available (Kelly *et al.* 1984 c). With this technique placement determination is carried out preoperatively. It is also possible, and less expensive, to enter the coordinates of a CT volume into a radiation treatment planning computer to attain superimposed theoretical isodose curves from radiation sources. During the stereotactic implantation itself great care must be taken in selecting the same target points in relation to the boundaries of the lesion on the CT console as those chosen at the treatment planning. The main restriction as to the applicability of this computer monitored stereotactic interstitial irradiation remains the uncertainty as to the true (highly irregular) tumor boundaries, which lie sometimes more than 1 cm beyond the tumor's outer edge as visualized on CT. NMR scanning, however, may become even more reliable than CT in determining tumor boundaries.

From these recent publications the reader may conclude that diagnostic stereotactics is in many instances linked to therapeutic stereotactics. Stereotactic biopsy alone (i.e. leaving the tumor for external irradiation or abstention because of its proven malignancy) will be performed less frequently with these therapeutic extrapolations of the stereotactic approach. Another fine example of combined diagnostic (identification of the lesion's nature) and therapeutic (lesion's removal) stereotactics is presented by Jacques (*et al.* 1980), who constructed an all-in-one stereotactic system based on the Riechert-Mundinger apparatus, which after biopsy allows the removal of small tumors through a small trephination with a newly designed tumorscope and specially designed instruments (Shelden *et al.* 1980). These authors also stress the great advantage of a three-dimensional reconstruction of the lesion in question to obtain what is considered to be a true removal. The newly designed Brown-Roberts-Wells (BRW) stereotactic system conveying rapid translation of CT derived data to the operating room (see for discussion chapter 4, sub II C) has been tested successfully by Apuzzo (and Sabshin 1983, *et al.* 1984 b). From their reports it is clear, that the BRW system has not only been constructed for CT guided stereotactics, but is also adaptable for utilization with magnetic resonance imaging (NMR, Fig. 212) and positron emission tomography (PET). Combination with laser endoscopy and its value for use with photodynamic agents via laser fiberoptics are also discussed.

The Leksell integrated system for CT and NMR (Fig. 213) guided stereotactic surgery has a newly constructed headframe leaving more room for open surgery (Leksell, personal communication 1985). With this frame craniotomy in stereotactic space is made more manageable and the

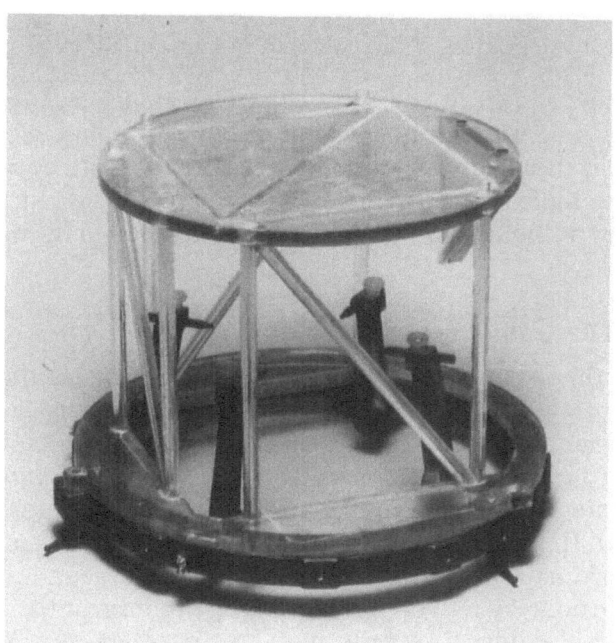

Fig. 212. The Nuclear Magnetic Resonance Adapter for use with the Brown-Roberts-Wells stereotactic system. Localizing rods (filled with a water solution) are mounted on the headring assembly (by courtesy of Dr. Cosman)

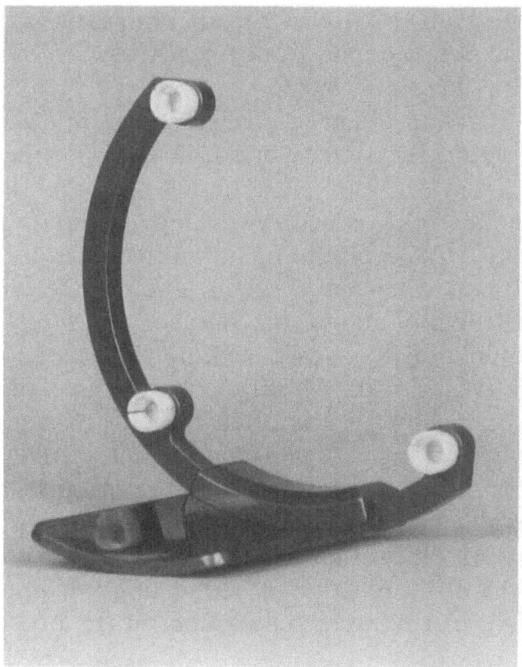

Fig. 213. The NMR Adapter for use with the Leksell stereotactic system (by courtesy of Prof. Leksell)

versatility of frame and head is guaranteed by a Mayfield adapter. Thus, with all types of modern instrumentation discussed in chapter 4 (sub II) stereotactic localization with subsequent open surgery in stereotactic space is made possible. Indications for this method of surgery (formerly called combined surgery, although now integrated) will increase in the near future.

## C. The Computer and Localizing Stereotactics

The value of the computer for general neurosurgery is clarified best by stressing its importance for calculating positions of targets inside the brain. Calculation is done in relationship to extracranial landmarks, which are provided for by the stereotactic apparatus. For example, in intracerebral hematoma stereotactic evacuation with an Archimedes screw (as described in chapter 11, sub III) is easily performed with computerized calculation of the lesion's coordinates from CT scan data. The evacuation may be completed by introducing a fiver optic endoscope to inspect the interior of the cavity. Acute bleeding, if present, may be controlled by a laser beam directed through the endoscope.

Even limited surgical procedures may be performed under direct visualization with the aid of an endoscopic stereotactic system after computer localization (Kelly 1983). The extraction of foreign bodies (Blacklock and Maxwell 1985), the resection of small vascular malformations, and vaporization of small tumors with the laser may be achieved (Kelly et al. 1983, Alker et al. 1983).

However, these techniques need precise, three-dimensional orientation as to the target within the stereotactic frame during the total length of surgery.

Particularly in the field of neuro-oncology computerized orientation becomes indispensable. Differentiating tumor from edema and surrounding brain is often difficult when the surgeon is relying on visual inspection. Computer reconstruction allows the surgeon to resect or vaporize a predetermined volume of tissue that is completely based on data derived from the preoperative CT scan. All surgeons will agree, that even in tumor resection during open surgery it is often difficult to assess the degree of resection when only working with two-dimensional scan films. Even in non-stereotactic surgery three-dimensional computer reconstruction may therefore be of considerable help in the prevention of a too conservative attitude during the extirpation of a tumor. Not only CT scan data but also NMR data, which may be of more value in delineating low grade malignancies (Laster et al. 1984), can be used successfully in the process of computer reconstruction.

In conclusion, a computer system dedicated to a stereotactic apparatus will become a most valuable and safe neurosurgical "instrument" in the

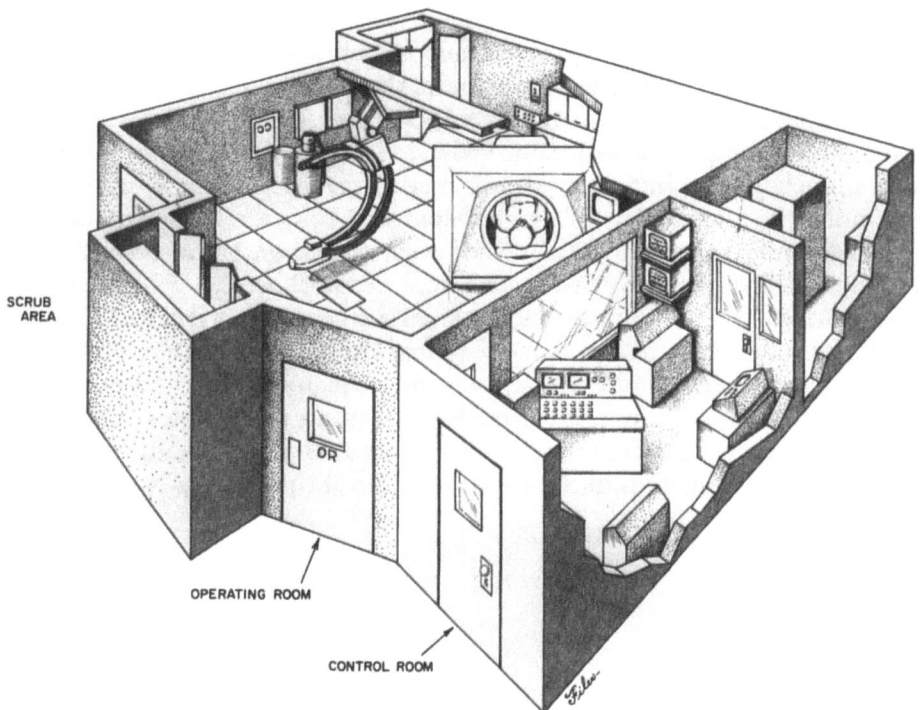

SCRUB
AREA

OPERATING ROOM

CONTROL ROOM

Fig. 214. Mock-up of operating room at Presbyterian-University Hospital, Pittsburgh, with a to surgery dedicated CT scan and ceiling mounted fluoroscope allowing intraoperative angiography (by courtesy of Dr. Lunsford; photograph published in Neurosurgery *15*, 559–561; 1984)

management of any intracerebral lesion. As Kelly (1983) states clearly, data from many sources (radiological investigations, scanning methods, neurophysiological information) may be collected and processed by the surgeon in order to "collate an anatomically correct picture of the patient's brain". To use the data effectively, these must then be translated into one reference system, i.e. the stereotactic instrument's coordinate system.

Computer hardware (already presented in the publications by Hardy *et al.* 1983, Kelly *et al.* 1984 b), is suited to serve as an operating room system, and can be fed with the computed tomographic data from the scanning unit. A similar construction can be made with NMR imaging. As few centers can afford the cost of a CT scanner in the theatre (dedicated to stereotactic surgery, Fig. 214), as in Pittsburgh (Lunsford *et al.* 1982, 1984 a), one may expect that stereotactic scan data stored on magnetic tape and transferred from the scan suite to a computer with display in the operating room will be a better alternative. At this stage a true integration of stereotactic in general neurosurgery will be a fact.

Finally, the reasons evident for a wide acceptance of computer monitored, and thus stereotactic, surgery may be summarized as follows. In the first place the treatment of intracerebral tumors, which is a main topic in neurosurgery, will progress rapidly with computer based information and three-dimensional reconstruction. From a technical point of view oncological surgery (i.e. controlled tumor resection) may become attainable. Secondly, the availability of a new theoretical basis for treatment of deep seated lesions in general, which often were not amenable to conventional surgery. In fact, one of various technical methods in the field of clinical neurosurgery (i.e. the stereotactic method) has become established as a full-grown methodology thanks to the ongoing research in and development of computer techniques. For this reason the computer and the stereotactic apparatus deserve an integrated position within neurosurgery. Out of all surgical disciplines neurosurgery in particular will benefit from the computer, because without its assistance spatial orientation is impossible.

Chapter 14

# Future Possibilities

## I. Introduction of Magnetic Resonance Imaging

The published literature on stereotactics taken over the last five years has brought an impressive amount of new data on localization techniques in general and in stereotactic space in particular. Decennia ago, stereotactics comprised of almost only functional surgery, and localization depended completely on radiographic methods. At the moment there is an almost exponential increase in interest for stereotactics. This is merely due to the availability of various sophisticated computerized imaging techniques, such as CT, MR, and PET scanning. It is obvious, that in the following years after a true integration of stereotactics in clinical neurosurgery has taken place, new developments will be reported. It should be emphasized that almost all publications on computerized scanning in stereotactic space rely on high resolution CT scanning, while reports on the validity of MR (Figs. 215 and 216) and PET scanning in various disorders are still awaited.

Preliminary evidence derived from MR scanning promises a better visualization of the histological boundaries of low grade malignancies (Laster *et al.* 1984). A problem, which is of the utmost importance in the treatment of such lesions. As these primary cerebral malignancies never give rise to metastasis, cure may be feasible with the advent of spatial reconstruction by computer and subsequent stereotactic debulking and interstitial irradiation, according to the best matching isodose curves (derived from simulation on the computer display).

Very recently, Leksell (*et al.* 1985 a, b) published reports on the application of magnetic resonance imaging to stereotactics. The authors stress some important advantages over X-ray imaging techniques, such as ventriculography, angiography, and computed tomography: clear contrast between grey and white matter and presentation of brain sections at any desired angle. With MR imaging very precise visualization is possible in axial, coronal and sagittal planes of scanning. With the use of plastic coordinate indicator discs (as in CT scanning, Leksell and Jernberg 1980), in which the indicator strips made from radio-opaque material are exchanged for liquid indicators (see Fig. 13), manual coordinate determination is possible using a ruler that is superimposed on the scan image. If desired, MR

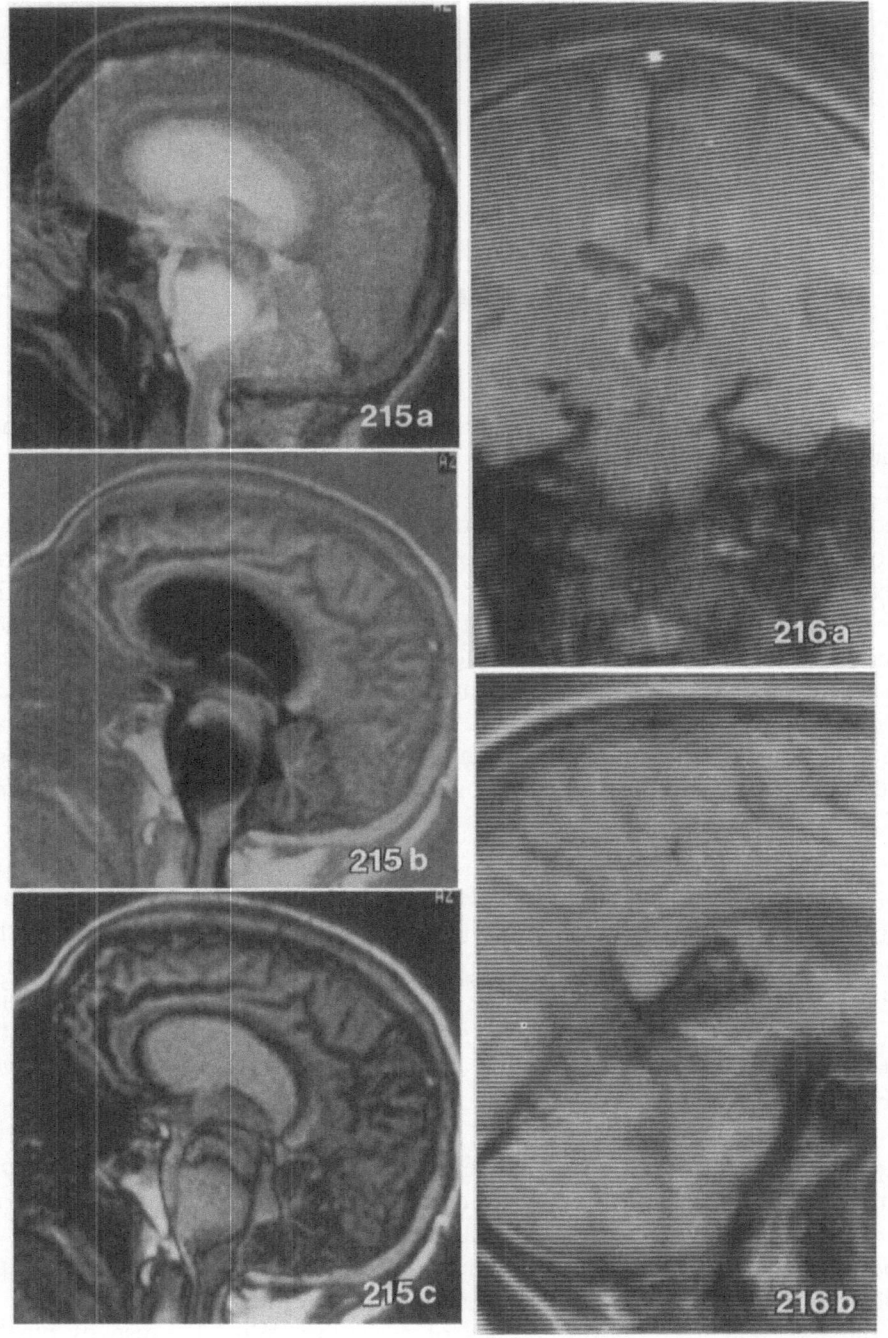

Fig. 215. Examples of NMR (a–c: different techniques) imaging in a case of a
brainstem tumor (male, 45 years)

Fig. 216. NMR scan pictures (coronal and sagittal view) showing a deep seated
arteriovenous malformation (posterior thalamus)

(as well as CT) localization may also be done directly on the screen of the scanner by means of the scanner's own software. A special MR adapter has become available for the Leksell headframe [that for use in MR scanning is mounted with non-magnetic feet (see Fig. 213)], allowing its use in all NMR machines fitted with a RF coil with a diameter of 30 cm or more. For performing MR scanning using the Brown-Roberts-Wells system (chapter 4, sub II C) a special MR localizer ring is available with hollow localizing rods that have to be filled with an appropriate water solution (see Fig. 212). The principle of target localization and coordinate calculation is identical for both CT and MR guided stereotactics. A major advantage over CT guided surgery will be the ease with which coronal and sagittal brain slices may be examined in MR stereotactics, including any angled section to simulate the probe trajectory towards the target. Extension of computer software for this purpose is not necessary for MR scanning.

Visualization of stereotactic radiolesions by MR is reported by Leksell (*et al.* 1985 b), in a case of psychosurgery by means of bilateral anterior capsulotomy (see chapters 3, sub I D, and 5, sub III C). The lesions made with stereotactic radiosurgery were clearly visible after only a 24 hour interval after surgery. MR imaging may well lead to a better understanding of both the method of stereotactic radiosurgery, which is based on a single dose target irradiation, and of the optimal dose of irradiation, needed to destroy brain tissue or certain brain lesions. Optimization of dosage might lead to selective destruction of white matter (for example fiber tracts), as suggested by Leksell (*et al.* 1985 b), because white matter seems to be more radiosensitive.

Shelden (*et al.* 1982) in discussing the value of his CT based microsurgical stereotactic system (chapter 4, sub II D 2) extrapolates the applicability of the algorithms developed for use with CT scanning to MR digital information output. Thus, similar computer based stereotactic surgery with MR guidance is achieved and (quote:) "the future of neurosurgical stereotaxis will soon include the ability to detect structures and metabolic defects almost at the single cell level" (Shelden *et al.* 1982). In similar words Leksell (*et al.* 1985 a) stresses the future possibilities with MR scanning, which gives (quote:) "the surgeon a kind of visual access to the depth of the brain which may be superior even to direct visual inspection".

## II. Future Applications of Stereotactics in Functional Disorders

Positron emission tomography (PET) is described by Fox (*et al.* 1985) as a physiological tomography, as opposed to CT and MR as structural tomographies. It permits quantitative in vivo measurements of local hemodynamics, metabolism, biochemistry, and pharmacokinetics in the human brain and may be of future use in functional stereotactic surgery.

Fox describes a stereotactic method to localize any point of interest from a PET image within the stereotactic atlas coordinate system. This approach is valuable for the study of behavior of specific brain regions under different physiological and pathophysiological conditions (for example on normal healthy volunteers and on persons with functional disorders, such as epilepsy and psychiatric disease). The authors (Fox *et al.* 1985) plea for anatomical localization of all areas of interest (whether structural via CT or MR, or physiological via PET) with a universally accepted stereotactic method, capable of giving reliable information on experimental data between various research centers.

Meyerson (*et al.* 1984) examined patients with focal epilepsy with PET in stereotactic circumstances. He stresses the usefulness of stereotactic PET studies for surgical treatment of epilepsy.

Functional stereotactic surgery using CT data and a computer generated stereotactic atlas is recently described by Kelly (*et al.* 1984 d), who discusses the average errors made in CT derived and ventriculography based target sites in tremor and pain surgery. Although these errors are small, they give additional information to the surgeon before a final decision as to the site of lesioning is made. In fact, microelectrode recording at both sites may add to the reliability of the information. Hitchcock and Cadavid (1984) conclude after a review of 111 sequential "normal" CT scans, that preoperative study of the thalamo-capsular distance (i.e. thalamic dimension) will greatly improve the accuracy of the otherwise empirical lateral coordinate value in stereotactic thalamotomy.

A very recent contribution to functional stereotactic research is given by Backlund (*et al.* 1985) with attempted amelioration of Parkinsonism symptoms by autologous transplantation of adrenal medullary tissue to the striatum with use of the stereotactic technique. This first clinical trial is based on extensive transplantation experiments on animals and has the aim to "internalize" the therapy for parkinsonism. Further clinical research seems justified to elaborate this new therapeutic approach.

Although general acceptance is poor, neuro-augmentative procedures might in the future play a role in functional pain surgery. In fact, this is a much spoken topic in functional stereotactic research and many papers have emphasized its value in the treatment of chronic intractable pain. In his introductory lecture on pain during the 6th Meeting of the European Society for Stereotactic and Functional Neurosurgery, Rome 1983, Gybels (1984) reviews the suggested mechanisms of chronic "intractable" pain and indications for neurosurgical treatment. Recently developed experimental models of chronic pain in animals may be subdivided in dysesthetic and somatic pain models. In the *dysesthetic* model damaged sensory axons (in experimentally induced neuroma) seem to become responsive to α-adrenergic stimulation and are therefore sensitive to sympathetic activity.

Blocking the sympathetic outflow, either by surgery or injection of the sympathetic chain with anesthetic drugs (or with guanethidine infusion) may result in pain relief in these chronic dysesthetic pain syndromes. Electrical stimulation at the site of nerve damage may stop the otherwise ongoing activity for a longer period and may lead to painfree episodes which last for various periods of time. In the *somatic* pain model (the arthritic rat) stimulation produced analgesia (SPA) was studied and proved to lead to suppression of pain behavior (scratching) in this specific situation.

On the other hand, too little experience has been gained to evaluate the preference for various stimulation sites (periaqueductal grey, nucleus raphe magnus) in SPA. However, it is generally believed that such pain suppression is at least partially mediated by endogenous opioids, because suppression is attenuated by the opiate antagonist naloxone as well as by morphine tolerance in experimental animals.

Therefore SPA might not be achieved in morphine-resistant pain syndromes and/or in morphine-tolerant patients. Indeed clinical evidence suggests that stimulation of the PAG or PVG regions is not beneficiary in most cancer pains. This is a major reason to continue with neuro-ablative procedures (such as stereotactic mesencephalotomy or extralemniscal myelotomy and percutaneous cervical cordotomy) for obtaining pain relief in cancer patients.

Recent investigations in experimental animals (Watkins and Mayer 1982) strongly suggest the existence of non-opiate pain suppression systems as well. Stimulation of such a system might be of use in the control of human pain that is morphine-resistant. Katayama and co-workers found that microinjection of a cholinergic agonist (carbachol) into the lateral part of the brachium conjunctivum produces profound analgesia in the cat (Desalles *et al.* 1985). This pontine parabrachial region appears to become an important target site for stereotactic electrical stimulation that aims to produce a non-opiate dependent form of pain suppression. Young (*et al.* 1985) reported on 5 years experience with stereotactic electrical stimulation of the opiate-dependent pain suppression systems in patients with chronic "intractable" pain. Their best results were obtained on patients whose pain was primarily of peripheral origin: from 16 with chronic pain due to the failed back syndrome 9 experienced excellent pain relief and 5 had partial relief. On the other hand only 1 out of 16 patients with pain of primarily central origin obtained excellent relief of pain. These data are very important, because of the follow-up period in Young's study (mean 20 months), indicating that deep brain stimulation in chronic pain of peripheral origin may lead to consistent results. When considering the patient population treated (totally disabled and treated at a multidisciplinary pain center with all appropriate forms of therapy prior to electrical stimulation) the results obtained are, in fact, very good. As compared with our previous discussion on pain suppression by stimulation (chapter 3, sub I B 2) results with SPA seem to become less inconsistent and improved in the last years. Future progress is awaited and may give more insight in the underlying pain mechanisms and systems.

In the field of otherwise intractable epilepsy major advances in treatment may become feasible with positron emission tomography in stereotactic space. Fox (*et al.* 1985) presented a method for integration of PET in the stereotactic study of the brain, and Meyerson (*et al.* 1984) studied cases with focal epilepsy with the aid of stereotactic PET scanning. It is logical to expect that with this tool areas of focal epileptic activity can be determined and delineated. These areas could then be resected with computer guided stereotactic techniques. Functional brain research as a whole might benefit considerably from PET studies. Even in psychiatric disease this technique might bring a better understanding of underlying pathology by studying and comparing patients and volunteers.

## III. Future Applications of Stereotactics in Mass Lesions

As a reduction of tumor bulk is the primary step to any successful therapeutic program, technological advances have been incorporated in stereotactic instrumentation, which include endoscopic laser instruments, to obtain stereotactic resection (Jacques *et al.* 1980, Kelly *et al.* 1982 a, b). In fact, nowadays few patients with intracerebral tumors will benefit more from conventional than from stereotactic resection. Perhaps only the large and superficially growing lesions do not require surgery in stereotactic space. In all other tumors visual control is insufficient and in these cases conventional craniotomies should be replaced by stereotactic procedures with CT guidance and computer reconstruction.

To proceed after debulking and laser vaporization with attempts to destroy the tumor cells left, various techniques are being tested out at the moment. These new techniques will be incorporated in the armentarium of the neuro-oncological surgeon to an extent yet to be confined. Shelden (*et al.* 1982) states, that stereotactic tumor localization and removal will soon be the procedure of choice. In addition these authors prelude on the various forms of adjuvant therapy (local forms of treatment to the tumor bed after stereotactic vaporization), and make a distinction between immediate and late forms of adjuvant therapy.

The immediate form, according to their view, would comprise temperature reduction to 20 °C at the site of the residual tumor cells to gain time for in vitro testing of immunological, chemical or other antitumor measures that react specifically against these cells.

The late form should be introduced after a period of several weeks and include antitumor chemicals. In the field of tumor immunology Shelden (*et al.* 1982) develops the idea of tagging the amino-acid sequence of monoclonal antibodies with drugs or photosensitizing agents.

Photo-irradiation (known from the publications of Dougherty *et al.* in 1978 and Laws *et al.* in 1981) could become a technique of great value after a suitable combination is found of maximum absorption of the dye by tumor cells and a high specificity to laser penetration. Even tumor cells that have infiltrated vital brain areas adjacent to the tumor bed could be destroyed effectively with red light of long wave length, that is still active at a depth of 1–2 cm (Shelden *et al.* 1982). Other immediate forms of adjuvant therapy are local heating and local drug delivery without previous sensitivity testing in vitro. Hyperthermic therapy for neoplasms has already been studied for a longer period by Storm and co-workers from the UCLA School of Medicine in Los Angeles (see for review: Storm *et al.* 1982). Radio-frequency hyperthermia by magnetic loop induction (Magnetrode™) was introduced as an experimental cancer therapy for solid human malignancies independent of their histology or size. The applicator employs a non-invasive circumferential electrode to produce hyperthermia at depth (42 °C, versus about 40 °C in normal surrounding brain) without significant heating of the skin. In these experiments temperature probes were introduced with stereotactic techniques. Silberman (*et al.* 1984) reports on combination of radiofrequency hyperthermia and chemotherapy (with BCNU) for brain malignancy and discusses animal experience and two case reports. In rabbits a mean survival after implantation of tumor of 18.6 days was found, compared with 9.3 days for the untreated controls. As to their two patients they conclude that no increase in chemotherapy toxicity was observed and that no normal tissue damage had occurred. Follow-up CT scans showed a dramatic improvement after four thermochemotherapy sessions (i.e. 1 month). The preliminary conclusion is, that non-invasive localized radiofrequency hyperthermia to the brain is feasible and can be performed safely in the presence of a solid brain tumor.

Boëthius (*et al.* 1984) presented a case of a small deep seated tumor treated with stereotactic cryosurgery in the CT scanner. During the freezing the tumor area could be seen and the event of ice formation controlled with consecutive scans. Intratumoral drug delivery after stereotactic biopsy in brain tumors has been reported only seldom. Bosch (*et al.* 1980) published a pilot study with intraneoplastic bleomycin in 3 patients, who underwent no tumor debulking. In only 1 case a 2 year survival was achieved; the other 2 patients died within 5 months. Morantz (*et al.* 1979) presented an evaluation of intratumoral bleomycin in a brain tumor model (rats), which proved to be more effective than the administration per intravenous route. Firth (*et al.* 1984) and Oliver (*et al.* 1985) studied the intracerebral injection of bleomycin and vincristine, entrapped within liposomes in the rat. They demonstrated a potential application of this "depot" therapy in the treatment of cerebral gliomas. Therefore, a study of the effects of bleomycin as adjuvant intratumoral therapy after stereotactic bulk resection might be most informative.

Intralesional and intraventricular administration of leukocyte interferon is discussed by Obbens (*et al.* 1985) in a Phase I clinical trial. Intraneoplastic interferon delivery showed, however, only a marginal effect on malignant astrocytomas. Although specific adjuvant therapy for brain tumors after stereotactic localization and removal of the tumor burden (up to 99% of tumor volume) is not yet clinically available, research is going on and may offer various approaches to kill the remaining tumor cells. In his letter to the editor on cerebral gliomas, Jacques (1981) complains about the therapeutic nihilism coming from many neurosurgeons and stresses that "the future of stereotactic neurosurgery with the advent of such technology as the positron computerized tomographic scanner and nuclear magnetic resonance is just on the verge of perhaps becoming the most important future technology in neurological surgery".

## IV. Conclusion

Over the last ten years a tremendous progress has been made in imaging neural structures. These imaging techniques not only comprise high resolution CT scanning, but also MR scanning with still better anatomical visualization, and PET scanning for physiological and physiopathological research. From the studies discussed in the previous chapter it is evident that all scanning methods available can be used with reference to a stereotactic coordinate system of axes erected inside the stereotactic apparatus in use. Prerequisite for studying the brain with scanning methods in stereotactic space is the availability of enough computer facilities, easy to handle in the surgical theatre. In the hands of some expert stereotactic surgeons computer technology has proven to be a most valuable tool in the study of deep brain structures and the penetration of overlying tissues with specially designed microsurgical instruments.

Therefore the way lies open to an integration of stereotactic methodology with its computer monitored and scan guided instrumentation into general neurosurgery. The impact on the clinician of these advances is not yet fully understood, but it is certain that it will abandon the therapeutic nihilism, still too often seen in neuro-oncology. Moreover, in our view stereotactic instrumentation will become incorporated into the daily armentarium of any neurosurgical center. Stereotactic surgery, years ago shrouded in mystery, will be one of the most important and daily used techniques in future neurosurgery.

Recapitulating our introductory comments on Clarke's idea, the suggested therapeutic possibilities of his invention are now within reach to an extent even Clarke could not have anticipated. Both imaging and computer techniques have brought about a reformation in stereotactic possibilities that is proved to be essential. Applying the stereotactic method depends on the understanding of his idea.

# References

Adams, J. E., Hosobuchi, Y., Fields, H. L.: Stimulation of internal capsule for relief of chronic pain. J. Neurosurg. *41*, 740—744 (1974).

— — Session on deep brain stimulation. Technique and technical problems. Neurosurgery *1*, 196—199 (1977).

Afshar, F., Watkins, E. S., Yap, J. C.: Stereotaxic Atlas of the Human Brainstem and Cerebellar Nuclei. A Variability Study. New York: Raven Press. 1978.

— Dykes, E.: A three-dimensional reconstruction of the human brain stem. J. Neurosurg. *57*, 491—495 (1982).

Albright, A. L., Price, R. A., Guthkelch, A. N.: Brainstem gliomas of children. Cancer (Philad.) *52*, 2313—2319 (1983).

Alker, G., Kelly, P. J., Kall, B., Goerss, S.: Stereotaxic laser ablation of intracranial lesions. AJNR *4*, 727—730 (1983).

— — An overview of CT based stereotactic systems for the localization of intracranial lesions. Comput. Radiol. *8*, 193—196 (1984).

Amano, K., Iseki, H., Notani, M., Kawabatake, H., Tanikawa, T., Kawamura, H., Kitamura, K.: Rostral mesencephalic reticulotomy for pain relief. Acta Neurochir. (Wien) Suppl. *30*, 391—393 (1980).

Andrew, J., Fowler, C. J., Harrison, M. J. G.: Tremor after head injury and its treatment by stereotactic surgery. J. Neurol. Neurosurg. Psychiat. *45*, 815—819 (1982).

— — — Stereotaxic thalamotomy in 55 cases of dystonia. Brain *106*, 981—1000 (1983).

Apuzzo, M. L. J., Sabshin, J. K.: Computed tomographic guidance stereotaxis in the management of intracranial mass lesions. Neurosurgery *12*, 277—285 (1983).

— Chandrasoma, P. T., Zelman, V., Giannotta, S. L., Weiss, M. H.: Computed tomographic guidance stereotaxis in the management of lesions of the third ventricular region. Neurosurgery *15*, 502—508 (1984 a).

— Zelman, V., Jepson, J., Chandrasoma, P.: Observations with the utilization of the Brown-Roberts-Wells stereotactic system in the management of intracranial mass lesions. Acta Neurochir. (Wien) Suppl. *33*, 261—263 (1984 b).

Archer, C. R., Ilinsky, I. A., Goldfader, P. R., Smith, K. R., Jr.: Aphasia in thalamic stroke: CT stereotactic localization. J. Comput. Assist. Tomogr. *5*, 427—432 (1981).

Backlund, E. O.: A new instrument for stereotaxic brain tumour biopsy. Acta chir. scand. *137*, 825—827 (1971).

— Studies on craniopharyngiomas. I. Treatment: past and present. Acta chir. scand. *138*, 743—748 (1972).

— Johansson, L., Sarby, B.: Studies on craniopharyngiomas. II. Treatment by stereotaxic and radiosurgery. Acta chir. scand. *138*, 749—759 (1972).

— Studies on craniopharyngiomas. III. Stereotaxic treatment with intracystic yttrium-90. Acta chir. scand. *139*, 237—247 (1973).

— Von Holst, H.: Controlled subtotal evacuation of intracerebral haematomas by stereotactic technique. Surg. Neurol. *9*, 99—101 (1978).

— Stereotactic radiosurgery in intracranial tumours and vascular malformations. In: Advances and Technical Standards in Neurosurgery 6 (Krayenbühl, H., *et al.*, eds.), pp. 3—37. Wien-New York: Springer. 1979.

— Granberg, P. O., Hamberger, B., Knutsson, E., Mårtensson, A., Sedvall, G., Seiger, Å., Olson, L.: Transplantation of adrenal medullary tissue to striatum in Parkinsonism. J. Neurosurg. *62*, 169—173 (1985).

Ballantine, H. Th., Jr., Cassidy, W. L., Flanagan, N. B., Marino, R., Jr.: Stereotaxic anterior cingulotomy for neuropsychiatric illness and intractable pain. J. Neurosurg. *26*, 488—495 (1967).

— Giriunas, I. E.: Advances in psychiatric surgery. In: Functional Neurosurgery (Rasmussen, Th., Marino, R., Jr., eds.), pp. 155—164. New York: Raven Press. 1979.

Barberá, J., Barcia-Salorio, J. L., Broseta, J.: Stereotaxic pontine spinothalamic tractotomy. Surg. Neurol. *11*, 111—114 (1979).

Beatty, R. M., Zervas, N. T.: Stereotactic aspiration of a brain stem hematoma. Neurosurgery *13*, 204—207 (1983).

Becker, D. H., Townsend, J. J., Kramer, R. A., Newton, Th. H.: Occult cerebrovascular malformations. Brain *102*, 249—287 (1979).

Bertrand, C., Molina-Negro, P., Martinez, S. N.: Combined stereotactic and peripheral surgical approach for spasmodic torticollis. Appl. Neurophysiol. *41*, 122—133 (1978).

Bertrand, G.: Computers in stereotaxic surgery. In: Stereotaxy of the Human Brain. Anatomical, Physiological and Clinical Applications, 2nd ed. (Schaltenbrand, G., Walker, A. E., eds.), pp. 364—371. Stuttgart-New York: G. Thieme. 1982.

Besson, J. M., Oliveras, J. L.: Analgesia induced by electrical stimulation of the brain stem in animals: involvement of serotoninergic mechanisms. Acta Neurochir. (Wien) Suppl. *30*, 201—217 (1980).

Bingley, T., Leksell, L., Meyerson, B. A., Rylander, G.: Stereotactic anterior capsulotomy in anxiety and obsessive-compulsive states. In: Surgical Approaches in Psychiatry (Laitinen, L. V., Livingston, K. E., eds.), pp. 96—100. Baltimore: University Park Press. 1973.

Birg, W., Mundinger, F.: Direct target point determination for stereotactic brain operations from CT data and the calculation of setting parameters for polar-coordinate stereotactic devices. Appl. Neurophysiol. *45*, 387—395 (1982).

Blacklock, J. B., Maxwell, R. E.: Stereotactic removal of a migrating ventricular catheter. Neurosurgery *16*, 230—231 (1985).

Boëthius, J., Bergström, M., Greitz, T.: Stereotaxic computerized tomography with a GE 8800 scanner. J. Neurosurg. *52*, 794—800 (1980).

— Greitz, T., Kuylenstierna, R., Lagerkranser, M., Lundquist, P. G., Ribbe, T., Wiksell, H.: Stereotactic cryosurgery in a CT scanner. Acta Neurochir. (Wien) Suppl. *33*, 553—557 (1984).

Bosch, D. A., Rähn, T., Backlund, E. O.: Treatment of colloid cysts of the third ventricle by stereotactic aspiration. Surg. Neurol. *9*, 15—18 (1978).

— Beekhuis, H.: Stereotactic application of $^{90}$Yttrium in cystic brain tumours. Neuropädiat. *10*, Suppl. 414—415 (1979).

— Indications for stereotactic biopsy in brain tumours. Acta Neurochir. (Wien) *54*, 167—179 (1980).

— Hindmarsch, T., Larsson, S., Backlund, E. O.: Intraneoplastic administration of bleomycin in intracerebral gliomas: a pilot study. Acta Neurochir. (Wien) Suppl. *30*, 441—444 (1980).

— Ebels, E. J., Vencken, L., Mooij, J. J. A., Beks, J. W. F.: Stereotactische biopsie van hersentumoren, verricht bij 100 patienten. Ned. T. Geneesk. *126*, 1765—1770 (1982).

— Pasmans, J., Lakke, J. P. W. F.: Caput selectum: Ervaringen met stereotaxie bij met levodopa behandelde Parkinson-patienten. Ned. T. Geneesk. *127*, 383—389 (1983).

— Beute, G. N.: Successful stereotaxic evacuation of an acute pontomedullary hematoma. Case report. J. Neurosurg. *62*, 153—156 (1985).

Bouchard, J.: Radiation Therapy of Tumors and Diseases of the Nervous System. London: Henry Kimpton. 1966.

Bowsher, D., Albe-Fessard, D.: Patterns of somatosensory organization within the central nervous system. In: The Assessment of Pain in Man and Animals. Proceedings International Symposium U.F.A.W., Middlesex 26–28 July, 1961 (Keele, C. A., Smith, R., eds.), pp. 107—122. Edinburgh: E. & S. Livingstone. 1963.

Bratislava: International Symposium on Functional and Stereotactic Neurosurgery; Brain Stimulation and Psychophysiology. Abstracta. 1983.

Brice, J., McLellan, L.: Suppression of intention tremor by contingent deep-brain stimulation. Lancet *1*, 1221—1222 (1980).

Britt, R. H., Silverberg, G. D., Enzmann, D. R., Hanberry, J. W.: Third ventricular choroid plexus arteriovenous malformation simulating a colloid cyst. J. Neurosurg. *52*, 246—250 (1980).

— Enzmann, D. R.: Clinical stages of human brain abscesses on serial CT scans after contrast infusion. Computerized tomographic, neuropathological and clinical correlations. J. Neurosurg. *59*, 972—989 (1983).

Broggi, G., Franzini, A.: Value of serial stereotactic biopsies and impedance monitoring in the treatment of deep brain tumours. J. Neurol. Neurosurg. Psychiat. *44*, 397—401 (1981).

Broseta, J., Gonzales-Darder, J., Barcia-Salorio, J. L.: Stereotactic evacuation of intracerebral hematomas. Appl. Neurophysiol. *45*, 443—448 (1982).

Brown, R. A.: A computerized tomography-computer graphics approach to stereotaxic localization. J. Neurosurg. *50*, 715—720 (1979).

— Roberts, T., Osborn, A. G.: Simplified CT-guided stereotaxic biopsy. AJNR *2*, 181—184 (1981).

Bryan, R., Weisberg, L.: Prolonged survival with good functional recovery in 3 patients with computed tomographic evidence of brainstem hemorrhage. Comput. Radiol. *6*, 43—48 (1982).

Bullard, D. E., Nashold, B. S., Jr.: Stereotaxic thalamotomy for treatment of posttraumatic movement disorders. J. Neurosurg. *61*, 316—321 (1984).

— — Osborne, D., Burger, P. C., Dubois, P.: CT-guided stereotactic biopsies using a modified frame and Gildenberg techniques. J. Neurol. Neurosurg. Psychiat. *47*, 590—595 (1984).

Burchiel, K. J., Ojemann, G. A., Bolender, N.: Localization of stereotaxic centers by computerized tomographic scanning. J. Neurosurg. *53*, 861—863 (1980).

Cahan, L. D., Rand, R. W.: Stereotaxic coagulation of a paraventricular arteriovenous malformation. Case report. J. Neurosurg. *39*, 770—774 (1973).

Carlsson, C. A., Leksell, L.: A diagram for determining space coordinates from two perpendicular roentgenograms. In: Stereotaxis and Radiosurgery. An Operative System (Leksell, L., ed.), Appendix I. Springfield, Ill.: Ch. C Thomas. 1971.

Carpenter, M. B., Whittier, J. R.: Study of methods for producing experimental lesions of the central nervous system with special reference to stereotaxic technique. J. comp. Neurol. *97*, 73—131 (1952).

Cavazzuti, V., Fischer, E. G., Welch, K., Belli, J. A., Winston, K. R.: Neurological and psychophysiological sequelae following different treatments of craniopharyngioma in children. J. Neurosurg. *59*, 409—417 (1983).

Caveness, W. F., Kato, M., Malamut, B. L., Hosokawa, S., Wakisaka, S., O'Neill, R. R.: Propagation of focal motor seizures in the pubescent monkey. Ann. Neurol. *7*, 213—221 (1980).

Chapman, P. H., Linggood, R. M.: The management of pineal area tumors: a recent reappraisal. Cancer (Philad.) *46*, 1253—1257 (1980).

Chernik, N. L., Armstrong, D., Posner, J. B.: Central nervous system infections in patients with cancer. Medicine (Baltimore) *52*, 563—581 (1973).

Clarke, R. H., Henderson, E. E.: Atlas of photographs of sections of the frozen cranium and brain of the cat (Felix domestica). Part I. Sagittal sections. J. Psychol. Neurol. (Lpz.) *18*, Suppl. 3, 391—409 (1911).

— — Atlas of photographs of sections of the frozen cranium and brain of the cat (Felix domestica). Part II. Frontal sections. J. Psychol. Neurol. (Lpz.) *21*, Suppl. 1, 273—277 (1914).

— — Investigation of the central nervous system. Part I. Methods and instruments. Part II. Atlas of photographs of the frontal sections of the cranium and brain of the rhesus monkey. John Hopk. Hosp. Rep. Special volume (1920).

— Investigation of the central nervous system: methods and instruments. John Hopk. Hosp. Rep. *1*, 1—159 (1921).

Conway, L. W., O'Foghludha, F. T., Collins, W. F.: Stereotactic treatment of acromegaly. J. Neurol. Neurosurg. Psychiat. *32*, 48—59 (1969).

— Stereotaxic diagnosis and treatment of intracranial tumors including an initial experience with cryosurgery for pinealomas. J. Neurosurg. *38*, 453—459 (1973).

— Stereotactic biopsy of deep intracranial tumors. In: Current Techniques in Operative Neurosurgery (Schmidek, H. H., Sweet, H., eds.), pp. 187—198. New York: Grune & Stratton. 1977.

Cook, A. W., Nathan, P. W., Smith, M. C.: Sensory consequences of commissural myelotomy. A challenge to traditional anatomical concepts. Brain *107*, 547—568 (1984).

Cooper, I. S., Bravo, G.: Chemopallidectomy and chemothalamectomy. J. Neurosurg. *15*, 244—250 (1958).
— Clinical and physiologic implications of thalamic surgery for disorders of sensory communication. Part 1. Thalamic surgery for intractable pain. J. neurol. Sci. *2*, 493—519 (1965 a).
— Clinical and physiologic implications of thalamic surgery for disorders of sensory communication. Part 2. Intention tremor, dystonia, Wilson's disease and torticollis. J. neurol. Sci. *2*, 520—553 (1965 b).
— Cerebellar Stimulation in Man. New York: Raven Press. 1978.
— Dystonia. In: Stereotaxy of the Human Brain. Anatomical, Physiological and Clinical Applications, 2nd ed. (Schaltenbrand, G., Walker, A. E., eds.), pp. 544—561. Stuttgart-New York: G. Thieme. 1982.
Cosman, E. R., Nashold, B. S., Bedenbaugh, P.: Stereotactic radiofrequency lesion making. Appl. Neurophysiol. *46*, 160—166 (1983).
Cotzias, G. C., Papavasiliou, P. S., Gellene, R.: Modification of Parkinsonism— chronic treatment with L-dopa. New Engl. J. Med. *280*, 337—345 (1969).
Crue, B. L., Jr., Todd, E. M., Carregal, E. J. A.: Percutaneous radiofrequency stereotactic tractotomy. In: Pain and Suffering. Selected Aspects (Crue, B. L., Jr., ed.), pp. 69—79. Springfield, Ill.: Ch. C Thomas. 1970.
Dashe, A. M., Solomon, D. H., Rand, R. W., Frasier, S. D., Brown, J., Spears, I.: Stereotaxic hypophyseal cryosurgery in acromegaly and other disorders. J. Amer. med. Ass. *198*, 591—596 (1966).
Deeley, T. J.: Central Nervous System Tumours. The Modern Radiotherapy and Oncology Series, pp. 131—152. Sevenoaks: Butterworth & Co. 1974.
Delgado, J. M. R., Obrador, S., Martin-Rodriguez, J. G.: Two-way radio communication with the brain in psychosurgical patients. In: Surgical Approaches in Psychiatry (Laitinen, L. V., Livingston, K. E., eds.), pp. 215— 223. Baltimore: University Park Press. 1973.
Desalles, A. A. F., Katayama, Y., Becker, D. P., Hayes, R. L.: Pain suppression induced by electrical stimulation of the pontine parabrachial region. Experimental study in cats. J. Neurosurg. *62*, 397—407 (1985).
Dettori, P., Colombo, F., Pinna, V., Benedetti, A.: CT control of stereotactic surgery in the diencephalon. Neuroradiology *23*, 91—94 (1982).
Dieckmann, G., Krainick, J. U.: Pain relief by chronic mediothalamic stimulation in man. In: Advances in Neurosurgery 7, Neurovascular Surgery. Specialized Neurosurgical Techniques (Marguth, F., Brock, M., Kazner, E., Klinger, M., Schmiedek, P., eds.), pp. 172—179. Berlin-New York: Springer. 1979.
Donat, J. F., Okazaki, H., Gomez, M. R., Reagan, Th. J., Baker, H. L., Laws, E. R.: Pineal tumors. A 53-year experience. Arch. Neurol. (Chic.) *35*, 736—740 (1978).
Dougherty, T. J., Kaufman, J. E., Goldfarb, A., Weishaupt, K. R., Boyle, D., Mittleman, A.: Photoradiation therapy for the treatment of malignant tumors. Cancer Res. *38*, 2628—2635 (1978).
Drake, C. G., McKenzie, K. G.: Mesencephalic tractotomy for pain. Experience with six cases. J. Neurosurg. *10*, 457—462 (1953).
— Cerebral arteriovenous malformations: considerations for and experience with

surgical treatment in 166 cases. In: Clinical Neurosurgery 26 (Carmel, P. W., ed.), pp. 145—208. Baltimore-London: Williams & Wilkins. 1979.

Durack, D. T.: Opportunistic infections and Kaposi's sarcoma in homosexual man. New Engl. J. Med. *305*, 1465—1467 (1981).

Durward, Q. J., Barnett, H. J. M., Barr, H. W. K.: Presentation and management of mesencephalic hematoma. Report of two cases. J. Neurosurg. *56*, 123—127 (1982).

Eccles, J. C., Ito, M., Szentágothai, J.: The Cerebellum as a Neuronal Machine. Berlin-Heidelberg-New York: Springer. 1967.

Edner, G.: Stereotactic biopsy of intracranial space occupying lesions. Acta Neurochir. (Wien) *57*, 213—234 (1981).

Edwards, M. S. B., Boggan, J. E., Fuller, T. A.: The laser in neurological surgery. J. Neurosurg. *59*, 555—566 (1983).

Eiras, J., Garcia, J., Gomez, J., Carcavilla, L. I., Ucar, S.: First results with extralemniscal myelotomy. Acta Neurochir. (Wien) Suppl. *30*, 377—381 (1980).

Emmers, R., Tasker, R. R.: The Human Somesthetic Thalamus, with Maps for Physiological Target Localization During Stereotactic Neurosurgery. New York: Raven Press. 1975.

Epstein, M.: Endoscopy: developments in optical instrumentation. Science *210*, 280—285 (1980).

Ferry, D. J., Kempe, L. G.: Colloid cyst of the third ventricle. Milit. Med. *133*, 734—737 (1968).

Fewer, D., Wilson, Ch. B., Levin, V. A.: Brain Tumor Chemotherapy. Springfield, Ill.: Ch. C Thomas. 1976.

Firth, G., Oliver, A. S., McKeran, R. O.: Studies on the intracerebral injection of bleomycin free and entrapped within liposomes in the rat. J. Neurol. Neurosurg. Psychiat. *47*, 585—589 (1984).

Foerster, O.: Über eine neue operative Methode der Behandlung spastischer Lähmungen durch Resektion hinterer Rückenmarkwurzeln. Z. orthop. Chir. *22*, 202—223 (1908).

Fox, J. L.: Selected Readings in Techniques of Stereotaxic Neurosurgery. A Bibliography Through 1968. Washington: Government Printing Office, 1969.

Fox, P. T., Perlmutter, J. S., Raichle, M. E.: A stereotactic method of anatomical localization for positron emission tomography. J. Comput. Assist. Tomogr. *9*, 141—153 (1985).

Frank, F., Tognetti, F., Gaist, G., Frank, G., Galassi, E., Sturiale, C.: Stereotaxic rostral mesencephalotomy in treatment of malignant faciothoracobrachial pain syndromes. J. Neurosurg. *56*, 807—811 (1982).

Gagliardi, F. M., Mercuri, S.: Single metastases in the brain: late results in 325 cases. Acta Neurochir. (Wien) *68*, 253—262 (1983).

Gahbauer, H., Sturm, V., Schlegel, W., Pastyr, O., Scharfenberg, H., Zabel, H. J., Van Kaick, G., Netzeband, G., Scheer, K. E., Schabbert, S.: Combined use of stereotaxic CT and angiography for brain biopsies and stereotaxic irradiation. AJNR *4*, 715—718 (1983).

Gajdusek, D. C., Gibbs, C. J., Asher, D. M., Brown, P., Diwan, A., Hoffman, P., Nemo, G., Rohwer, R., White, L.: Precautions in medical care of, and in handling materials from, patients with transmissible virus dementia (Creutzfeldt-Jakob disease). New Engl. J. Med. *297*, 1253—1258 (1977).

Garcia de Sola, R., Cabezudo, J., Areitio, E., Bravo, G.: Combined approach (stereotactic-microsurgical) to a paraventricular arteriovenous malformation. Case report. Acta Neurochir. (Wien) Suppl. *30*, 413—416 (1980).

Garfield, J., Dayan, A. D., Weller, R. O.: Postoperative intracavitary chemotherapy of malignant supratentorial astrocytomas using BCNU. Clin. Oncol. *1*, 213—222 (1975).

Geissinger, J. D., Bucy, P. C.: Astrocytomas of the cerebellum in children. Long-term study. Arch. Neurol. (Chic.) *24*, 125—135 (1971).

Georgi, P., Strauss, L., Sturm, V., Ostertag, H., Sinn, H., Rommel, T.: Prä- und intraoperative Volumenbestimmung bei Craniopharyngiomcysten. Nucl. Med. (Amst.) *19*, 187—190 (1980).

Gildenberg, P. L., Marino, R., Jr. (eds.): Advances in Stereoencephalotomy 8, 7th Symposium of the International Society for Research in Stereoencephalotomy, São Paulo, June 1977. Basel: S. Karger. 1978.

— Spinal stereotaxic procedures. In: Stereotaxy of the Human Brain. Anatomical, Physiological and Clinical Applications, 2nd ed. (Schaltenbrand, G., Walker, A. E., eds.), pp. 467—474. Stuttgart-New York: G. Thieme. 1982 a.

— Computerized tomography and stereotactic surgery. In: Guided Brain Operations. Methodological and Clinical Developments in Stereotactic Surgery. Contributions to the Physiology of Subcortical Structures (Spiegel, E. A. ed.), pp. 24—34. Basel-New York: S. Karger. 1982 b.

— Kaufman, H. H., Krisna Murthy, K. S.: Calculation of stereotactic coordinates from the computed tomographic scan. Neurosurgery *10*, 580—586 (1982).

— Stereotactic neurosurgery and computerized tomographic scanning. Appl. Neurophysiol. *46*, 170—179 (1983).

— The present role of stereotactic surgery in the management of Parkinson's disease. In: Advances in Neurology 40. Parkinson-Specific Motor and Mental Disorders. Role of the Pallidum: Pathophysiological, Biochemical, and Therapeutic Aspects (Hassler, R. G., Christ, J. F., eds.), pp. 447—452. New York: Raven Press. 1984.

Gillingham, F. J., Watson, W. S., Donaldson, A. A., Naughton, J. A. L.: The surgical treatment of Parkinsonism. Brit. med. J. *2*, 1395—1402 (1960).

— — — Cairns, V. M.: Stereotactic lesions for the control of intractable epilepsy. Acta Neurochir. (Wien) Suppl. *23*, 263—269 (1976).

— Campbell, D.: Surgical interruption of the conduction pathways for the control of intractable epilepsy. Acta Neurochir. (Wien) Suppl. *30*, 67—74 (1980).

— Gybels, J., Hitchcock, E. R., Rossi, G. F., Szikla, G. (eds.): Advances in Stereotactic and Functional Neurosurgery 4. Acta Neurochir. (Wien) Suppl. 30. Wien-New York: Springer. 1980.

Gleason, C. A., Wise, B. L., Feinstein, B.: Stereotactic localization (with computerized tomographic scanning), biopsy and radiofrequency treatment of deep brain lesions. Neurosurgery *2*, 217—222 (1978).

Graf, C. J., Perret, G. E., Torner, J. C.: Bleeding from cerebral arteriovenous malformations as part of their natural history. J. Neurosurg. *58*, 331—337 (1983).

Grand, W., Kinkel, W. R., Glasauer, F. E., Hopkins, L. N.: Ring formation on computerized tomography in the postoperative patient. Neurosurgery 2, 107—109 (1978).

Greenblatt, S. H., Rayport, M., Savolaine, E. R., Harris, J. H., Hitchins, M. W.: Computed tomography-guided intracranial biopsy and cyst aspiration. Neurosurgery 11, 589—598 (1982).

Gros, C., Ouaknine, G., Vlahovitch, B., Frerebeau, P.: La radicotomie sélective postérieure dans le traitement neuro-chirurgical de l'hypertonie pyramidale. Neuro-chirurgie 13, 505—518 (1967).

Guiot, G., Rougerie, J., Sachs, M., Herzog, E., Molina, P.: Repérage stéréotaxique de malformations vasculaires profondes intracérébrales. Sem. Hôp. Paris 36, 1134—1143 (1960).

— Derome, P., Robert, G.: La chirurgie stéréotaxique des tremblements. Neuro-chirurgie 22, 532—535 (1976).

Gutierrez-Lara, F., Patino, R., Hakim, S.: Treatment of tumors of the third ventricle: a new and simple technique. Surg. Neurol. 3, 323—325 (1975).

Gutin, P. H., Klemme, W. M., Lagger, R. L., MacKay, A. R., Pitts, L. H., Hosobuchi, Y.: Management of the unresectable cystic craniopharyngioma by aspiration through an Ommaya reservoir drainage system. J. Neurosurg. 52, 36—40 (1980).

— Hosobuchi, Y., Phillips, T. L., Stupar, T. A.: Stereotactic interstitial irradiation for the treatment of brain tumors. Cancer Treatm. Rep. 65, Suppl. 2, 103—106 (1981).

Gybels, J. M.: The Neural Mechanism of Parkinsonian Tremor. Thesis. Brussels: Editions Arscia S.A. 1963.

— The suggested mechanisms of chronic pain and the rationale of neurosurgical treatment. Acta Neurochir. (Wien) Suppl. 33, 397—406 (1984).

— Hitchcock, E. R., Ostertag, C., Rossi, G. F., Siegfried, J., Szikla, G. (eds.): Advances in Stereotactic and Functional Neurosurgery 6. Acta Neurochir. (Wien) Suppl. 33. Wien-New York: Springer. 1984.

Hagan, R. E.: Early complications following penetrating wounds of the brain. J. Neurosurg. 34, 132—141 (1971).

Hahn, G. M.: Hyperthermia and Cancer. New York-London: Plenum Publishing Corporation. 1982.

Handler, M., Ho, V., Whelan, M., Budzilovich, G.: Intracerebral toxoplasmosis in patients with acquired immune deficiency syndrome. J. Neurosurg. 59, 994—1001 (1983).

Hara, M., Takeuchi, K., Okada, J., Takizawa, T., Matsumoto, M.: Evaluation of brain tumour laser surgery. Acta Neurochir. (Wien) 53, 141—149 (1980).

Hardy, T. L., Bertrand, G., Thompson, C. J.: Position of the medial internal capsular border in relation to third ventricular width. Appl. Neurophysiol. 42, 234—247 (1979).

— Koch, J., Lassiter, A.: Computer graphics with computerized tomography for functional neurosurgery. Appl. Neurophysiol. 46, 217—226 (1983).

Hassler, R.: The pathological and pathophysiological basis of tremor and Parkinsonism. In: Proceedings of the Second International Congress on

Neuropathology, London, 1955. Part 1, pp. 29—40. Amsterdam: Excerpta Medica Foundation. 1955 a.

Hassler, R.: The influence of stimulations and coagulations in the human thalamus on the tremor at rest and its physiopathologic mechanism. In: Proceedings of the Second International Congress on Neuropathology, London, 1955. Part 2, pp. 637—642. Amsterdam: Excerpta Medica Foundation. 1955 b.

— Anatomie du thalamus. In: Actas y Trabajos del VI Congreso Latinoamericano de Neurocirugía (Arana-Iñíguez, R., ed.), pp. 754—787. Montevideo: Imprenta Rosgal-Hilario Rosillo. 1955 c.

— Die zentralen Systeme des Schmerzes. Acta Neurochir. (Wien) 8, 353—423 (1960).

— Dieckmann, G.: Stereotactic treatment of different kinds of spasmodic torticollis. Confin. neurol. (Basel) 32, 135—143 (1970).

— Mundinger, F., Riechert, T.: Stereotaxis in Parkinson Syndrome. Clinical-Anatomical Contributions to its Pathophysiology. Berlin-Heidelberg-New York: Springer. 1979.

— Dieckmann, G.: Stereotaxic treatment for spasmodic torticollis. In: Stereotaxy of the Human Brain. Anatomical, Physiological and Clinical Applications, 2nd ed. (Schaltenbrand, G., Walker, A. E., eds.), pp. 522—531. Stuttgart-New York: G. Thieme. 1982.

Heilbrun, M. P., Roberts, T. S., Apuzzo, M. L. J., Wells, T. H., Jr., Sabshin, J. K.: Preliminary experience with Brown-Roberts-Wells (BRW) computerized tomography stereotaxic guidance system. J. Neurosurg. 59, 217—222 (1983).

Heimburger, R. F., Small, I. F., Small, J. G., Milstein, V., Moore, D.: Stereotactic amygdalotomy for convulsive and behavioural disorders. Long-term follow-up study. Appl. Neurophysiol. 41, 43—51 (1978).

Henry, J. M., Heffner, R. R., Dillard, S. H., Earle, K. M., Davis, R. L.: Primary malignant lymphomas of the central nervous system. Cancer (Philad.) 34, 1293—1302 (1974).

Higgins, A. C., Nashold, B. S., Cosman, E.: Stereotactic evacuation of primary intracerebral hematomas: new instrumentation. Appl. Neurophysiol. 45, 438—442 (1982).

Hildebrand, J.: Treatment of brain and spinal metastases. In: Developments in Oncology 3. Neuro-Oncology. Clinical and Experimental Aspects (Ongerboer de Visser, B. W., Bosch, D. A., Van Woerkom-Eykenboom, W. M. H., eds.), pp. 73—86. The Hague-Boston-London: Martinus Nijhoff Publishers. 1980.

Hirano, A., Ghatak, N. R.: The fine structure of colloid cysts of the third ventricle. J. Neuropath. exp. Neurol. 33, 333—341 (1974).

Hitchcock, E. R.: Stereotaxic spinal surgery. J. Neurosurg. 31, 386—392 (1969).

— Stereotactic trigeminal tractotomy. Ann. clin. Res. 2, 131—135 (1970 a).

— Stereotactic cervical myelotomy. J. Neurol. Neurosurg. Psychiat. 33, 224—230 (1970 b).

— Stereotaxic pontine spinothalamic tractotomy. J. Neurosurg. 39, 746—752 (1973).

— Stereotactic myelotomy. Proc. roy. Soc. Med. 67, 771—772 (1974).

— Oppitz, P., Donaldson, A. A.: Relationship between portions of the third and fourth ventricles; an aid to stereotactic accuracy for posterior fossa stereotaxy. Neuroradiology *15*, 197—199 (1978).

— Cowie, R.: Stereotactic removal of intracranial foreign bodies: review and case report. Injury *14*, 471—475 (1983).

— Cadavid, J.: Third ventricular width and thalamo-capsular laterality. Acta Neurochir. (Wien) Suppl. *33*, 547—551 (1984).

Hoehn, M. M., Yahr, M. D.: Parkinsonism: onset, progression, and mortality. Neurology (Minneap.) *17*, 427—442 (1967).

Hornykiewicz, O.: Dopamine (3-hydroxytyramine) and brain function. Pharmacol. Rev. *18*, 925—962 (1966).

Horsley, V., Clarke, R. H.: The structure and functions of the cerebellum examined by a new method. Brain *31*, 45—124 (1908).

Hosobuchi, Y., Adams, J. E., Rutkin, B.: Chronic thalamic stimulation for the control of facial anesthesia dolorosa. Arch. Neurol. (Chic.) *29*, 158—161 (1973).

— The current status of analgesic brain stimulation. Acta Neurochir. (Wien) Suppl. *30*, 219—227 (1980).

Hounsfield, G. N., Ambrose, J., Perry, B. J., Bridges, C.: Computerized transverse axial scanning (tomography). Brit. J. Radiol. *46*, 1016—1051 (1973).

Huang, Y. P., Robbins, A., Patel, S. C., Chaudhary, M.: Cerebral venous malformations and a new classification of cerebral vascular malformations. In: The Cerebral Venous System and Its Disorders (Kapp, J. P., Schmidek, H. H., eds.), pp. 373—474. New York: Grune & Stratton. 1984.

Hughes, R. C., Polgar, J. G., Weightman, D., Walton, J. N.: L-dopa in Parkinsonism and the influence of previous thalamotomy. Brit. med. J. *1*, 7—13 (1971).

Huk, W. J., Mahlstedt, J.: Intracystic radiotherapy ($^{90}$Y) of craniopharyngiomas: CT-guided stereotaxic implantation of indwelling drainage system. AJNR *4*, 803—806 (1983).

Inoue, Y., Takeuchi, T., Tamaki, M., Nin, K., Hakuba, A., Nishimura, S.: Sequential CT observations of irradiated intracranial germinomas. Amer. J. Roentgenol. *132*, 361—365 (1979).

Ischia, S., Luzzani, A., Ischia, A., Maffezzoli, G.: Bilateral percutaneous cervical cordotomy: immediate and long-term results in 36 patients with neoplastic disease. J. Neurol. Neurosurg. Psychiat. *47*, 141—147 (1984).

Jacques, S., Shelden, C. H., McCann, G. D., Freshwater, D. B., Rand, R.: Computerized three-dimensional stereotaxic removal of small central nervous system lesions in patients. J. Neurosurg. *53*, 816—820 (1980).

— Letter to the editor: cerebral gliomas. Surg. Neurol. *16*, 25 (1981).

Jankovic, J.: Treatment of hyperkinetic movement disorders with tetrabenazine: a double-blind crossover study. Ann. Neurol. *11*, 41—47 (1982).

Jefferson, D., Jenner, P., Marsden, C. D.: Relationship between plasma propanolol concentration and relief of essential tremor. J. Neurol. Neurosurg. Psychiat. *42*, 831—837 (1979 a).

— — — Bèta-adrenoreceptor antagonists in essential tremor. J. Neurol. Neurosurg. Psychiat. *42*, 904—909 (1979 b).

Jefferson, G.: Sir Victor Horsley 1857—1916. Brit. med. J. *1*, 903—910 (1957).

Jones, A.: Supervoltage X-ray therapy of intra-cranial tumours. Ann. roy. Coll. Surg. Engl. *27*, 310—354 (1960).

Juel-Jensen, B.: Superimposed viral infection. The behaviour of herpes viruses in immunosuppressed patients. In: Developments in Oncology 3. Neuro-Oncology. Clinical and Experimental Aspects (Ongerboer de Visser, B. W., Bosch, D. A., Van Woerkom-Eykenboom, W. M. H., eds.), pp. 133—139. The Hague-Boston-London: Martinus Nijhoff Publishers. 1980.

Kanaka, T. S., Balasubramaniam, V.: Stereotactic cingulotomy for drug addiction. Appl. Neurophysiol. *41*, 86—92 (1978).

Kanaya, H., Yukawa, H., Itoh, Z., Kagawa, M., Kanno, T., Kuwabara, T., Mizukami, M.: A neurological grading for patients with hypertensive intracerebral hemorrhage and a classification for hematoma location on computed tomography (Japanese). In: Proceedings of the 7th Conference of Surgical Treatment of Stroke, pp. 265—270. Tokyo: Neuron. 1978.

Kandel, E. I., Schavinsky, Y. V.: Stereotaxic apparatus and operations in Russia in the 19th century. J. Neurosurg. *37*, 407—411 (1972).

— Peresedov, V. V.: Stereotaxic clipping of arterial aneurysms and arteriovenous malformations. J. Neurosurg. *46*, 12—23 (1977).

— Peresedov, V. V.: Stereotaxic evacuation of spontaneous intracerebral hematomas. J. Neurosurg. *62*, 206—213 (1985).

Kaneko, M., Koba, T., Yokoyama, T.: Early surgical treatment for hypertensive intracerebral hemorrhage. J. Neurosurg. *46*, 579—583 (1977).

— Tanaka, K., Shimada, T., Sato, K., Uemura, K.: Long-term evaluation of ultra-early operation for hypertensive intracerebral hemorrhage in 100 cases. J. Neurosurg. *58*, 838—842 (1983).

Kase, C. S., Williams, J. P., Wyatt, D. A., Mohr, J. P.: Lobar intracerebral hematomas: clinical and CT analysis of 22 cases. Neurology (Minneap.) *32*, 1146—1150 (1982).

Katz, J., Levin, A. B.: Treatment of diffuse metastatic cancer pain by instillation of alcohol into the sella turcica. Anesthesiology *46*, 115—121 (1977).

Kelly, P. J., Olson, M. H., Wright, A. E.: Stereotactic implantation of Iridium[192] into CNS neoplasms. Surg. Neurol. *10*, 349—354 (1978).

— Gillingham, F. J.: The long-term results of stereotaxic surgery and L-dopa therapy in patients with Parkinson's disease. A 10-year follow-up study. J. Neurosurg. *53*, 332—337 (1980).

— Alker, G. J., Jr., Goerss, S.: Computer-assisted stereotactic laser microsurgery for the treatment of intracranial neoplasms. Neurosurgery *10*, 324—331 (1982 a).

— — Zoll, J. G.: A microstereotactic approach to deep-seated arteriovenous malformations. Surg. Neurol. *17*, 260—262 (1982 b).

— Future possibilities in stereotactic neurosurgery. Special article. Surg. Neurol. *19*, 4—9 (1983).

— Kall, B., Goerss, S., Alker, G. J., Jr.: Precision resection of intra-axial CNS lesions by CT-based stereotactic craniotomy and computer monitored $CO_2$ laser. Acta Neurochir. (Wien) *68*, 1—9 (1983).

— Alker, G. J., Jr., Kall, B. A., Goerss, S.: Method of computed tomography-based stereotactic biopsy with arteriographic control. Neurosurgery *14*, 172—177 (1984 a).

— Kall, B. A., Goerss, S.: Transposition of volumetric information derived from computed tomography scanning into stereotactic space. Surg. Neurol. *21*, 463—471 (1984 b).

— — — Computer simulation for the stereotactic placement of interstitial radionuclide sources into computed tomography-defined tumor volumes. Neurosurgery *14*, 442—448 (1984 c).

— — — Functional stereotactic surgery utilizing CT data and computer generated stereotactic atlas. Acta Neurochir. (Wien) Suppl. *33*, 577—583 (1984 d).

Kirschner, M.: Die Punktionstechnik und die Elektrokoagulation des Ganglion Gasseri. Über „gezielte" Operationen. Arch. klin. Chir. *176*, 581—620 (1933).

Kjellberg, R. N., Koehler, A. M., Preston, W. M., Sweet, W. H.: Intracranial lesions made by the Bragg peak of a proton beam. In: Response of the Nervous System to Ionizing Radiation (Haley, T. J., Snider, R. S., eds.), pp. 36—53. Boston: Little, Brown and Company, Inc. 1964.

— Stereotactic Bragg peak proton radiosurgery results. In: INSERM Symposia-12. Stereotactic Cerebral Irradiation (Szikla, G., ed.), pp. 233—240. Amsterdam-New York-Oxford: Elsevier/North-Holland Biomedical Press. 1979.

— Hanamura, T., Davis, K. R., Lyons, S. L., Adams, R. D.: Bragg-peak proton-beam therapy for arteriovenous malformations of the brain. New Engl. J. Med. *309*, 269—274 (1983).

Klawans, H. L., Goetz, C. G., Perlik, S.: Tardive dyskinesia: review and update. Amer. J. Psychiat. *37*, 900—908 (1980).

Kleihues, P., Volk, B., Anagnostopoulos, J., Kiessling, M.: Morphologic evaluation of stereotactic brain tumour biopsies. Acta Neurochir. (Wien) Suppl. *33*, 171—181 (1984).

Koide, O., Watanabe, Y., Sato, K.: A pathological survey of intracranial germinoma and pinealoma in Japan. Cancer (Philad.) *45*, 2119—2130 (1980).

Krayenbühl, H., Wyss, O. A. M., Yaşargil, M. G.: Bilateral thalamotomy and pallidotomy as treatment for bilateral Parkinsonism. J. Neurosurg. *18*, 429—444 (1961).

Kroin, J. S., Penn, R. D.: Intracerebral chemotherapy: chronic microinfusion of cisplatin. Neurosurgery *10*, 349—354 (1982).

Laitinen, L. V., Nilsson, S., Fugl-Meyer, A. R.: Selective posterior rhizotomy for treatment of spasticity. J. Neurosurg. *58*, 895—899 (1983).

— Brain targets in surgery for Parkinson's disease. Results of a survey of neurosurgeons. J. Neurosurg. *62*, 349—351 (1985).

Laster, D. W., Ball, M. R., Moody, D. M., Witcofski, R. L., Kelly, D. L.: Results of nuclear magnetic resonance with cerebral glioma. Comparison with computed tomography. Surg. Neurol. *22*, 113—122 (1984).

Lawrence, J. H., Tobias, C. A., Born, J. L., Wang, C. C., Linfoot, J. H.: Heavy-particle irradiation in neoplastic and neurologic disease. J. Neurosurg. *19*, 717—722 (1962).

Laws, E. R., Jr., Cortese, D. A., Kinsey, J. H., Eaton, R. T., Anderson, R. E.: Photoradiation therapy in the treatment of malignant brain tumors: a Phase I (feasibility) study. Neurosurgery *9*, 672—678 (1981).

Leksell, L.: A stereotaxic apparatus for intracerebral surgery. Acta chir. scand. *99*, 229—233 (1949).
— The stereotaxic method and radiosurgery of the brain. Acta chir. scand. *102*, 316—319 (1951).
— Lidén, K.: A therapeutic trial with radioactive isotopes in cystic brain tumour. In: Radioisotope Techniques. Vol. I: Medical and Physiological Applications. Proceedings of the Isotope Techniques Conference, Oxford, July 1951, pp. 1—4. London: H. M. Stationery Office. 1953.
— Gezielte Hirnoperationen. In: Handbuch der Neurochirurgie, 6. Band. Chirurgie der Hirnnerven und der Hirnbahnen (Olivecrona, H., Tönnis, W., eds.), pp. 178—218. Berlin-Göttingen-Heidelberg: Springer. 1957.
— Some principles and technical aspects of stereotaxic surgery. In: Pain. Henry Ford Hospital International Symposium (Knighton, R. S., Dumke, P. R., eds.), pp. 493—502. Boston: Little, Brown and Company, Inc. 1966.
— Stereotaxis and Radiosurgery. An Operative System. Springfield, Ill.: Ch. C Thomas. 1971.
— Jernberg, B.: Stereotaxis and tomography. A technical note. Acta Neurochir. (Wien) *52*, 1—7 (1980).
— Leksell, D., Schwebel, J.: Stereotaxis and nuclear magnetic resonance. J. Neurol. Neurosurg. Psychiat. *48*, 14—18 (1985 a).
— Herner, T., Leksell, D., Persson, B., Lindquist, C.: Visualisation of stereotactic radiolesions by nuclear magnetic resonance. J. Neurol. Neurosurg. Psychiat. *48*, 19—20 (1985 b).
Levin, A. B., Katz, J., Benson, R. G.: Treatment of pain of diffuse metastatic cancer by stereotactic chemical hypophysectomy: long term results and observations on mechanism of action. Neurosurgery *6*, 258—262 (1980).
— Ramirez, L. F., Katz, J.: The use of stereotaxic chemical hypophysectomy in the treatment of thalamic pain syndrome. J. Neurosurg. *59*, 1002—1006 (1983).
Levy, R. M., Pons, V. G., Rosenblum, M. L.: Central nervous system mass lesions in the acquired immunodeficiency syndrome (AIDS). J. Neurosurg. *61*, 9—16 (1984).
— Bredesen, D. E., Rosenblum, M. L.: Neurological manifestations of the acquired immunodeficiency syndrome (AIDS): experience at UCSF and review of the literature. Review article. J. Neurosurg. *62*, 475—495 (1985).
Luessenhop, A. J., Rosa, L.: Cerebral arteriovenous malformations. J. Neurosurg. *60*, 14—22 (1984).
Lunsford, L. D., Nelson, P. B.: Stereotactic aspiration of a brain abscess using the "therapeutic" CT scanner. Acta Neurochir. (Wien) *62*, 25—29 (1982).
— Rosenbaum, A. E., Perry, J.: Stereotactic surgery using the "therapeutic" CT scanner. Surg. Neurol. *18*, 116—122 (1982).
— Leksell, L., Jernberg, B.: Probe holder for stereotactic surgery in the CT scanner. A technical note. Acta Neurochir. (Wien) *69*, 297—304 (1983).
— Martinez, A. J.: Stereotactic exploration of the brain in the era of computed tomography. Surg. Neurol. *22*, 222—230 (1984).
— Parrish, R., Albright, L.: Intraoperative imaging with a therapeutic computed tomographic scanner. Neurosurgery *15*, 559—561 (1984 a).

— Martinez, A. J., Latchaw, R. E., Pazin, G. J.: Rapid and accurate diagnosis of herpes simplex encephalitis with computed tomography stereotaxic biopsy. Surg. Neurol. *21*, 249—257 (1984 b).

Mackay, A. R., Gutin, P. H., Hosobuchi, Y., Norman, D.: Computed tomography-directed stereotaxy for biopsy and interstitial irradiation of brain tumors: technical note. Neurosurgery *11*, 38—41 (1982).

Mann, K. S., Yue, C. P., Ong, G. B.: Percutaneous sump drainage: a palliation for oft-recurring intracranial cystic lesions. Surg. Neurol. *19*, 86—90 (1983).

Matsumoto, K., Hondo, H.: CT-guided stereotaxic evacuation of hypertensive intracerebral hematomas. J. Neurosurg. *61*, 440—448 (1984).

— Schichijo, F., Fukami, T.: Long-term follow-up review of cases of Parkinson's disease after unilateral or bilateral thalamotomy. J. Neurosurg. *60*, 1033—1044 (1984).

Mattos Pimenta, L. H., Mattos Pimenta, A., Zuckerman, E.: Pontine haematoma: successful removal of two cases with review of 22 cases previously described in accessible literature. Neurosurg. Rev. *4*, 139—142 (1981).

Mazars, G. L., Merienne, L., Ciolocca, C.: Stimulations thalamiques intermittentes. Note préliminaire. Rev. neurol. *128*, 273—279 (1973).

McKissock, W.: The surgical treatment of colloid cyst of the third ventricle. A report based on 21 personal cases. Brain *74*, 1—9 (1951).

— Richardson, A., Taylor, J.: Primary intracerebral hemorrhage: a controlled trial of surgical and conservative treatment in 180 unselected cases. Lancet *2*, 221—226 (1961).

Melzack, R., Wall, P. D.: Pain mechanisms: a new theory. Science *150*, 971—979 (1965).

Mendenhall, N. P., Thar, T. L., Agee, O. F., Harty-Golder, B., Ballinger, W. E., Jr., Million, R. R.: Primary lymphoma of the central nervous system. Computerized tomography scan characteristics and treatment results for 12 cases. Cancer (Philad.) *52*, 1993—2000 (1983).

Meyers, R.: The modification of alternating tremors, rigidity and festination by surgery of the basal ganglia. Res. Publ. Ass. nerv. ment. Dis. *21*, 602—665 (1941).

— Sweeney, D. B., Schwidde, J. T.: Hemiballismus: etiology and surgical treatment. J. Neurol. Neurosurg. Psychiat. *13*, 115—126 (1950).

Meyerson, B. A.: Biochemistry of pain relief with intracerebral stimulation. Few facts and many hypotheses. Acta Neurochir. (Wien) Suppl. *30*, 229—237 (1980).

— Widén, L., Greitz, T., Blomquist, G., Ehrin, E.: Positron emission tomographic studies in focal epilepsy. Acta Neurochir. (Wien) Suppl. *33*, 105—112 (1984).

Molina-Negro, P.: Functional surgery of abnormal movements. In: Functional Neurosurgery (Rasmussen, Th., Marino, R., Jr., eds.), pp. 89—121. New York: Raven Press. 1979.

Moniz, E.: Essai d'un traitement chirurgical de certaines psychoses. Bull. Acad. Méd. (Paris) *115*, 385—392 (1936).

Mooij, J. J. A., Bosch, D. A., Beks, J. W. F.: The cause of failure in high cervical percutaneous cordotomy: an analysis. Acta Neurochir. (Wien) *72*, 1—14 (1984).

Morantz, R. A., Vats, T. S., Tilzer, S.: An evaluation of systemic and intratumor bleomycin in a brain tumor model. AANS Annual Meeting 1979: Scientific Manuscripts, pp. 160—161. 1979.

Mullan, S., Harper, P. V., Hekmatpanah, J., Torres, H., Dobbin, G.: Percutaneous interruption of spinal-pain tracts by means of a strontium[90] needle. J. Neurosurg. 20, 931—938 (1963).

— Mailis, M., Karasick, J., Vailati, G., Beckman, B. A.: A reappraisal of the unipolar anodal electrolytic lesion. J. Neurosurg. 22, 531—538 (1965).

— Experiences with surgical thrombosis of intracranial berry aneurysms and carotid cavernous fistulas. J. Neurosurg. 41, 657—670 (1974).

Mundinger, F.: Beitrag zur Dosimetrie und Applikation Radio-Tantal (Ta[128]) zur Langzeitbestrahlung von Hirngeschwülsten. Fortschr. Röntgenstr. 89, 86—91 (1958).

— Riechert, T., Gabriel, E.: Untersuchungen zu den physikalischen und technischen Voraussetzungen einer dosierten Hochfrequenzkoagulation bei stereotaktischen Hirnoperationen. Zbl. Chir. 85, 1051—1063 (1960).

— Die interstitielle Radio-Isotopen-Bestrahlung von Hirntumoren mit vergleichenden Langzeitergebnissen zur Röntgentiefentherapie. Acta Neurochir. (Wien) 11, 89—109 (1963).

— The treatment of brain tumors with radioisotopes. In: Progress in Neurological Surgery-1 (Krayenbühl, H., Maspes, P. E., Sweet, W. H., eds.), pp. 202—257. Basel-New York: S. Karger. 1966.

— The treatment of brain tumors with interstitially applied radioactive isotopes. In: Radionuclide Applications in Neurology and Neurosurgery (Wang, Y., Paoletti, P., eds.), pp. 199—265. Springfield, Ill.: Ch. C Thomas. 1970.

— Metzel, E.: Interstitial radioisotope therapy of intractable diencephalic tumors by the stereotaxic permanent implantation of Iridium[192], including bioptic control. Confin. neurol. (Basel) 32, 195—202 (1970).

— Birg, W., Klar, M.: Computer-assisted stereotactic brain operations by means including computerized axial tomography. Appl. Neurophysiol. 41, 169—182 (1978 a).

— — Ostertag, C. B.: Treatment of small cerebral gliomas with CT-aided stereotaxic curietherapy. Neuroradiology 16, 564—567 (1978 b).

— Busam, B., Birg, W., Schildge, J.: Results of interstitial Iridium-192 brachycurie therapy and Iridium-192 protracted long term irradiation. In: INSERM Symposia-12. Stereotactic Cerebral Irradiation (Szikla, G., ed.), pp. 303—319. Amsterdam-New York-Oxford: Elsevier/North-Holland Biomedical Press. 1979.

— Implantation of radioisotopes (Curie-therapy). In: Stereotaxy of the Human Brain. Anatomical, Physiological and Clinical Applications, 2nd ed. (Schaltenbrand, G., Walker, A. E., eds.), pp. 410—435. Stuttgart-New York: G. Thieme. 1982 a.

— Stereotactic interstitial therapy of non-resectable intracranial tumours with Iridium-192 and Iodine-125. In: Progress in Radio-Oncology-2 (Kärcher, K. H., Kogelnik, H. D., Reinartz, G., eds.), pp. 371—380. New York: Raven Press. 1982 b.

— Birg, W.: CT-stereotaxy in the clinical routine. Neurosurg. Rev. 7, 219—224 (1984).

Nádvorník, P., Sramka, M., Gajdosova, D.: Critical remarks on stereotaxic treatment of epilepsy. J. Neurosurg. Sci. *18*, 133—135 (1974).

— Frohlich, J., Galanda, M.: Spinal cord stereotaxy in the treatment of pain and spasticity. In: Abstracta International Symposium on Functional ,and Stereotactic Neurosurgery; Brain Stimulation and Psychophysiology. Bratislava. 1983.

Narabayashi, H.: Stereotaxic amygdalotomy. In: Advances in Behavoral Biology-2: The Neurobiology of the Amygdala (Eleftheriou, B. E., ed.), pp. 459—483. New York: Plenum Publishing Corporation. 1972.

— Ohye, Ch.: Parkinsonian tremor and nucleus ventralis intermedius (Vim) of the human thalamus. In: Progress in Clinical Neurophysiology-5: Physiological Tremor, Pathological Tremors and Clonus (Desmedt, J. E., ed.), pp. 165—172. Basel: S. Karger. 1978.

— From experiences of medial amygdalotomy on epileptics. Acta Neurochir. (Wien) Suppl. *30*, 75—81 (1980).

— Choreoathetosis and spasticity. In: Stereotaxy of the Human Brain. Anatomical, Physiological and Clinical Applications, 2nd ed. (Schaltenbrand, G., Walker, A. E., eds.), pp. 532—543. Stuttgart-New York: G. Thieme. 1982.

— Recent status of stereotaxic surgery. Special article. Surg. Neurol. *19*, 493—496 (1983).

— Yokochi, F., Nakajima, Y.: Levodopa-induced dyskinesia and thalamotomy. J. Neurol. Neurosurg. Psychiat. *47*, 831—839 (1984).

Nashold, B. S., Jr., Wilson, W. P., Slaughter, D. G.: Sensations evoked by stimulation in the midbrain of man. J. Neurosurg. *30*, 14—24 (1969).

— Mesencephalotomy. A current appraisal. In: Treatment of Pain (Voris, H. C., Whisler, W. W., eds.), pp. 121—131. Springfield, Ill.: Ch. C Thomas. 1975.

— Ostdahl, R. H.: Dorsal root entry zone lesions for pain relief. J. Neurosurg. *51*, 59—70 (1979).

— Brainstem stereotaxic procedures. In: Stereotaxy of the Human Brain. Anatomical, Physiological and Clinical Applications, 2nd ed. (Schaltenbrand, G., Walker, A. E., eds.), pp. 475—483. Stuttgart-New York: G. Thieme. 1982.

Nauta, H. J. W., Guinto, F. C., Pisharodi, M.: Arterial bolus contrast medium enhancement for computed tomographically guided stereotactic biopsy. Surg. Neurol. *22*, 559—564 (1984).

Neuwelt, E. A., Glasberg, M., Frenkel, E., Clark, W. K.: Malignant pineal region tumors. A clinico-pathological study. J. Neurosurg. *51*, 597—607 (1979).

— Balaban, E., Diehl, J., Hill, S., Frenkel, E.: Successful treatment of primary central nervous system lymphomas with chemotherapy after osmotic blood-brain barrier opening. Neurosurgery *12*, 662—671 (1983).

Noordenbos, W.: Pain: Problems Pertaining to the Transmission of Nerve Impulses Which Give Rise to Pain. Amsterdam-London-New York: Elsevier Publishing Company. 1959.

Obbens, E. A. M. T., Feun, L. G., Leavens, M. E., Savaraj, N., Stewart, D. J., Gutterman, J. U.: Phase I clinical trial of intralesional or intraventricular leukocyte interferon for intracranial malignancies. J. Neuro-Oncol. *3*, 61—67 (1985).

O'Brien, M. D., Upton, A. R., Toseland, P. A.: Benign familial tremor treated with primidone. Brit. med. J. *282*, 178—180 (1981).

O'Laoire, S. A., Crockard, H. A., Thomas, D. G. T., Gordon, D. S.: Brainstem hematoma. A report of six surgically treated cases. J. Neurosurg. *56*, 222—227 (1982).

Olivecrona, H.: The surgical treatment of intracranial tumors. In: Handbuch der Neurochirurgie, 4. Band, 4. Teil. Klinik und Behandlung der raumbeengenden intrakraniellen Prozesse (Olivecrona, H., Tönnis, W., eds.), pp. 1—301. Berlin-Heidelberg-New York: Springer. 1967.

Oliver, A. S., Firth, G., McKeran, R. O.: Studies on the intracerebral injection of vincristine free and entrapped within liposomes in the rat. J. neurol. Sci. *68*, 25—30 (1985).

Ommaya, A. K., Wood, J. H., Walters, C. L., Reed, J., Sadowski, D.: Intracerebral 8-azaguanine: a ten year follow-up study of a novel technique for local chemotherapy of malignant gliomas. AANS Annual Meeting 1979: Scientific Manuscripts, pp. 19—20. 1979.

Orthner, H.: Sexual disorders. In: Stereotaxy of the Human Brain. Anatomical, Physiological and Clinical Applications, 2nd ed. (Schaltenbrand, G., Walker, A. E., eds.), pp. 600—616. Stuttgart-New York: G. Thieme. 1982.

Ostertag, C. B., Mennek, H. D., Kiessling, M.: Stereotactic biopsy of brain tumors. Surg. Neurol. *14*, 275—283 (1980).

Passerini, A., Broggi, G., Giorgi, C., Savoiardo, M.: CT studies in patients operated with stereotaxic thalamotomies. Neuroradiology *16*, 561—563 (1978).

Pecker, J., Scarabin, J. M., Brucher, J. M., Vallée, B.: Apport des techniques stéréotaxiques au diagnostic et au traitement des tumeurs de la région pinéale. Rev. neurol. *134*, 287—294 (1978).

— — — — Démarche Stéréotaxique en Neurochirurgie Tumorale. Paris: Laboratoires Pierre Fabre. 1979 a.

— — Vallée, B., Brucher, J. M.: Treatment in tumours of the pineal region: value of stereotaxic biopsy. Surg. Neurol. *12*, 341—348 (1979 b).

Penn, I.: Chemical immunosuppression and human cancer. Cancer (Philad.) *34*, 1474—1480 (1974).

— Second malignant neoplasms associated with immunosuppressive medications. Cancer (Philad.) *37*, 1024—1032 (1976).

Penning, L., Front, D.: Brain Scintigraphy, a Neuroradiological Approach. Amsterdam-New York: Excerpta Medica. 1975.

Petrovici, J. N.: Speech disturbances following stereotaxic surgery in ventrolateral thalamus. Neurosurg. Rev. *3*, 189—195 (1980).

Picard, C., Olivier, A., Bertrand, G.: The first human stereotaxic apparatus. The contribution of Aubrey Mussen to the field of stereotaxis. J. Neurosurg. *59*, 673—676 (1983).

Porter, R. J., Penry, J. K., Lacy, J. R.: Diagnostic and therapeutic reevaluation of patients with intractable epilepsy. Neurology (Minneap.) *27*, 1006—1011 (1977).

Rähn, T.: Stereotactic Radiosurgery in Cushing's Disease. Stockholm: Thesis. 1980.

Rasmussen, Th.: Cortical resection for medically refractory focal epilepsy: results, lessons, and questions. In: Functional Neurosurgery (Rasmussen, Th., Marino, R., Jr., eds.), pp. 253—269. New York: Raven Press. 1979.

— Marino, R., Jr.: Functional Neurosurgery. New York: Raven Press. 1979.

— Surgical aspects of temporal lobe epilepsy. Results and problems. Acta Neurochir. (Wien) Suppl. *30*, 13—24 (1980).

Reynolds, D. V.: Surgery in the rat during electrical analgesia induced by focal brain stimulation. Science *164*, 444—445 (1969).

Riechert, T.: Die Entfernung von tiefsitzenden Hirnstecksplittern mit Hilfe des stereotaktischen Operationsverfahrens. Zbl. Neurochir. *15*, 159—164 (1955 a).

— Die stereotaktische Hypophysenoperation. Acta Neurochir. (Wien) Suppl. *3*, 90—97 (1955 b).

— Mundinger, F.: Beschreibung und Anwendung eines Zielgerätes für stereotaktische Hirnoperationen. Acta Neurochir. (Wien) Suppl. *3*, 308—337 (1955).

— — Stereotaxic instruments. In: Introduction to Stereotaxis with an Atlas of the Human Brain (Schaltenbrand, G., Bailey, P., eds.), pp. 437—472. Stuttgart: G. Thieme. 1959.

— Die chirurgische Behandlung der zentralen Schmerzzustände, einschließlich der stereotaktischen Operationen im Thalamus und Mesencephalon. Acta Neurochir. (Wien) *8*, 136—152 (1960).

— Eine neue Methode zur Behandlung bisher inoperabler arterio-venöser Angiome: die Operation auf stereotaktischem Wege. Presented at Czechoslovakian Medical Congress, Prague, November 12–17, 1962.

— Mundinger, F.: Combined stereotaxic operation for treatment of deep-seated angiomas and aneurysms. J. Neurosurg. *21*, 358—363 (1964).

— Relief of certain types of intractable pain. Pain *39*, 519—529 (1966).

— Gisinger, M. A., Mölbert, E.: Biopsien während stereotaktischer Operationen beim Parkinsonsyndrom. Neurochirurgia (Stuttgart) *10*, 106—118 (1967).

— Stereotactic Brain Operations. Methods, Clinical Aspects, Indications. Bern: Hans Huber Publishers. 1980.

Rivas, J. J., Lobato, R. D.: CT-assisted stereotaxic aspiration of colloid cysts of the third ventricle. J. Neurosurg. *62*, 238—242 (1985).

Rosomoff, H. L., Carroll, F., Brown, J., Sheptak, P.: Percutaneous radiofrequency cervical cordotomy: technique. J. Neurosurg. *23*, 639—644 (1965).

Rylander, G.: The renaissance of psychosurgery. In: Surgical Approaches in Psychiatry (Laitinen, L., Livingston, K., eds.), pp. 3—12. Lancaster: MTP Press Limited. 1973.

Sackett, J. F., Messina, A. V., Petito, C. K.: Computed tomography and magnification vertebral angiotomography in the diagnosis of colloid cysts of the third ventricle. Radiology *116*, 95—100 (1975).

Sagar, H. J., Warlow, C. P., Sheldon, P. W. E., Esiri, M. M.: Multiple sclerosis with clinical and radiological features of cerebral tumour. J. Neurol. Neurosurg. Psychiat. *45*, 802—808 (1982).

Sano, K., Ochiai, C.: Brainstem haematomas. Clinical aspects with reference to indications for treatment. In: Spontaneous Intracerebral Haematomas. Advances in Diagnosis and Therapy (Pia, H. W., Langmaid, C., Zierski, J., eds.), pp. 366—371. Berlin-Heidelberg-New York: Springer. 1980.

Saris, S. C., Iacono, R. P., Nashold, B. S., Jr.: Dorsal root entry zone lesions for post-amputation pain. J. Neurosurg. *62*, 72—76 (1985).

Scarabin, J. M., Pecker, J., Brucher, J. M., Vallée, B., Guagan, Y., Faivre, J., Simon, J.: Stereotaxic exploration in 200 supratentorial brain tumors. Its value in addition to computerized tomography. Neuroradiology *16*, 591—593 (1978).

Scerrati, M., Fiorentino, A., Fiorentino, M., Pola, P.: Stereotaxic device for polar approaches in orthogonal systems. Technical note. J. Neurosurg. *61*, 1146—1147 (1984).

Schaltenbrand, G., Bailey, P.: Introduction to Stereotaxis with an Atlas of the Human Brain. Stuttgart: G. Thieme. 1959.

— Wahren, W.: Atlas for Stereotaxy of the Human Brain, 2nd ed. Stuttgart: G. Thieme. 1977.

— Walker, A. E.: Stereotaxy of the Human Brain. Anatomical, Physiological and Clinical Applications, 2nd ed. Stuttgart-New York: G. Thieme. 1982.

Schaub, C., Bluet-Pajot, M. T., Videau-Lornet, C., Askienazy, S., Szikla, G.: Endocavitary bèta irradiation of glioma cysts with colloidal 186-Rhenium. In: INSERM Symposium-12. Stereotactic Cerebral Irradiation (Szikla, G., ed.), pp. 293—302. Amsterdam-New York-Oxford: Elsevier/North-Holland Biomedical Press. 1979.

Schneck, S. A., Penn, I.: De-novo brain tumours in renal-transplant recipients. Lancet *1*, 983—986 (1971).

Schoenberg, B. S., Christine, B. W., Whisnant, J. P.: Nervous system neoplasms and primary malignancies of other sites. Neurology (Minneap.) *25*, 705—712 (1975).

Schurr, P. H., Merrington, W. R.: The Horsley-Clarke stereotaxic apparatus. Brit. J. Surg. *65*, 33—36 (1978).

Schvarcz, J. R.: Stereotactic extralemniscal myelotomy. J. Neurol. Neurosurg. Psychiat. *39*, 53—57 (1976).

— Spinal cord stereotactic techniques re trigeminal nucleotomy and extralemniscal myelotomy. In: Advances in Stereoencephalotomy-8, 7th Symposium of the International Society for Research in Stereoencephalotomy, São Paulo, June 1977 (Gildenberg, P. L., Marino, R., Jr., eds.), pp. 99—112. Basel: S. Karger. 1978.

Scoville, W. B., Bettis, D. B.: Results of orbital undercutting today: A personal series. In: Neurosurgical Treatment in Psychiatry, Pain, and Epilepsy (Sweet, W. H., Obrador, S., Martin-Rodriguez, J. G., eds.), pp. 189—202. Baltimore: University Park Press. 1977.

Sedan, R., Lazorthes, Y.: La Neurostimulation Électrique Thérapeutique. Monographies des Périodiques Masson, Série Médecine, No. 17. Paris-New York: Masson. 1978.

Shelden, C. H., McCann, G., Jacques, S., Lutes, H. R., Frazier, R. E., Kutz, R., Kuki, R.: Development of a computerized microstereotaxic method for localization and removal of minute CNS lesions under direct 3-D vision. Technical report. J. Neurosurg. *52*, 21—27 (1980).

— Jacques, S., McCann, G.: The Shelden CT-based microneurosurgical stereotactic system: its application to CNS pathology. Appl. Neurophysiol. *45*, 341—346 (1982).

Sheline, G. E.: Radiation therapy of primary tumors. Semin. Oncol. 2, 29—42 (1975).

Sheptak, P. E., Zanetti, P. H., Susen, A. F.: The treatment of intracranial aneurysms by injection with a tissue adhesive. Neurosurgery 1, 25—29 (1977).

Shillito, J.: Craniopharyngiomas: the subfrontal approach, or none at all? Clin. Neurosurg. 27, 188—205 (1980).

Shinn-Zong Lin, Chun-Jen Shih, Yeou-Chih Wang, Shin-Han Tsai: Intracerebral hematoma simulating a new growth. Surg. Neurol. 21, 459—464 (1984).

Siegfried, J.: Neurosurgical treatment of spasticity. In: Functional Neurosurgery (Rasmussen, Th., Marino, R., Jr., eds.), pp. 123—128. New York: Raven Press. 1979.

— Is the neurosurgical treatment of Parkinson's disease still indicated? J. Neural Transm. Suppl. 16, 195—198 (1980).

— Stereotaxic cerebellar surgery for spasticity. In: Stereotaxy of the Human Brain. Anatomical, Physiological and Clinical Applications, 2nd ed. (Schaltenbrand, G., Walker, A. E., eds.), pp. 562—564. Stuttgart-New York: G. Thieme. 1982.

Silberman, A. W., Morgan, D. F., Storm, F. K., Rand, R. W., Benz, M., Drury, B., Morton, D. L.: Combination radiofrequency hyperthermia and chemotherapy (BCNU) for brain malignancy. Animal experience and two case reports. J. Neuro-Oncol. 2, 19—29 (1984).

Sjöquist, O.: Studies on pain conduction in the trigeminal nerve. A contribution to the surgical treatment of facial pain. Acta psychiat. scand. 17, 1—138 (1938).

Smith, R. W., Alksne, J. F.: Stereotaxic thrombosis of inaccessible intracranial aneurysms. J. Neurosurg. 47, 833—839 (1977).

Speelman, J. D., Van Manen, J.: Stereotactic thalamotomy for the relief of intention tremor of multiple sclerosis. J. Neurol. Neurosurg. Psychiat. 47, 596—599 (1984).

Spiegel, E. A., Wycis, H. T., Marks, M., Lee, A.: Stereotaxic apparatus for operations on the human brain. Science 106, 349—350 (1947).

— — Mesencephalotomy for relief of pain: principles of the method. In: Anniversary Volume for O. Pötzl, p. 438. Vienna: 1948.

— — Stereoencephalotomy: Thalamotomy and Related Procedures. Part I: Methods and Stereotaxic Atlas of the Human Brain. New York: Grune & Stratton. 1952.

— — Stereoencephalotomy: Thalamotomy and Related Procedures. Part II: Clinical and Physiological Applications. New York: Grune & Stratton. 1962.

— Guided Brain Operations. Methodological and Clinical Developments in Stereotactic Surgery. Contributions to the Physiology of Subcortical Structures. Basel-New York: S. Karger. 1982.

Stein, B. M.: Special article. Supracerebellar-infratentorial approach to pineal tumors. Surg. Neurol. 11, 331—337 (1979).

Steiner, L., Leksell, L., Forster, D. M. C., Greitz, T., Backlund, E. O.: Stereotactic radiosurgery in intracranial arteriovenous malformations. Acta Neurochir. (Wien) Suppl. 21, 195—209 (1974).

Storm, F. K., Morton, D. L., Kaiser, L. R., Harrison, W. H., Elliott, R. S., Weisenburger, T. H., Parker, R. G., Haskell, C. M.: Clinical radiofrequency hyperthermia: a review. J. nat. Cancer Inst. Monogr. 61, 343—350 (1982).

Suetens, P., Gybels, J., Jansen, P., Oosterlinck, A., Hagemans, A., Dierckx, P.: A global 3-D image of the blood vessels, tumor and simulated electrode. Acta Neurochir. (Wien) Suppl. *33*, 225—232 (1984).

Sugita, K., Doi, T., Sato, O., Takaoka, Y., Mutsuga, N., Tsugane, R.: Successful removal of intracranial air-gun bullet with stereotactic apparatus: case report. J. Neurosurg. *30*, 177—181 (1969).

— Mutsuga, N., Takaoka, Y., Hirota, T., Shibuya, M., Doi, T.: Stereotaxic exploration of para-third ventricle tumors. Confin. neurol. (Basel) *37*, 156—162 (1975).

Sung, D. I., Harisiadis, L., Chang, Ch. H.: Midline pineal tumors and suprasellar germinomas: highly curable by irradiation. Radiology *128*, 745—751 (1978).

Sweet, W. H., Mark, V. H.: Unipolar anodal electrolytic lesions in the brain of man and cat. Arch. Neurol. Psychiat. (Chic.) *70*, 224—234 (1953).

Szikla, G. (ed.): INSERM-Symposium-12. Stereotactic Cerebral Irradiation. Amsterdam-New York-Oxford: Elsevier/North-Holland Biomedical Press. 1979 a.

— Stereotactic neuroradiology and functional neurosurgery: localization of cortical structures by three-dimensional angiography. In: Functional Neurosurgery (Rasmussen, Th., Marino, R., Jr., eds.), pp. 197—217. New York: Raven Press. 1979 b.

Talairach, J., Hecaen, H., David, M., Monnier, M., De Ajuriaguerra, J.: Recherches sur la coagulation thérapeutique des structures sous-corticales chez l'homme. Rev. neurol. *81*, 4—24 (1949).

— Chirurgie stéréotaxique du thalamus. In: Actas y Trabajos del VI Congreso Latinoamericano de Neurocirugía (Arana-Iñíguez, R., ed.), pp. 865—925. Montevideo: Imprenta Rosgal-Hilario Rosillo. 1955.

— David, M., Tournoux, P., Corredor, H., Kvasina, T.: Atlas d'Anatomie Stéréotaxique. Repérage Radiologique Indirect des Noyaux Gris Centraux des Régions Mésencéphalo-Sous-Optique et Hypothalamique de l'Homme. Paris: Masson et Cie. 1957.

— Szikla, G.: Applications of stereotactic concepts to the surgery of epilepsy. Acta Neurochir. (Wien) Suppl. *30*, 35—54 (1980).

Tampieri, D., Bergstrand, G.: Postural displacements of the brain—on the feasibility of using CT for determination of stereotactic coordinates. Neuroradiology *24*, 167—168 (1983).

Tasker, R. R.: Thalamic stereotaxic procedures. In: Stereotaxy of the Human Brain. Anatomical, Physiological and Clinical Applications, 2nd ed. (Schaltenbrand, G., Walker, A. E., eds.), pp. 484—497. Stuttgart-New York: G. Thieme. 1982.

Tator, C. H.: Intraneoplastic injection of CCNU for experimental brain tumor chemotherapy. Surg. Neurol. *7*, 73—77 (1977).

Teuber, H. L., Corkin, S. H., Twitchell, T. E.: Study of cingulotomy in man: a summary. In: Neurosurgical Treatment in Psychiatry, Pain, and Epilepsy (Sweet, W. H., Obrador, S., Martin-Rodriguez, J. G., eds.), pp. 355—362. Baltimore: University Park Press. 1977.

Thomas, D. G. T., Anderson, R. E., Du Boulay, G. H.: CT-guided stereotactic neurosurgery: experience in 24 cases with a new stereotactic system. J. Neurol. Neurosurg. Psychiat. *47*, 9—16 (1984).

Tindall, G. T., Payne, N. S., Nixon, D. W.: Transsphenoidal hypophysectomy for disseminated carcinoma of the prostate gland. Results in 53 patients. J. Neurosurg. *50*, 275—282 (1979).

Todd, E. M.: Todd-Wells Manual of Stereotaxic Procedures. Randolph: Codman & Shurtleff. 1967.

Valentine, A. R., Kendall, B. E., Harding, B. N.: Computed tomography in acute haemorrhagic leukoencephalitis. Neuroradiology *22*, 215—219 (1982).

Van den Berg, J. W., Van Manen, J.: Graded coagulation of brain tissue. Acta physiol. pharmacol. neerl. *10*, 353—377 (1962).

Van Manen, J.: Stereotactic Methods and Their Applications in Disorder of the Motor System. Assen: Van Gorcum. 1967.

— Stereotaxic operation in cases of hereditary and intention tremor. Acta Neurochir. (Wien) Suppl. *21*, 49—50 (1974).

— Speelman, J. D., Tans, R. J. J.: Indications for surgical treatment of Parkinson's disease after levodopa therapy. Clin. Neurol. Neurosurg. *86*, 207—212 (1984).

Vaquero, J., Carrillo, R., Cabezudo, J., Leunda, G., Villoria, F., Bravo, G.: Cavernous angiomas of the pineal region. J. Neurosurg. *53*, 833—835 (1980).

Voris, H. C., Whisler, W. W.: Results of stereotaxic surgery for intractable pain. Confin. neurol. (Basel) *37*, 86—96 (1975).

Walker, A. E.: Classification of movement disorders. In: Stereotaxy of the Human Brain. Anatomical, Physiological and Clinical Applications, 2nd ed. (Schaltenbrand, G., Walker, A. E., eds.), pp. 503—509. Stuttgart-New York: G. Thieme. 1982 a.

— Stereotaxic surgery for tremor. In: Stereotaxy of the Human Brain. Anatomical, Physiological and Clinical Applications, 2nd ed. (Schaltenbrand, G., Walker, A. E., eds.), pp. 515—521. Stuttgart-New York: G. Thieme. 1982 b.

Waltimo, O.: The relationship of size, density and localization of intracranial arteriovenous malformations to the type of initial symptom. J. neurol. Sci. *19*, 13—19 (1973).

Wang, A. M., Morris, J. H., Hickey, W. F., Hammerschlag, S. B., O'Reilly, G. V., Rumbaugh, C. L.: Unusual CT patterns of multiple sclerosis. AJNR *4*, 47—50 (1983).

Watkins, L. R., Mayer, D. J.: Organization of endogenous opiate and nonopiate pain control systems. Science *216*, 1185—1192 (1982).

Whisler, W. W., Voris, H. C.: Mesencephalotomy for intractable pain due to malignant disease. Appl. Neurophysiol. *41*, 52—56 (1978).

Whitley, R. J., Soong, S. J., Hirsch, M. S., Karchmer, A. W., Dolin, R., Galasso, G., Dunnick, J. K., Alford, C. A., NIAID Collaborative Antiviral Study Group: Herpes simplex encephalitis. Vidarabine therapy and diagnostic problems. New Engl. J. Med. *304*, 313—318 (1981).

Whyte, T. R., Colby, M. Y., Layton, D. D.: Radiation therapy of brainstem tumors. Radiology *93*, 413—416 (1969).

Wilson, Ch. B., Hoi Sang U, Domingue, J.: Microsurgical treatment of intracranial vascular malformations. J. Neurosurg. *51*, 446—454 (1979).

Wise, B. L., Gleason, C. A.: CT-directed stereotactic surgery in the management of brain abscess. Ann. Neurol. *6*, 457 (1979).

Wycis, H. T., Spiegel, E. A.: Long range results in the treatment of intractable pain by stereotaxic midbrain surgery. J. Neurosurg. *19*, 101—107 (1962).

— The role of stereotaxic surgery in the compulsive state. In: Psychosurgery. Proceedings of the 2nd International Conference on Psychosurgery, Copenhagen, Denmark, 1972 (Hitchcock, E., Laitinen, L. V., Vaernet, K., eds.), pp. 115—116. Springfield, Ill.: Ch. C Thomas. 1972.

Yamada, S., Ritland, S., Knierim, D.: Stereotactic localization of deep-seated arteriovenous malformations in the functional area. Appl. Neurophysiol. *46*, 231—235 (1983).

Young, R. F., Kroening, R., Fulton, W., Feldman, R. A., Chambi, I.: Electrical stimulation of the brain in treatment of chronic pain. Experience over 5 years. J. Neurosurg. *62*, 389—396 (1985).

Zervas, N. T.: Long-term review of dentatectomy in dystonia musculorum deformans and cerebral palsy. Acta Neurochir. (Wien) Suppl. *24*, 49—51 (1977).

Zlatos, J., Cierny, G.: Statistical model map of the spinal cord and its use. Appl. Neurophysiol. *38*, 225—239 (1975).

# Subject Index

G. Pendl

# Pineal and Midbrain Lesions

By **Gerhard Pendl**, M. D.,
Associate Professor of Neurosurgery, Department of Neurosurgery, University of Vienna Medical School, Vienna

1985. 206 partly colored figures. XI, 269 pages.
Cloth DM 158,–, öS 1110,–
ISBN 3-211-81858-8

This book presents extensive microanatomical and topographical investigations relevant to the surgery of pineal and midbrain lesions. By taking into account a variety of approaches and pointing out their pitfalls—especially with regard to the area of the great vein of Galen and its tributaries—the author develops a more rational surgical approach to these tumors.

In addition to covering clinical signs and symptoms, the neuropathology and neuroimaging of numerous lesions encountered in the midbrain are also discussed. Moreover, many clinical cases are utilized to demonstrate the potential for microsurgery of the pineal and midbrain region.

**Contents:** Topography and Microanatomy of the Pineal and Midbrain Region. — The Pathology of Pineal Region Lesions. — Clinical Diagnosis. — Neuroimaging of Lesions of the Pineal and Midbrain Region. — Stereotactic Biopsy. — History of the Surgical Approach to Pineal and Midbrain Lesions. — Microsurgical Approaches to the Pineal and Midbrain Region. — Indication and Principles of Surgical Treatment. — Case Material. — References. — Subject Index.

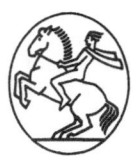

Springer-Verlag
Wien New York

# Differential Approaches in Microsurgery of the Brain

By Professor **W. Seeger,** M. D., Medical Director
of the Department of General Neurosurgery
and Chairman of Neurosurgery of the
Neurosurgical Clinic,
University of Freiburg i. Br.

In Collaboration with
**W. Mann**

1985. 201 figures.
VII, 414 pages.
Format: 23,7 cm × 32 cm
Cloth DM 268,–, öS 1880,–
ISBN 3-211-81857-X

In this book the various possible approaches to the same target are presented with their advantages and disadvantages for the first time. The normal anatomical variations seen pre-operatively and the specific processes which are similar but never identical may require different operative procedures even for the same target area. This problem concerns almost exclusively the deep lying processes in the area of the brainstem and ventricular system. In most routine interventions in the cerebrum and cerebellum this problem is not present, so that one can limit the operative approaches according to the cisterns. The dorsal cisternal area of the brainstem is especially important and has only in recent years been increasingly operated on. Here the danger of psychological disturbances due to damage of the limbic system is particularly great. Until now a systematic review of this area from the micro-surgical aspect has been absent.

As in his previous volumes Professor Seeger proves once again to be not only an extremely experienced and gifted specialist in his field but also a man with rare artistic talents.

The book presents highly valuable information to specialists working in the fields of neurosurgery, neuro-rhinootology, neurology, neuroradiology, neuropathology, anatomy, pathology, ophthalmology, microvascular surgery, oral surgery, and plastic surgery.

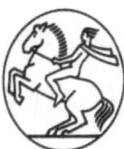

# Springer-Verlag Wien New York

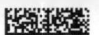